Medical Terminology
a systems approach

Holly Mason

SECOND EDITION

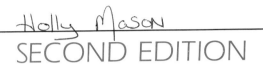
BARBARA A. GYLYS, B.S., M.Ed., C.M.A.-A.
Professor of Health and Human Services
Coordinator of Medical Assisting Technology
University of Toledo Community and Technical College
Toledo, Ohio

MARY ELLEN WEDDING, B.S., M.T. (A.S.C.P.), M.Ed., C.M.A.
Associate Professor of Health and Human Services
University of Toledo Community and Technical College
Toledo, Ohio

F. A. DAVIS COMPANY 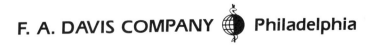 Philadelphia

Library of Congress Cataloging-in-Publication Data
Gylys, Barbara A.
    Medical terminology.

    Includes index.
    1. Medicine—Terminology.   I. Wedding, Mary Ellen.
II. Title.   [DNLM: 1. Nomenclature—problems.
W 15 G996m]
R123.G94   1987   610'.14   87-13732
ISBN 0-8036-4495-7

This book is dedicated with love

to my husband, Julius A. Gylys
        and
to my children, Regina Maria and Julius A., II

                                    B.G.

to my sister, Sr. M. Adele Karwacki
        and
to my children, Carol Ann, Don II, Vicki, and Daniel
        and
to my husband, Don

                                    M.E.W.

Foreword

It is always a pleasure to write a foreword for a well-prepared book that meets the needs of readers in an ever-growing field, and that accomplishes the purposes of the authors.

The publication of a second edition indicates that the book has been successful in its usefulness and has been well received by those it intends to serve, despite the rapidly increasing number of publications of the same nature. The success of books dealing with etymology, word formation, or word building may be related to the recent reduction in courses in Latin and Greek, which are so necessary for both humanistic studies and education in general. Our everchanging world, as has happened periodically, is requiring a revival of the study of the so-called dead languages, the knowledge of which is essential to learn modern vocabularies and understand neologisms, proposed by scholars, scientists, technologists, educators, and others. Knowledge of the origin of each word is one of the clues to understanding, learning, and remembering ideas and concepts. However, the revival of courses in Latin at the undergraduate level will not, by itself, dispense with books such as *Medical Terminology: A Systems Approach*, which is especially dedicated to those interested in the health field. Books such as this will be needed in each specific field as the basic vocabulary for the corresponding scientific and technological language.

A key to the success of *Medical Terminology: A Systems Approach* is certainly the competence of the authors, Barbara A. Gylys and Mary Ellen Wedding. Their expertise and approach have been applied to the preparation of a well-organized book, which allows for pleasant reading and effective learning of the material.

Medical Terminology: A Systems Approach provides a sound basis for those who plan to be involved or are already engaged in the medical, dental, nursing, veterinary, anthropological, or allied health fields, helping them to become familiar with the most important words, with their derivatives, and with the formation of related terms. It provides a working tool for those dealing with health or health-related sciences, at present characterized by outstanding development and progress.

The authors can be congratulated for their second edition. They can expect to be more and more successful as they expand the book to match the fast-paced, extraordinary advances in the scientific and technological fields, both of which are continuously creating new terms, many based on old linguistic roots.

Liberato J.A. DiDio, M.D., Ph.D., D.Sc.
Chairman and Professor, Department of Anatomy
Medical College of Ohio
July 13, 1987

Acknowledgments

We wish to acknowledge the untiring assistance of Dr. Julius Gylys, who reviewed the manuscript of the second edition. His valuable input and editorial skills are evident in each chapter.

Special thanks are given to our colleague, Professor Donna Adler, who helped with the review of the entire manuscript. The authors also acknowledge the assistance and expertise of the following people, who likewise reviewed and edited the manuscript: Deborah Anthony, Temple University; Margaret Bobo, Medical University of South Carolina; Pamela Buccelli, Hahnemann University; Elsie Campbell, Bakersfield College; George Downs, Philadelphia College of Pharmacy; Marti Hitchcock, Gwinnett Area Technical College; Angela Klice, Kansas City College of Medical and Dental Careers; Martha Leonard, Midlands Technical College; Anne Lilly, Santa Rosa Community College; Sarah-Lu Mitchell, Mira Loma, CA; Mary Jean-Paxton, Jacksonville State University; Martha Rouland, Community College of Philadelphia; Cheryl K. Smith, National Education Centers; Gretchen Spence, Cencor Career Colleges; Shirley Zeitter, Davenport College. Their attention to detail, as well as their technical competence, made many mundane tasks more bearable.

We extend our appreciation to Stephen Bazeley, M.D., Steven Selman, M.D., Professors Cathy Bazeley, Philip Geronimo, Regina Hoffman, Lori Lupe, Margaret Traband, and Dawn Wetmore, as well as to Lorraine Nelson, R.Ph., who willingly reviewed and edited selected chapters or sections of the manuscript.

We wish to thank the editorial staff of F. A. Davis Company, especially Zena Sandler Gordon, for their assistance in the production of this book. We are also especially grateful to Jean François Vilain, Allied Health Editor, for his endless encouragement and support. His understanding and innovative suggestions are most appreciated.

Last, our present and future students deserve an acknowledgment in their own right. It is for them and because of them that we undertook the writing of this book.

Preface

The second edition of *Medical Terminology: A Systems Approach* is designed to provide basic principles of medical word building. The underlying pedagogy consists of a textbook/workbook approach. The accompanying *Instructor's Guide To Medical Terminology: A Systems Approach* explains how the textbook is structured to meet the criteria of a competency-based curriculum.

Just as in the first edition, the authors have directed their efforts to meet the needs of students in medical, biological, and health-oriented programs. Among the students specifically served by this text are nurses, medical laboratory technologists, radiologic technologists, medical assistants, medical secretaries, cardiovascular technicians, respiratory therapists, dental assistants, physical therapists, medical record keepers, pre-medical students, medical transcriptionists, medical librarians, and hospital personnel. The non-professional who is interested in becoming acquainted with the most current medical terminology will also find the book both rewarding and helpful.

Thanks to suggestions from numerous medical terminology instructors, the second edition includes additional suffixes, prefixes, and directional terms. Also, medical terms that are uncommon or are currently used infrequently have been deleted. As a result, students using the second edition are exposed not only to a more up-to-date background in medical vocabulary but also to one that is considerably more comprehensive in nature.

The principal objectives of the textbook are twofold. The first objective is to provide the student with basic principles of medical word building. These principles, once learned, can readily be applied to building an extensive medical vocabulary. The book is basically designed as a classroom teaching text for programs that require medical terminology. Yet, its organization incorporates self-teaching features that allow a student to work through the chapters at his or her own pace without any outside guidance. The authors have taken into account the needs of both the students who want to proceed at their own pace and those of an instructor who employs the traditional lecture and recitation method.

The second objective is to present the material at a level that the average student would have no problems in following. Thus, no previous knowledge of anatomy, physiology, or biology is necessary (although upon completion of the course, the student will have acquired a solid basic knowledge of anatomy and physiology). Even a competent high-school-level student should readily understand the contents of this textbook.

Those who have used the first edition will find that the format of the book is unchanged. The basic rules of medical word building are established in the text's Introduction. Chapters 1 and 2 are devoted to the identification of the major suffixes. It is recommended that these two chapters be introduced at the initial stages of the course. Chapter 3 covers prefixes, and the structure of its contents allows it to be taught either after the suffix chapters or in segments as subsequent chapters are covered. Chapter 4 is concerned with an orientation to the body as a whole.

Each of the body system's chapters, Chapters 5 to 15, has a similar format and is organized as follows:

       Anatomy and physiology of the body system
       Word roots/combining forms of the body system
       Suffixes related to the body system
       Pathology of the body system
       Other terms related to the body system

Special procedures related to the body system
    Radiographic and Clinical Procedures
    Endoscopic Procedures
    Surgical Procedures
    Laboratory Procedures
Pharmacology related to the body system
Abbreviations related to the body system
Worksheets

Chapter 16 presents current oncology (cancer) terminology.

In Appendix A, an answer key to the Worksheets is provided to generate immediate feedback. Appendix B provides a list of common medical abbreviations. Appendix C consists of a list of genetic disorders and the corresponding page number in the text. Appendix D is a complete index of the medical word elements and English terms presented in the book, including pronunciations, meanings, and corresponding page numbers.

The *Instructor's Guide To Medical Terminology: A Systems Approach* was developed to meet the requirements for competency-based education. There is an extensive test bank for each chapter and a comprehensive test bank for the entire textbook. Numerous teaching suggestions have been incorporated to assist the instructor in classroom presentations.

Taber's Cyclopedic Medical Dictionary is a highly recommended companion reference, since it provides etymologies for nearly all of the main entries presented in this book.

A *Computer Software Program* that provides approximately 30 student-interactive hours on a microcomputer can be utilized as a supplemental teaching aide or as a completely self-tutorial program. The software can be obtained from F. A. Davis Company.

Audio Cassettes to accompany the text are also available and are highly recommended by the authors.

B.A.G.
M.E.W.

Contents

CHAPTER 15.

CHAPTER 16.

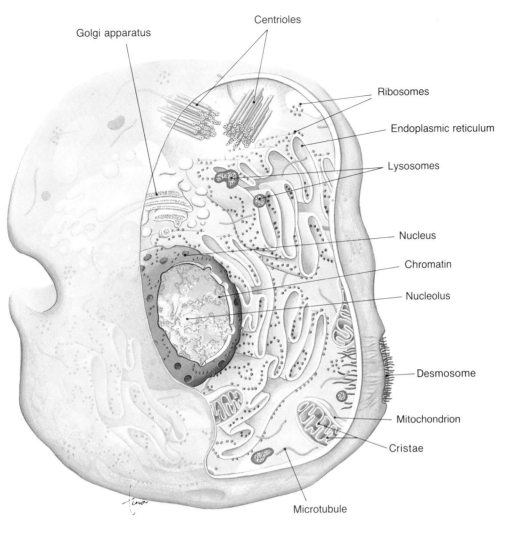

Golgi apparatus

Centrioles

Ribosomes

Endoplasmic reticulum

Lysosomes

Nucleus

Chromatin

Nucleolus

Desmosome

Mitochondrion

Cristae

Microtubule

Plate 1.   The Cell.

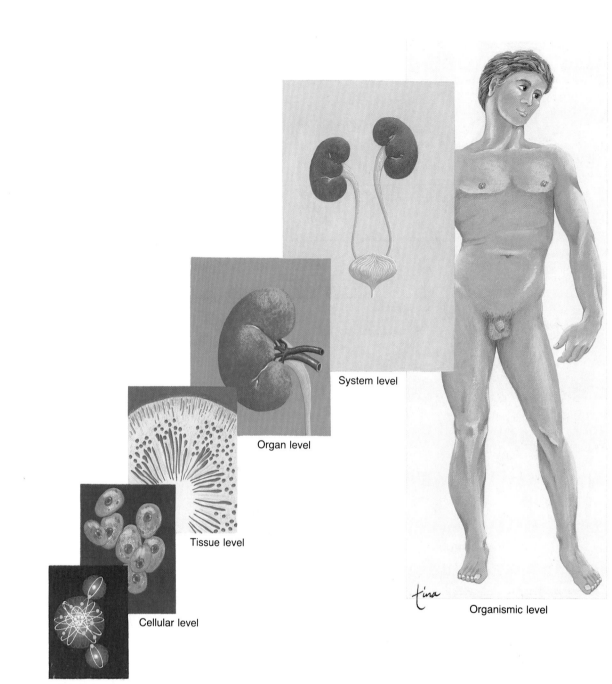

Atomic level

Cellular level

Tissue level

Organ level

System level

Organismic level

Plate 2.   Levels of Organization of the Body.

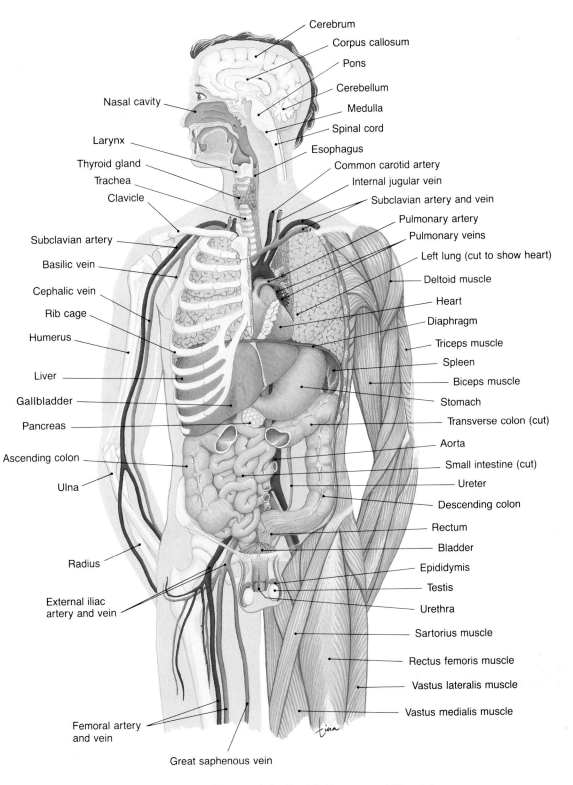

Cerebrum
Corpus callosum
Pons
Cerebellum
Medulla
Spinal cord
Esophagus
Common carotid artery
Internal jugular vein
Subclavian artery and vein
Pulmonary artery
Pulmonary veins
Left lung (cut to show heart)
Deltoid muscle
Heart
Diaphragm
Triceps muscle
Spleen
Biceps muscle
Stomach
Transverse colon (cut)
Aorta
Small intestine (cut)
Ureter
Descending colon
Rectum
Bladder
Epididymis
Testis
Urethra
Sartorius muscle
Rectus femoris muscle
Vastus lateralis muscle
Vastus medialis muscle

Nasal cavity
Larynx
Thyroid gland
Trachea
Clavicle
Subclavian artery
Basilic vein
Cephalic vein
Rib cage
Humerus
Liver
Gallbladder
Pancreas
Ascending colon
Ulna
Radius
External iliac artery and vein
Femoral artery and vein
Great saphenous vein

Plate 3.   Overview of Some of the Body's Organs and Structures.

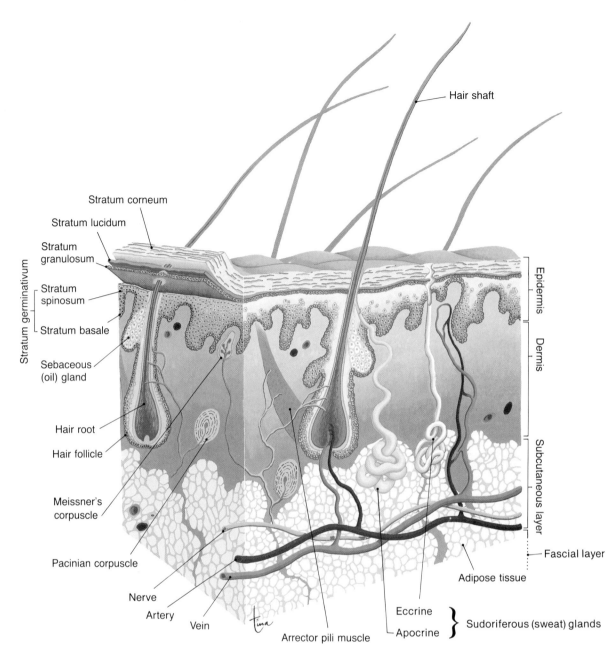

Stratum corneum

Stratum lucidum

Stratum granulosum

Stratum germinativum

Stratum spinosum

Stratum basale

Sebaceous (oil) gland

Hair root

Hair follicle

Meissner's corpuscle

Pacinian corpuscle

Nerve

Artery

Vein

Arrector pili muscle

Eccrine

Apocrine

Sudoriferous (sweat) glands

Adipose tissue

Fascial layer

Subcutaneous layer

Dermis

Epidermis

Hair shaft

Plate 4.   Cross-Section of the Skin.

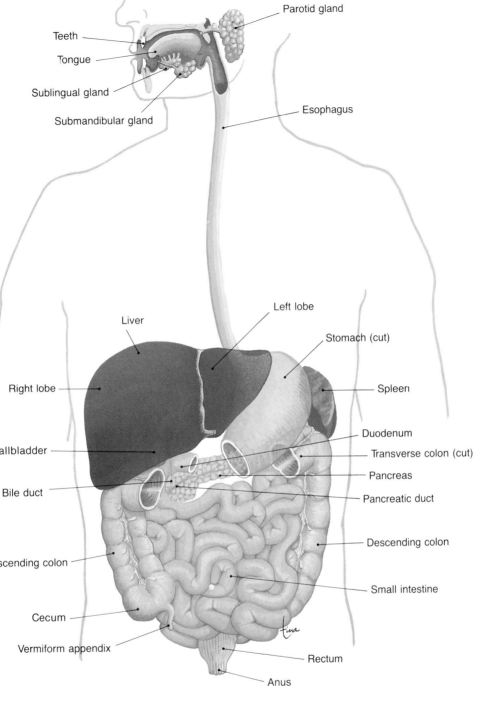
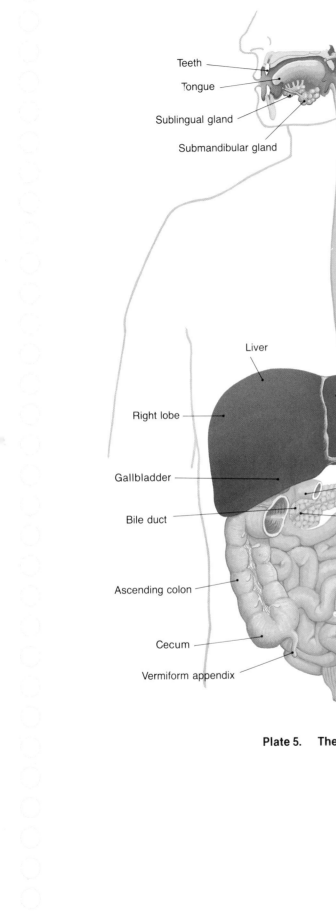

Teeth

Tongue

Sublingual gland

Submandibular gland

Parotid gland

Esophagus

Left lobe

Liver

Stomach (cut)

Right lobe

Spleen

Duodenum

Gallbladder

Transverse colon (cut)

Pancreas

Bile duct

Pancreatic duct

Descending colon

Ascending colon

Small intestine

Cecum

Vermiform appendix

Rectum

Anus

Plate 5.   The Digestive System.

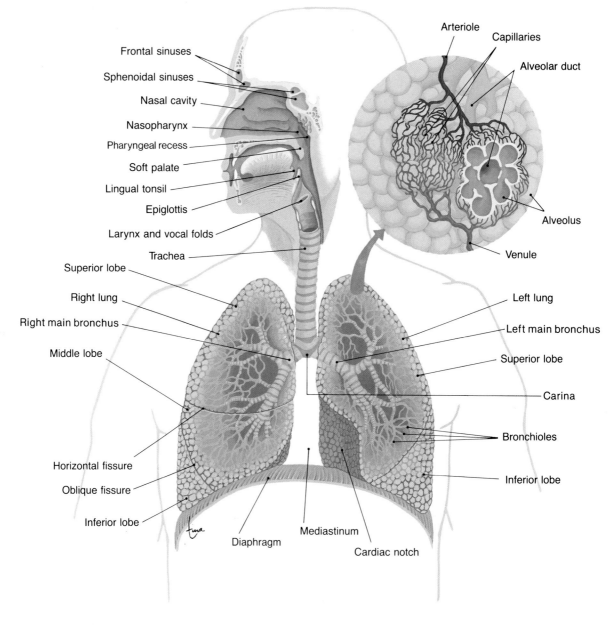

Frontal sinuses

Sphenoidal sinuses

Nasal cavity

Nasopharynx

Pharyngeal recess

Soft palate

Lingual tonsil

Epiglottis

Larynx and vocal folds

Trachea

Superior lobe

Right lung

Right main bronchus

Middle lobe

Horizontal fissure

Oblique fissure

Inferior lobe

Diaphragm

Mediastinum

Cardiac notch

Arteriole

Capillaries

Alveolar duct

Alveolus

Venule

Left lung

Left main bronchus

Superior lobe

Carina

Bronchioles

Inferior lobe

Plate 6.   The Respiratory System.

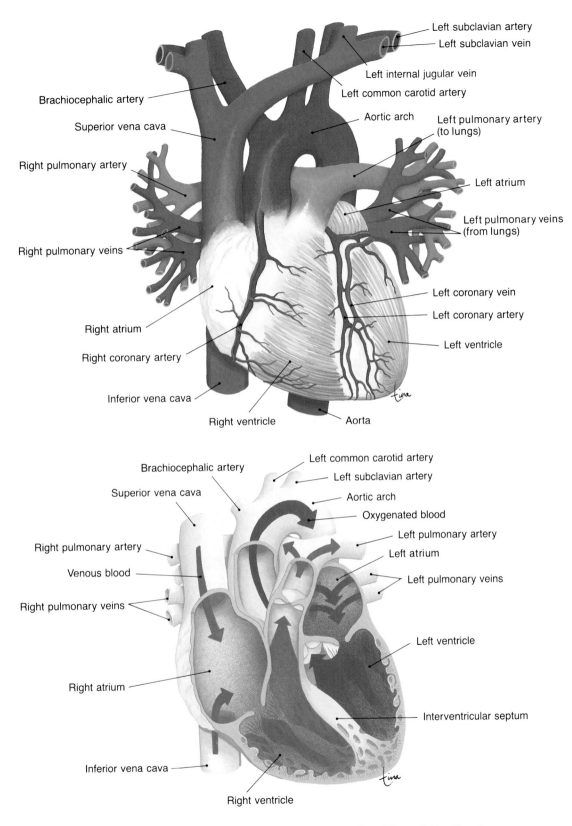

Left subclavian artery

Left subclavian vein

Left internal jugular vein

Left common carotid artery

Brachiocephalic artery

Superior vena cava

Aortic arch

Left pulmonary artery (to lungs)

Right pulmonary artery

Left atrium

Right pulmonary veins

Left pulmonary veins (from lungs)

Left coronary vein

Left coronary artery

Right atrium

Left ventricle

Right coronary artery

Inferior vena cava

Right ventricle

Aorta

Brachiocephalic artery

Left common carotid artery

Superior vena cava

Left subclavian artery

Aortic arch

Oxygenated blood

Right pulmonary artery

Left pulmonary artery

Venous blood

Left atrium

Right pulmonary veins

Left pulmonary veins

Left ventricle

Right atrium

Interventricular septum

Inferior vena cava

Right ventricle

Plate 7.   The Exterior of the Heart, and Blood Flow Through the Heart.

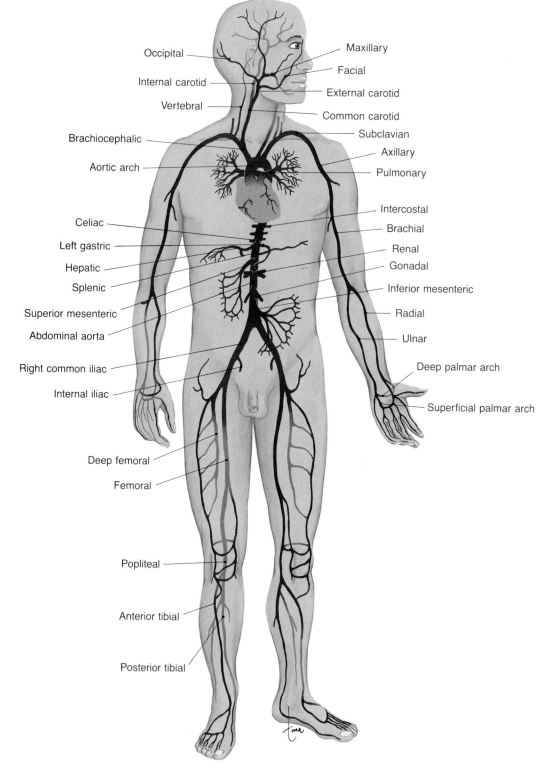

Occipital

Maxillary

Facial

Internal carotid

External carotid

Vertebral

Common carotid

Brachiocephalic

Subclavian

Aortic arch

Axillary

Pulmonary

Celiac

Intercostal

Left gastric

Brachial

Hepatic

Renal

Splenic

Gonadal

Superior mesenteric

Inferior mesenteric

Abdominal aorta

Radial

Right common iliac

Ulnar

Internal iliac

Deep palmar arch

Superficial palmar arch

Deep femoral

Femoral

Popliteal

Anterior tibial

Posterior tibial

Plate 8.   The Arteries.

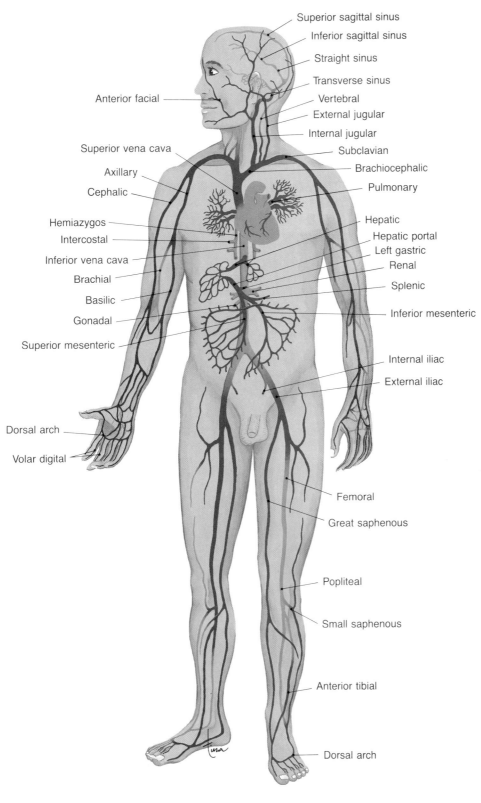

Superior sagittal sinus
Inferior sagittal sinus
Straight sinus
Transverse sinus
Anterior facial
Vertebral
External jugular
Internal jugular
Superior vena cava
Subclavian
Axillary
Brachiocephalic
Cephalic
Pulmonary
Hemiazygos
Hepatic
Intercostal
Hepatic portal
Inferior vena cava
Left gastric
Brachial
Renal
Basilic
Splenic
Gonadal
Inferior mesenteric
Superior mesenteric
Internal iliac
External iliac
Dorsal arch
Volar digital
Femoral
Great saphenous
Popliteal
Small saphenous
Anterior tibial
Dorsal arch

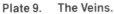

Plate 9.   The Veins.

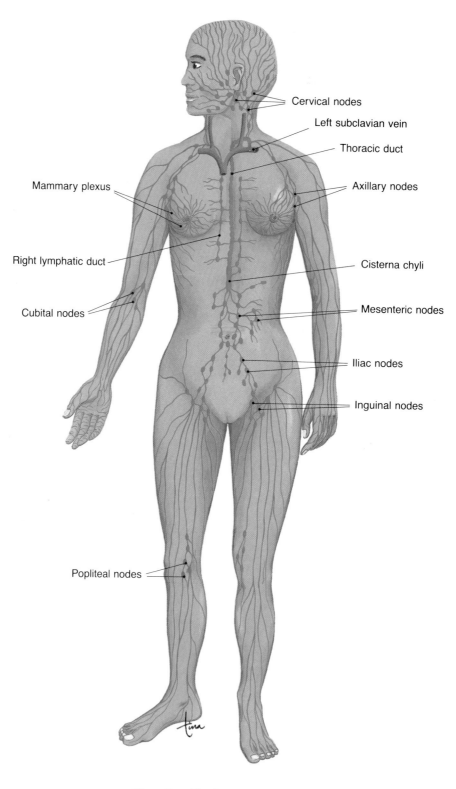

Cervical nodes

Left subclavian vein

Thoracic duct

Mammary plexus

Axillary nodes

Right lymphatic duct

Cisterna chyli

Cubital nodes

Mesenteric nodes

Iliac nodes

Inguinal nodes

Popliteal nodes

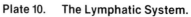

Plate 10.   The Lymphatic System.

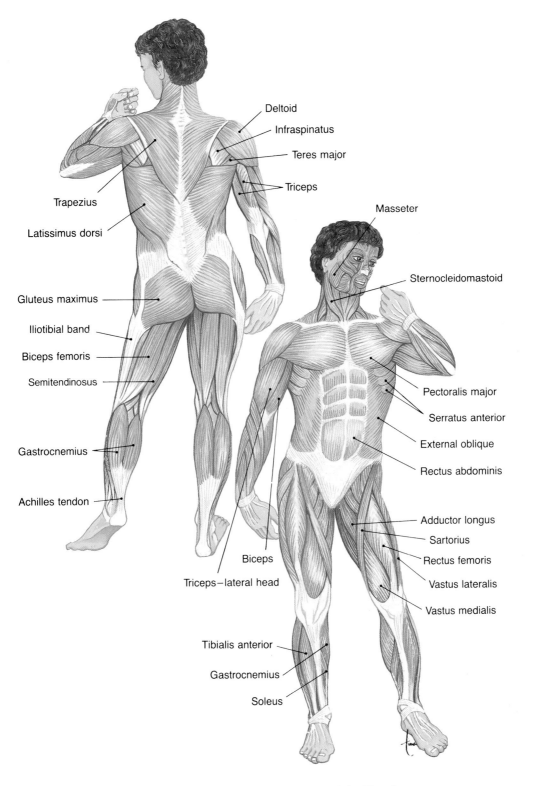

Deltoid

Infraspinatus

Teres major

Triceps

Masseter

Trapezius

Sternocleidomastoid

Latissimus dorsi

Gluteus maximus

Iliotibial band

Pectoralis major

Biceps femoris

Serratus anterior

Semitendinosus

External oblique

Rectus abdominis

Adductor longus

Sartorius

Rectus femoris

Vastus lateralis

Vastus medialis

Gastrocnemius

Achilles tendon

Biceps

Triceps—lateral head

Tibialis anterior

Gastrocnemius

Soleus

Plate 11.   Posterior and Anterior Views of the Muscles.

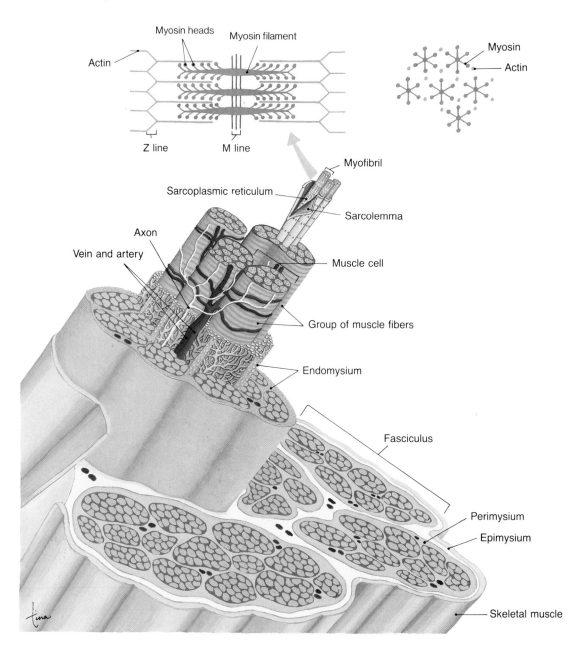

Plate 12. Cross-Section of Skeletal Muscle.

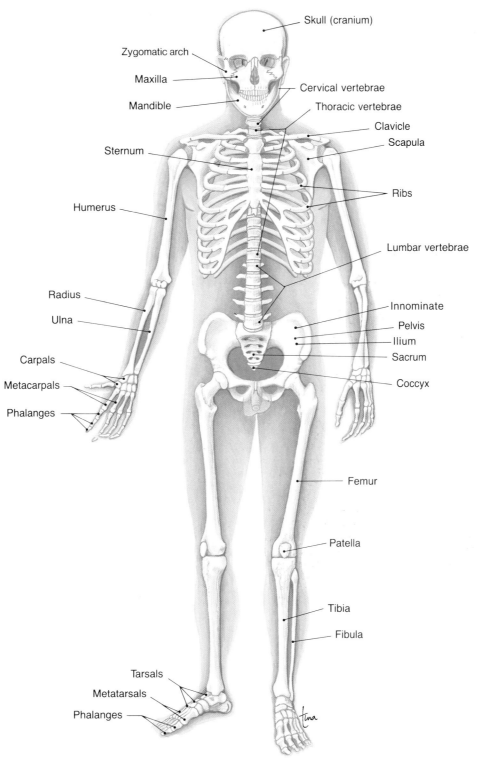

Skull (cranium)

Zygomatic arch

Maxilla

Mandible

Cervical vertebrae

Thoracic vertebrae

Clavicle

Scapula

Sternum

Ribs

Humerus

Lumbar vertebrae

Radius

Ulna

Innominate

Pelvis

Ilium

Sacrum

Carpals

Coccyx

Metacarpals

Phalanges

Femur

Patella

Tibia

Fibula

Tarsals

Metatarsals

Phalanges

Plate 13.   Anterior View of the Skeleton.

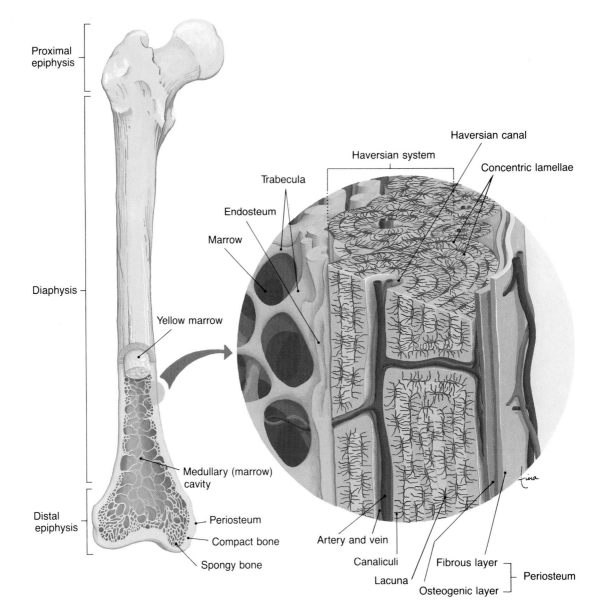

Plate 14.   Longitudinal Section of a Long Bone.

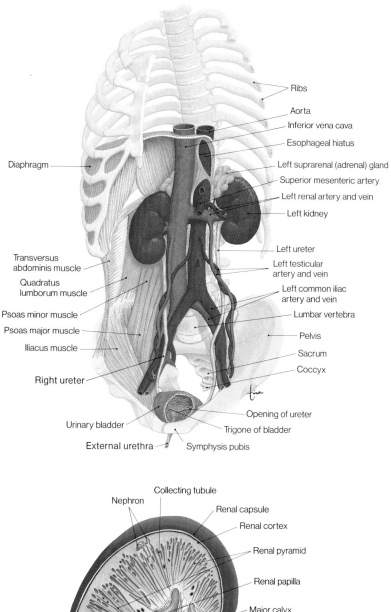

Ribs
Aorta
Inferior vena cava
Esophageal hiatus
Diaphragm
Left suprarenal (adrenal) gland
Superior mesenteric artery
Left renal artery and vein
Left kidney
Left ureter
Transversus abdominis muscle
Left testicular artery and vein
Quadratus lumborum muscle
Left common iliac artery and vein
Psoas minor muscle
Lumbar vertebra
Psoas major muscle
Pelvis
Iliacus muscle
Sacrum
Right ureter
Coccyx
Opening of ureter
Urinary bladder
Trigone of bladder
External urethra
Symphysis pubis

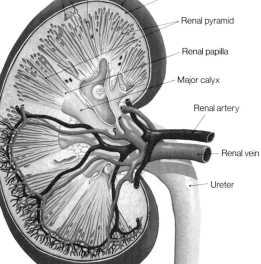

Collecting tubule
Nephron
Renal capsule
Renal cortex
Renal pyramid
Renal papilla
Major calyx
Renal artery
Renal vein
Ureter

Plate 15.   The Urinary System, and the Kidney.

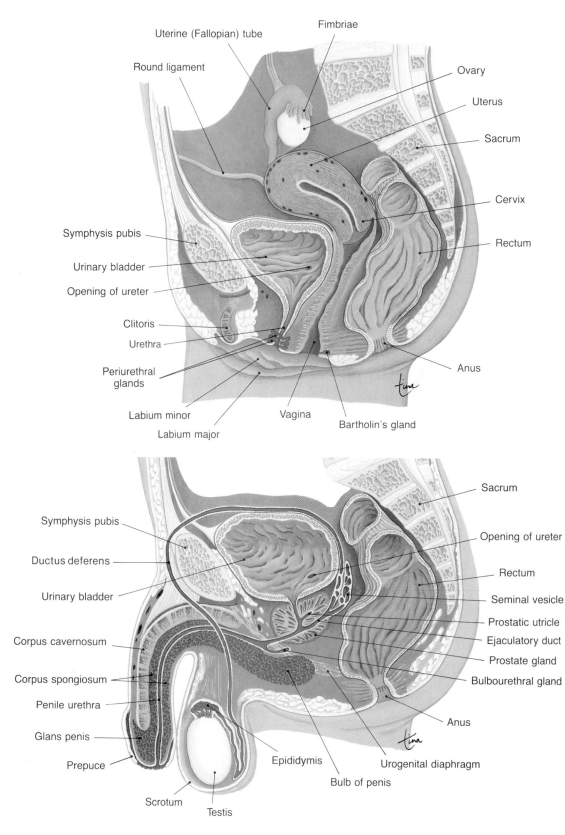

Plate 16. **The Female and Male Reproductive Systems.**

Uterine (Fallopian) tube

Fimbriae

Round ligament

Ovary

Uterus

Sacrum

Cervix

Symphysis pubis

Rectum

Urinary bladder

Opening of ureter

Clitoris

Urethra

Periurethral glands

Anus

Labium minor

Vagina

Bartholin's gland

Labium major

Sacrum

Symphysis pubis

Opening of ureter

Ductus deferens

Rectum

Urinary bladder

Seminal vesicle

Prostatic utricle

Corpus cavernosum

Ejaculatory duct

Prostate gland

Corpus spongiosum

Bulbourethral gland

Penile urethra

Glans penis

Anus

Prepuce

Urogenital diaphragm

Epididymis

Bulb of penis

Scrotum

Testis

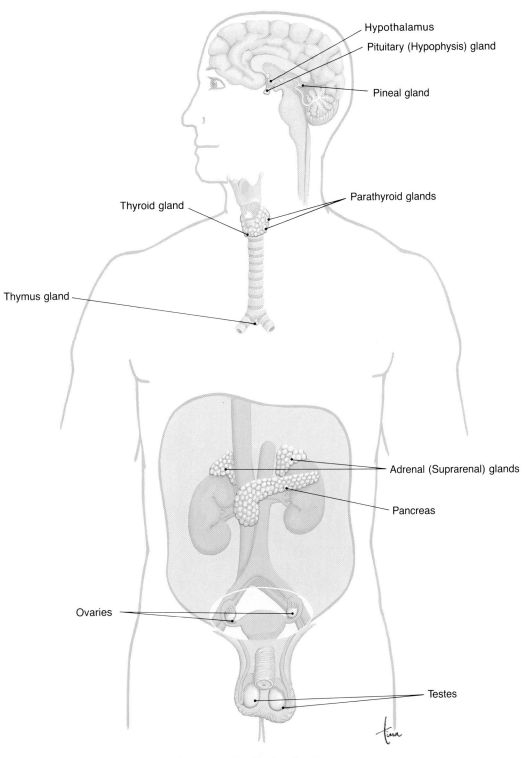

Hypothalamus

Pituitary (Hypophysis) gland

Pineal gland

Thyroid gland

Parathyroid glands

Thymus gland

Adrenal (Suprarenal) glands

Pancreas

Ovaries

Testes

Plate 17.   The Endocrine System.

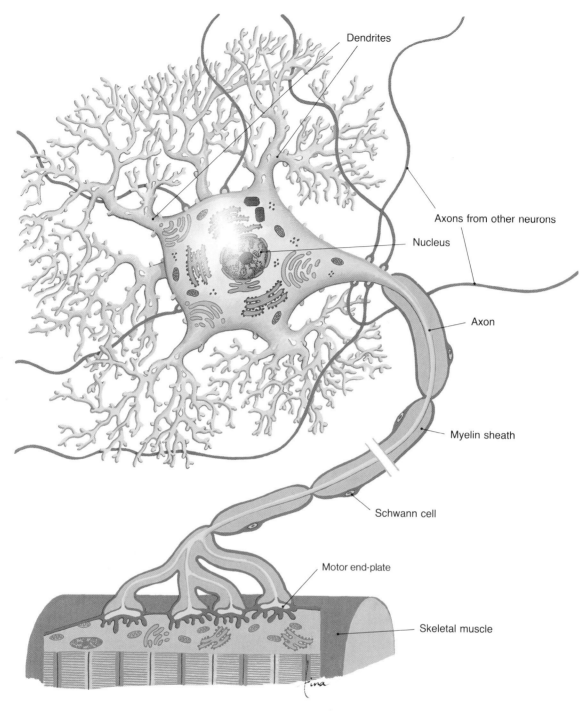

Dendrites

Axons from other neurons

Nucleus

Axon

Myelin sheath

Schwann cell

Motor end-plate

Skeletal muscle

Plate 18.   A Motor Neuron.

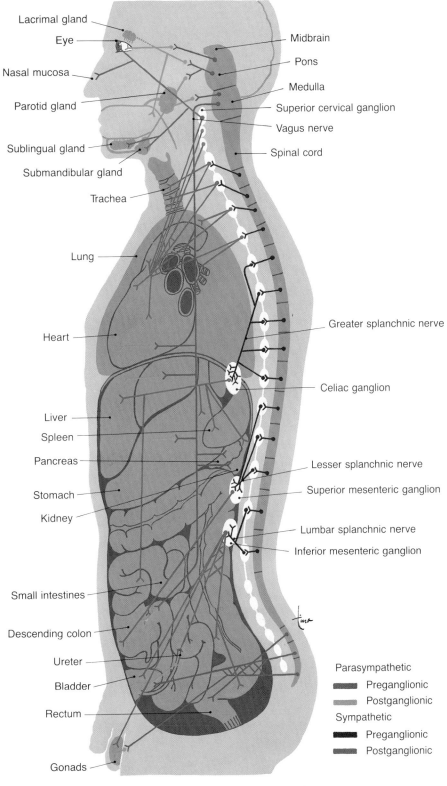

Lacrimal gland

Eye

Nasal mucosa

Parotid gland

Sublingual gland

Submandibular gland

Trachea

Lung

Heart

Liver

Spleen

Pancreas

Stomach

Kidney

Small intestines

Descending colon

Ureter

Bladder

Rectum

Gonads

Midbrain

Pons

Medulla

Superior cervical ganglion

Vagus nerve

Spinal cord

Greater splanchnic nerve

Celiac ganglion

Lesser splanchnic nerve

Superior mesenteric ganglion

Lumbar splanchnic nerve

Inferior mesenteric ganglion

Parasympathetic
Preganglionic
Postganglionic
Sympathetic
Preganglionic
Postganglionic

Plate 19.   The Autonomic Nervous System.

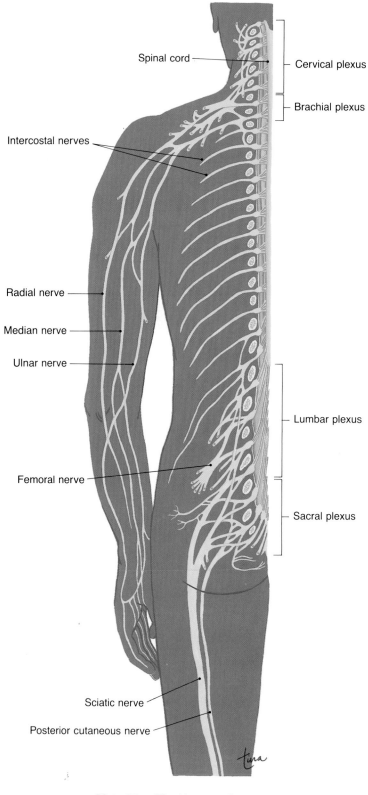

Spinal cord

Cervical plexus

Brachial plexus

Intercostal nerves

Radial nerve

Median nerve

Ulnar nerve

Lumbar plexus

Femoral nerve

Sacral plexus

Sciatic nerve

Posterior cutaneous nerve

tina

Plate 20. The Nervous System.

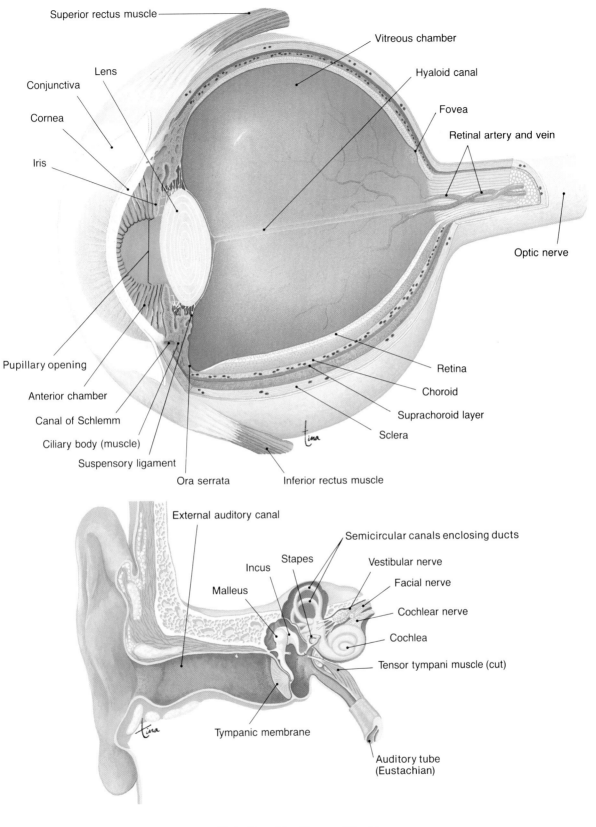

Superior rectus muscle

Vitreous chamber

Hyaloid canal

Lens

Conjunctiva

Fovea

Cornea

Retinal artery and vein

Iris

Optic nerve

Pupillary opening

Retina

Anterior chamber

Choroid

Canal of Schlemm

Suprachoroid layer

Ciliary body (muscle)

Sclera

Suspensory ligament

Ora serrata

Inferior rectus muscle

External auditory canal

Semicircular canals enclosing ducts

Stapes

Vestibular nerve

Incus

Facial nerve

Malleus

Cochlear nerve

Cochlea

Tensor tympani muscle (cut)

Tympanic membrane

Auditory tube (Eustachian)

Plate 21.   The Eye, and the Ear.

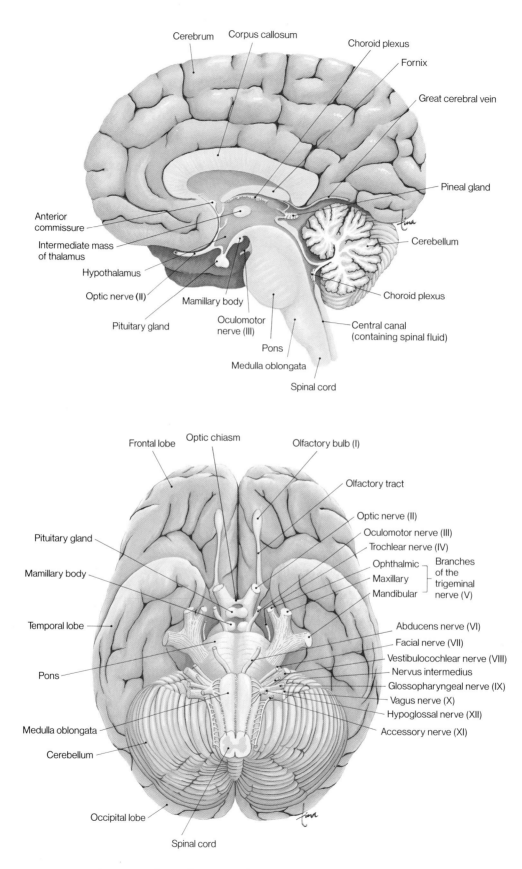

Plate 22.   Cross-Sections of the Brain, and the Cranial Nerves.

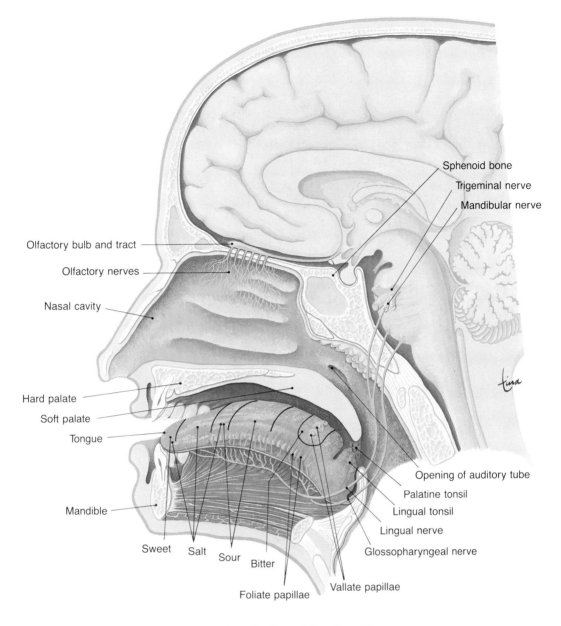

Olfactory bulb and tract

Olfactory nerves

Nasal cavity

Hard palate

Soft palate

Tongue

Mandible

Sweet

Salt

Sour

Bitter

Foliate papillae

Sphenoid bone

Trigeminal nerve

Mandibular nerve

Opening of auditory tube

Palatine tonsil

Lingual tonsil

Lingual nerve

Glossopharyngeal nerve

Vallate papillae

Plate 23.   The Centers of Smell and Taste.

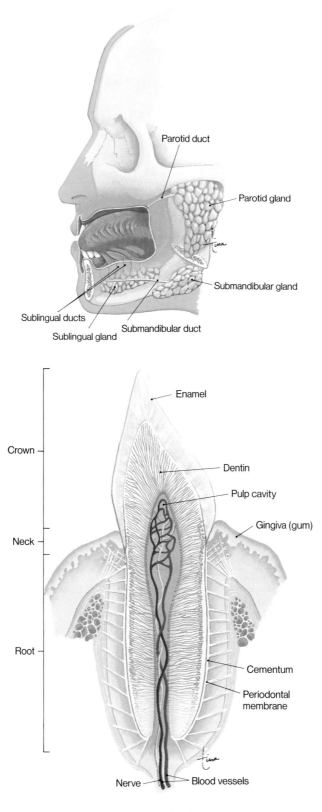

Parotid duct

Parotid gland

Submandibular gland

Sublingual ducts

Sublingual gland

Submandibular duct

Enamel

Crown

Dentin

Pulp cavity

Gingiva (gum)

Neck

Root

Cementum

Periodontal membrane

Nerve

Blood vessels

Plate 24.   The Salivary Glands, and the Tooth.

Introduction

Medical terminology is the study of words that pertain to body systems, anatomical structures, medical processes and procedures, and a variety of diseases. It provides a specialized language for the health care team so they may communicate in a concise and accurate way. Thus, medical terminology is a language created exclusively for the convenience of those who work in the health care industry.

There are no indications that the rapid growth of the health care industry will subside. This means that a steadily increasing demand for individuals skilled in the language of medicine will continue in the years to come. The growth of the health care industry manifests itself in various ways, including the proliferation of numerous health occupations, the explosive growth of the insurance industry offering various new types of health insurance plans, and the rapid expansion of biotechnical engineering firms, to mention only a few. In order for health professional teams to function effectively in all these areas, there is a need for individuals who are skilled in medical terminology.

The basic purpose of this book is to equip members of the health care industry with a working knowledge of medical vocabulary. Every chapter is structured to serve as both a text and a student workbook. Chapter 1 introduces the majority of suffixes used in the formation of medical vocabulary. In many cases, the pronunciations are included along with the definitions. Chapter 2 presents suffixes that denote adjective, noun, and singular and plural forms. Chapter 3 provides an analysis of prefixes for many medical words found in subsequent chapters. Chapter 4 presents the general structure of the body as a whole. The remainder of the text is dedicated to an analysis of medical terms that apply to the various body systems. In every body system chapter, the combining forms, prefixes, suffixes, and pathology are developed. The body system chapters also include common diagnostic, laboratory, and surgical procedures, as well as pharmacology and abbreviation sections.

Worksheets are included to provide you not only with a means of thorough self-testing, but also with exercises that will help you to formulate operative, diagnostic, and symptomatic terms that relate to the specific body system covered in the chapter. Successful completion of the worksheets will enrich your medical vocabulary and amplify the essentials of word-building skills.

In order to facilitate the self-testing and word-forming capabilities of the student, answers are provided in the back of the textbook in Appendix A. This permits the use of the worksheets for either independent study or for formal classroom instruction.

For the most part, the methodology of medical word building follows simple rules. Once these rules are learned, a variety of new medical terms can be built and defined. As in all languages, there are some words that are exceptions to such rules. Fortunately, in medicine there are few words subject to irregularities.

Word Root (WR) is a basic stem word, usually derived from the Greek or Latin language. Word roots are the building blocks for many prefixes, suffixes, anatomical words, medical procedures, laboratory techniques, and abbreviations.

EXAMPLES OF WORD ROOTS

GREEK WORD	WORD ROOT (WR)
kardia (heart)	cardi
osteon (bone)	oste
nephros (kidney)	nephr
erythros (red)	erythr
gastros (stomach)	gastr

Combining Form (CF) is a word root to which you add a combining vowel (usually an ''o''). In this text, a combining form will be represented by the following: word root (WR), a slash (/), and a vowel. More simply: word root/vowel = a combining form (WR/o = CF).

EXAMPLES OF COMBINING FORMS

WR	+ /o (combining vowel)	=	CF	MEANING
cardi	+ /o	=	cardi/o	heart
cyt	+ /o	=	cyt/o	cell
oste	+ /o	=	oste/o	bone
erythr	+ /o	=	erythr/o	red
nephr	+ /o	=	nephr/o	kidney
gastr	+ /o	=	gastr/o	stomach

We recommend that you memorize the combining form rather than the word root because the combining form provides ease of pronunciation for many words. For example, the word roots for kidney, red, and stomach (listed above) are difficult to pronounce, while the combining forms for these word elements are not.

There are three basic rules to follow when building medical terms. They are:

1. In building words with more than one root (compound words), retain the combin-

ing vowel when the second word root begins with a consonant. (See example below.)

therm /   o   / meter = instrument to measure heat
   ↓   ↓   ↓
  WR   combining   suffix
           vowel

2. The combining vowel is usually retained between two roots even if the second root begins with a vowel. (See examples below.)

gastr /   o   / enter /   itis   = inflammation of the stomach and intestines
   ↓   ↓   ↓   ↓
  WR   combining   WR   suffix
           vowel

dacry /   o   / aden /   itis   = inflammation of the lacrimal gland
   ↓   ↓   ↓   ↓   (tear duct)
  WR   combining   WR   suffix
           vowel

3. The combining vowel is usually dropped before a **suffix** that begins with a vowel. However, it is usually retained if the suffix begins with a consonant. (See examples below.)

nephr /   o   / scler /   osis   = abnormal condition of hardening
   ↓   ↓   ↓   ↓   of the kidney
  WR   combining   WR   suffix
           vowel

oste /   o   / tome = instrument used to cut bone
   ↓   ↓   ↓
  WR   combining   suffix
           vowel

When defining medical terms, read the definition as follows:
1. Define the **suffix**.
2. Define the **prefix**, or first part of the word.
3. Define the **middle part** of the word.

Example

gastr / o / enter / itis
   ↓   ↓   ↓
  (2)   (3)   (1)

Read as follows:
1. Inflammation.
2. Stomach.
3. Intestines (usually small intestine).
The definition is inflammation (of) stomach (and) intestines.

4 PRONUNCIATION

Medical terms may be difficult to pronounce when you first encounter them. Here are some general rules you will find helpful:

- ae and oe, pronounce only the second vowel. Examples: bursae, pleurae.
- c and g have a hard sound before other letters. Examples: cardiac, cast, gastric, gonad.
- c and g are given the soft sound of s and j, respectively, before e, i, and y in words of both Greek and Latin origins. Examples: gingivitis, giant, cytometer, cycle.
- e and es, when forming the final letter or letters of a word, are often pronounced as separate syllables. Examples: nares, rete.
- ch is sometimes pronounced like k. Examples: cholesterol, cholera, cholemia.
- i at the end of a word (to form a plural) is pronounced "eye." Examples: bronchi, fungi, nuclei.
- pn at the beginning of a word is pronounced with only the n sound. Examples: pneumonia, pneumotoxin.
- pn in the middle of the word is pronounced with a hard p and a hard n. Examples: orthopnea, hyperpnea.
- ps is pronounced like s. Examples: psychology, psychosis.
- All other vowels and consonants have ordinary English sounds.

More than 95 percent of the medical words in this textbook are spelled phonetically. Pronunciations are included throughout, using diacritical marks to indicate most of the long and short vowels. Diacritics are marks over or under vowels. In this text, only two diacritics are used. The macron (‾) indicates the long sound of vowels, as in the following:

ā in rate
ē in rebirth
ī in isle
ō in over
ū in unite

The breve (˘) indicates the short sound of vowels, as in the following:

ă in apple
ĕ in ever
ĭ in it
ŏ in not
ŭ in cut

To indicate stress on certain syllables, these syllables are capitalized, as in LĔT - ter.

WORKSHEET 1

Complete the following statements.

1. Basic stem words that act as building blocks for many prefixes, suffixes, anatomical words, medical procedures, laboratory techniques, and abbreviations are called ___word___ ___roots___ .

2. Many word roots are derived from the ___Greek___ or _____ language.

3. A ___combining___ ___form___ is a word root to which a final vowel is added.

4. The combining form vowel is usually a/an ___o___ .

5. In building compound words, the combining form vowel is retained when the second word root begins with a/an ___consonant___ .

6 WORKSHEET 2

Underline all combining forms in the following list.

1. cardi

2. cardi/o

3. gastr/o

4. cyt

5. erythr/o

6. oste

7. oste/o

8. gastr

9. nephr

10. erythr

WORKSHEET 3

In the space provided, build combining forms for the following word roots.

1. mast (breast) _____mast/o_____

2. hepat (liver) _____hepat/o_____

3. arthr (joint) _____arthr/o_____

4. cyst (bladder) _____cyst/o_____

5. phleb (vein) _____phleb/o_____

6. thorac (chest) _____thorac/o_____

7. abdomin (abdomen) _____abdomin/o_____

8. trache (trachea) _____trache/o_____

8   ## WORKSHEET 4

Express each of the following combining forms as word roots.

1. rhin/o (nose) _____ rhin _____

2. splen/o (spleen) _____ splen _____

3. hyster/o (uterus) _____ hyster _____

4. enter/o (intestines) _____ enter _____

5. neur/o (nerve) _____ neur _____

6. ot/o (ear) _____ ot _____

7. dermat/o (skin) _____ dermat _____

8. hydr/o (water) _____ hydr _____

WORKSHEET 5

Place a slash between compound words, then list the combining form in the space provided. Place parentheses around the combining vowel.

COMPOUND WORD	COMBINING FORM
1. gastro/enteritis	gastr(o)
2. enteroanastomosis	enter(o)
3. nephrosclerosis	nephr(o)
4. ileocolic	ile(o)
5. gastrointestinal	gastr(o)
6. nephroabdominal	nephr(o)
7. microscope	micr(o)
8. thermometer	therm(o)
9. leukoderma	leuk(o)
10. hydrochloride	hydr(o)

CHAPTER 1

Suffixes: Surgical, Diagnostic, Symptomatic

STUDENT OBJECTIVES

Upon completion of this chapter, you will be able to do the following:

Define and give several examples of word roots, combining forms, and suffixes.

Describe how medical words are formed from word roots, combining forms, and suffixes. Apply this knowledge by completing worksheet exercises.

Build medical words for surgical, diagnostic, and symptomatic suffixes by completing the worksheets.

A suffix is a word element that serves to form a new word when it is placed at the end of a word. Some of the more familiar examples of suffixes used in ordinary speech are: -ness, -ing, -ism. You can observe how variations of the words are formed by placing these suffixes at the ends of words.

EXAMPLES

dark darkness
sing singing
patriot patriotism

Similarly, by adding a suffix to a medical word, a new medical word can be formed.
Medical vocabulary is a concise language and has a multitude of suffixes. For instance, there are suffixes that indicate parts of speech or singular or plural word forms.

Formation of a new word by suffix addition gives it a meaning that often takes several words to communicate in ordinary language. For example, the medical term tonsillectomy means ''surgical excision or removal of the tonsils.'' It can be broken down into component parts as follows:

tonsill / ectomy

↓   ↓

tonsil   excision

From this example, it is evident that, in the field of medicine, medical terminology provides an exact and accurate form of communication. Most suffixes in medical terminology are derived from the **Greek** or **Latin** language.

Three basic rules for building medical words were listed in the introduction of the textbook. You might wish to review the third rule before proceeding with the suffix chapter. Nevertheless, a few examples can be summarized as follows:

The first example applies when the suffix begins with a vowel: -itis (inflammation); -algia (pain); -ectomy (excision). In most cases, when building medical words with suffixes that begin with a vowel, add the word root directly to the suffix. In most instances, no combining vowel is needed.

EXAMPLES OF SUFFIXES BEGINNING WITH VOWELS

WR	+	SUFFIX	=	MEDICAL WORD
gastr (stomach)	+	itis (inflammation)	=	gastritis
cephal (head)	+	algia (pain)	=	cephalalgia
mast (breast)	+	ectomy (excision)	=	mastectomy

The second example governs suffixes that begin with a consonant: -tomy (incision); -scopy (visual examination). In this situation, a combining form is needed to form the medical word. In most instances, the combining vowel is an "o." However, it can also be another vowel, as in the word pelvimeter, which has the connecting vowel "i."

EXAMPLES OF SUFFIXES BEGINNING WITH CONSONANTS

COMBINING FORM		+ SUFFIX	= MEDICAL WORD
WR	+ o		
phleb (vein)	+ o	+ tomy (incision)	= phlebotomy
colon (colon)	+ o	+ scopy (visual examination)	= colonoscopy
arthr (joint)	+ o	+ centesis (surgical puncture)	= arthrocentesis
pelv (pelvis)	+ i	+ meter (instrument to measure)	= pelvimeter

SUMMARY OF RULES

Build medical words by following three rules:

RULE 1. In building words with more than one root, the combining vowel is retained when the second word root begins with a consonant.

RULE 2. The combining vowel is usually retained between two roots even if the second root begins with a vowel.

RULE 3. The combining vowel is usually dropped before a suffix that begins with a vowel. However, it is usually retained if the suffix begins with a consonant.

All of the major medical suffixes in this text are classified by categories and are presented in this chapter. They are designated as Surgical Procedure, Diagnostic, Symptomatic, and Miscellaneous Suffixes.

SURGICAL PROCEDURE SUFFIXES

Suffixes Denoting Incisions

Some of the surgical suffixes denoting incisions are:

SUFFIX	MEANING	EXAMPLE	PRONUNCIATION
-ectomy	excision, removal	append/ectomy appendix	ăp - ĕn - DĔK - tŏ - mē
-centesis	surgical puncture	arthr/o/centesis joint	ăr - thrō - sĕn - TĒ - sĭs
-stomy	mouth, forming a new opening	col/o/stomy colon	kŏ - LŎS - tō - mē
-tome	instrument to cut	oste/o/tome bone	ŎS - tē - ō - tōm
-tomy	incision, cut into	phleb/o/tomy vein	flĕ - BŎT - ō - mē

Suffixes Denoting Reconstructive Surgeries

The surgical suffixes that can be classified in terms of reconstructive surgeries (repair, rebuild, or bind) include:

SUFFIX	MEANING	EXAMPLE	PRONUNCIATION
-desis	binding, stabilization, fusion	arthr/o/desis joint	ăr - thrō - DĒ - sĭs
-rrhaphy	suture	colp/o/rrhaphy vagina	kŏl - POR - ă - fē
-pexy	fixation, suspension	gastr/o/pexy stomach	GAS - trō - pĕk - sē
-plasty	formation, plastic repair, surgical repair	rhin/o/plasty nose	RĪ - nō - plăs - tē

14 Suffixes Denoting Refracturing, Loosening, or Crushing

The surgical suffixes employed for refracturing, loosening, or crushing are:

SUFFIX	MEANING	EXAMPLE	PRONUNCIATION
-clasis	a breaking (of), refracture	oste/o/clasis bone	ŏs - tē - ŎK - lăh - sĭs
-lysis	separate, destroy, break down	enter/o/lysis intestines (usually small)	ĕn - tĕr - ŎL - ĭ - sĭs
-tripsy	crush	lith/o/tripsy stone	LĪTH - ō - trĭp - sē

DIAGNOSTIC AND SYMPTOMATIC SUFFIXES

The following suffixes indicate a disease or a condition or a change in the body or its functions.

SUFFIX	MEANING	EXAMPLE	PRONUNCIATION
-algia	pain	cephal/algia head	sĕf - ăh - LĂL - jē - ăh
-cele	hernia, swelling	hepat/o/cele liver	HĔP - ă - tō - sĕl
-dynia	pain	gastr/o/dynia stomach	găs - trō - DĬN - ē - ăh
-ectasis	dilation, expansion	bronchi/ectasis bronchus	brŏng - kē - ĔK - tăh - sĭs
-emia	blood condition (of)	leuk/emia white	loo - KĒ - mē - ăh
-gen	to produce	carcin/o/gen cancer	kăr - SIN - ō - jĕn
-gram	a writing, record	electr/o/cardi/o/gram heart	ē - lĕk - trō - KĂR - dē - ō - grăm
-graph	instrument for recording	electr/o/cardi/o/graph heart	ē - lĕk - trō - KĂR - dē - ŏ - grăf
-graphy	process of recording	electr/o/cardi/o/graphy heart record	ē - lĕk - trō - KĂR - dē - ŏ - gră - fē
-iasis	condition, formation of, presence of	chole/lith/iasis gall stone	kō - lē - lĭ - THĪ - ăh - sĭs

Continued on following page

SUFFIX	MEANING	EXAMPLE	PRONUNCIATION
-itis	inflammation	gastr/<u>itis</u> stomach	găs - TRĪ - tĭs
-logy	study of	psych/o/<u>logy</u> mind	sī - KŎL - ō - jē
-malacia	softening	oste/o/<u>malacia</u> bone	ŏs - tē - ō - măh - LĀ - shē - ăh
-megaly	enlargement	hepat/o/<u>megaly</u> liver	hĕp - ăh - tō - MEG - ăh - lē
-meter	measure, instrument for measuring	therm/o/<u>meter</u> heat	thĕr - MŎM - ĕ - tĕr
-metry	act of measuring, to measure	pelv/i/<u>metry</u> pelvis	pĕl - VĬM - ĕt - rē
-oid	resemble	lip/<u>oid</u> fat	LĬP - oid
-oma	tumor	aden/<u>oma</u> gland	ăd - ĕ - NŌ - măh
-osis	abnormal condition, increase (used primarily with blood cells)	dermat/<u>osis</u> skin, abnormal condition (of) erythr/o/cyt/ <u>osis</u> red cell increase	dĕr - măh - TŌ - sĭs ĕ - rĭth - rō - sī - TŌ - sĭs
-pathy	disease	nephr/o/<u>pathy</u> kidney	nē - FRŎP - ăh - thē
-penia	decrease, deficiency, lack of	leuk/o/<u>penia</u> white (cell)	loo - kō - PĒ - nē - ăh
-phagia	eating, ingesting, swallowing	dys/<u>phagia</u> difficult	dĭs - FĀ - jē - ăh
-phasia	speech	a/<u>phasia</u> without	ăh - FĀ - zē - ăh
-paresis	partial or incomplete paralysis	hemi/<u>paresis</u> half	hĕm - ē - PĂR - ĕ - sĭs
-plegia	paralysis, stroke	hemi/<u>plegia</u> half	hĕm - ē - PLĒ - jē - ăh
-phobia	fear (of)	claustr/o/<u>phobia</u> confined place	klaws - trō - FŌ - bē - ăh

Continued on following page

16

SUFFIX	MEANING	EXAMPLE	PRONUNCIATION
-ptosis	prolapse, falling, dropping	hyster/o/ptosis uterus	hĭs - tĕr - ŏp - TŌ - sĭs
-rrhage -rrhagia }	burst forth (of)	hem/o/rrhage blood	HĔM - or -ĭj
-rrhea	discharge, flow	men/o/rrhea menses	mĕn - ō - RĒ - ăh
-rrhexis	rupture	angi/o/rrhexis vessel	ăn - jĭ - o - REK - sĭs
-sclerosis	abnormal condition (of) hardening	arteri/o/sclerosis artery	ăr - tē - rē - ō - sklĕ - RŌ - sĭs
-scope	instrument to view or examine	gastr/o/scope stomach	GĂS - trō - skōp
-scopy	visual examination	ot/o/scopy ear	ō - TŎS - kō - pē
-spasm	involuntary contraction, twitching	blephar/o/spasm eyelid	BLĔF - ăh - rō - spăzm
-stasis	standing still	hemo/stasis blood	hē - mō - STĀ - sĭs

MISCELLANEOUS SUFFIXES

SUFFIX	MEANING	EXAMPLE	PRONUNCIATION
-lith	stone, calculus	chole/lith gall	KŌ - lē - lĭth
-philia	attraction for, to love	hem/o/philia blood	hē - mō - FĬL - ē - ăh
-plasia	formation, development, growth	hyper/plasia excessive	hĭ - pĕr - PLĀ - zē - ăh
-poiesis	formation, production	hem/o/poiesis blood	hē - mō - poy - Ē - sĭs
-stenosis	constriction, narrowing	angi/o/stenosis vessel	ăn - jē - ō - stĕ - NŌ - sĭs
-toxic	poison	thyr/o/toxic thyroid	thĭ - rō - TŎKS - ĭk

GENERAL REVIEW

Recall the rules for building a medical word. The combining form is used when a suffix begins with a consonant. (See examples below.) (There are some exceptions to this rule.)

erythr / o / cyte = red blood cell
   ↓   ↓
  CF   suffix

men / o / rrhea
   ↓   ↓
  CF   suffix

leuk / o / cyte = white blood cell
   ↓   ↓
  CF   suffix

oste / o / cyte
   ↓   ↓
  CF   suffix

However, when the suffix begins with a vowel, the root is joined directly to the suffix. No combining vowel is needed. (See examples below.)

mast / ectomy = excision of a breast
  ↓   ↓
WR suffix

neur / algia = pain of a nerve
  ↓   ↓
WR suffix

dermat / osis = abnormal condition
  ↓   ↓   of the skin
WR suffix

nephr / oma = tumor of the kidney
  ↓   ↓
WR suffix

18

WORKSHEET 1

Surgical Suffixes Denoting Incisions

Complete the following exercise. Note that the word root is underlined.

INCOMPLETE WORD	MEANING
1. cyst/o/ t o m y	Incision of the bladder
2. col e c t o m y	Excision (of part or all) of the colon
3. arthr/o/ c e n t e s i s	Puncture of a joint
4. splen e c t o m y	Excision of the spleen
5. col/o/ s t o m y	New permanent opening into the colon
6. derma t o m e	Instrument to cut skin
7. myring o t o m y	Incision of the tympanic membrane
8. trache/o/ s t o m y	New permanent opening into the trachea
9. lith/o/ t o m y	Incision to remove a stone or calculus
10. phleb/o/ t o m	Incision of a vein
11. mast e c t o m y	Excision of a breast
12. hemorrhoid e c t o m y	Excision of hemorrhoids
13. trache/o/ t o m y	Incision of the trachea

Using the above list, build a medical term that means:

14. Excision of a breast ___mastectomy___

15. Excision of part of the colon ___colectomy___

16. Incision of the tympanic membrane ___myringotomy___

17. New permanent opening into the colon ___colostomy___

18. Incision of the trachea ___tracheotomy___

19. Removal of the spleen ___slenectomy___

20. Instrument to cut skin ___dermatome___

21. Creation of a permanent opening into the trachea _tracheostomy_

22. Incision to remove a stone or calculus _litho tomy_

23. Puncture of a joint _arthrocentesis_

24. Removal of hemorrhoids _hemorrhoidectomy_

25. Incision of a vein _phlebotomy_

20

WORKSHEET 2

Surgical Suffixes Denoting Reconstructive Surgeries (Repair, Rebuild, or Bind)

Complete the following exercise. Note that the word root is underlined. Each suffix begins with a consonant; therefore, a connecting vowel is needed to change the word root to a combining form.

INCOMPLETE WORD	MEANING
1. episi /o/ t o m y	Incision of perineum
2. mast /o/ p e x y	Surgical fixation of a (pendulous) breast
3. nephr /o/ p e x y	Surgical fixation of a (floating) kidney
4. gastr /o/ r r h a p h y	Suture of the stomach (wall)
5. hyster /o/ p e x y	Surgical fixation of the uterus
6. rhin /o/ p l a s t y	Plastic surgery of the nose
7. arthr /o/ d e s i s	Fusion of a joint
8. splen /o/ p e x y	Fixation of a (movable) spleen

Using the above list, build a medical term that means:

9. Surgical fixation of the uterus hysteropexy

10. Surgical fixation of the stomach gastropexy

11. Plastic repair of the nose rhinoplasty

12. Fusion of a joint arthrodesis

13. Surgical fixation of a breast mastopexy

14. Suture of the spleen splenorrhaphy

15. Surgical puncture of a joint arthrocentesis

WORKSHEET 3

Surgical Suffixes Denoting Refracturing, Loosening, or Crushing

Complete the following exercise.

INCOMPLETE WORD	MEANING
1. oste/o/_c_l_a_s_i_s	Surgical breaking or refracturing of a bone
2. lith/o/_t_r_i_p_s_y	Crushing of a stone or calculus
3. hem/o/_l_y_s_i_s	Destruction of blood
4. neur/o/_t_r_i_p_s_y	Crushing of a nerve

5. Write the word root found in osteoclasis. _oste_

6. Write the combining form found in neurotripsy. _neuro_

7. Write the word root found in nephropexy. _nephr_

8. Write the combining form found in gastroscopy. _gastro_

Build medical words that mean:

9. Destruction of blood _hematolysis_

10. Refracturing of a bone _osteoclasis_

11. Crushing of calculi or stones _lithotripsy_

12. Surgical crushing of a nerve _neurotripsy_

13. Freeing the intestines from adhesions _enterolysis_

WORSHEET 4

22

WORKSHEET 4

Diagnostic and Symptomatic Suffixes

Complete the following exercise.

INCOMPLETE WORD	MEANING
1. bronchi_ectasis_	Dilation of a bronchus
2. gastr_odynia_	Pain in the stomach
3. neur_algia_	Pain (along the course) of a nerve
4. gastr_itis_	Inflammation of the stomach
5. cephal_algia_	Headache; pain in the head
6. leuk_emia_	Abnormal condition (of) white blood
7. carcin_ogen_	To produce cancer
8. dermat_osis_	Abnormal condition of skin
9. lip_oid_	Resembling fat
10. carcin_oid_	Resembling cancer
11. cyt_openia_	Decrease of cellular elements (in the blood)
12. leuk_openia_	Decrease in number of white cells in the blood
13. oto_rrhea_	Discharge or flow from the ear
14. leuk_orrhea_	White mucus discharge (from vagina or cervical canal)
15. gastr_ospasm_	Spasm or twitching of the stomach
16. blephar_ospasm_	Spasm or twitching of the eyelid
17. neur_olysis_	Destruction or dissolution of nerve tissue
18. my_olysis_	Destruction or degeneration of muscle tissue
19. osteo_gen_	To produce bone
20. hemi_paresis_	Partial or incomplete paralysis

WORKSHEET 5

Symptomatic and Miscellaneous Suffixes

Complete the following exercise. Remember to use the word root if the suffix begins with a vowel. If the suffix begins with a consonant, use a combining form.

INCOMPLETE WORD	MEANING
1. cyst_ocele_	Hernia of the bladder
2. quadri_plegia_	Paralysis of all four extremities and usually the trunk
3. myel_ocele_	Herniation of the spinal cord
4. lith_iasis_	Formation of a stone
5. nephr_olithiasis_	Presence of a kidney stone
6. hemi_paresis_	Paralysis affecting one side
7. leuko_poiesis_	Production of white cells
8. hepato_megaly_	Enlargement (of the) liver
9. _gastr_itis	Inflammation of the stomach
10. oste_omalacia_	Softening of bone
11. nephr_omalacia_	Softening of the kidney
12. nephr_omegaly_	Enlarged kidney
13. cardi_omegaly_	Enlarged heart
14. erythr_openia_	Deficiency in number of red (blood cells)
15. splen_omegaly_	Enlarged spleen
16. nephr_oma_	Tumor of the kidney
17. nephr_osis_	Abnormal condition of the kidney
18. _scler_osis	Condition of hardening
19. gastr_opathy_	Disease of the stomach
20. _nephro_pathy	Disease of a kidney

24

21. gastr <u>optosis</u>   Dropped or displaced stomach

22. nephr <u>optosis</u>   Dropped or displaced kidney

23. angi <u>orrhexis</u>   Rupture of a (blood) vessel

24. hyster <u>orrhexis</u>   Rupture of the uterus

25. <u>dermat</u> itis   Inflammation of the skin

WORKSHEET 6

Test your overall knowledge by filling in the meanings for the following suffixes.

1. -itis _inflammation of_
2. -o/megaly _enlargement_
3. -o/pathy _disease_
4. -o/centesis _puncture_
5. -o/plasty _plastic surgery_
6. -o/lysis _destroy_
7. -o/rrhaphy _suture_
8. -emia _blood condition_
9. -algia _pain_
10. -o/rrhea _flow_
11. -o/spasm _involuntary twitch_
12. -o/malacia _softening_
13. -o/plegia _partial paralysis_
14. -o/rrhexis _rupture_
15. -o/cele _hernia_

16. -ectasis _dilation_
17. -iasis _formation of_
18. -o/rrhage _burst forth_
19. -o/ptosis _dropping_
20. -oma _tumor_
21. -o/gen _to produce_
22. -stasis _stand still_
23. -o/penia _decrease_
24. -o/stomy _mouth_
25. -o/tomy _incision_
26. -phasia _speech_
27. -poiesis _formation_
28. -phagia _ingesting_
29. -penia _decrease_
30. -stenosis _constricting_

CHAPTER 2

Suffixes: Adjective, Noun, Diminutive, Singular, Plural

STUDENT OBJECTIVES

Upon completion of this chapter, you will be able to do the following:

List and define suffixes for adjective endings, and apply this knowledge by completing Worksheet 1.

List and define suffixes for noun endings, and apply this knowledge by completing Worksheet 2.

List and define suffixes for diminutive endings.

Define the rules for changing singular words to plural words, and apply this knowledge by completing Worksheet 3.

The suffixes discussed in this chapter are added to word roots to indicate either a part of speech or a singular or plural form.

ADJECTIVE ENDINGS

The adjective endings that mean "pertaining to" and/or "relating to" are:

ADJECTIVE ENDING	EXAMPLE
-ac*	cardi/ac heart
-al	neur/al nerve
-ar	muscul/ar muscle
-ary	saliv/ary saliva
-ic	hypo/ derm/ic under skin
-ical†	med/ical medicine
-ous‡	sub/ cutane/ous under skin
-ory	audit/ory hearing
-tic	paraly/tic paralysis

*—ac ending is rarely used
†—ical is a combination of -ic and -al
‡—ous also means composed of, producing

NOUN ENDINGS

The suffixes that are added to word roots to indicate a noun are:

NOUN ENDING	MEANING	EXAMPLE
-er	one who	paint/er
-ia	condition (of), process	pneumon/ia lung
-is	forms the noun from the root	cut/is skin
-ism	condition, state of being	alcohol/ism alcohol

Continued on following page

NOUN ENDING	MEANING	EXAMPLE	
-ist	one who specializes	uro/ urology	log/ist study of
-y	condition, process	myo/ muscle	path/ y disease

DIMINUTIVE ENDINGS

A diminutive ending forms a word designating a small version of the thing indicated by the main stem of the word.

DIMINUTIVE ENDING	MEANING	EXAMPLE
-ole		arteri/ole artery
-icle	small, little, minute	part/icle piece
-ula		mac/ula spot
-ule		ven/ule vein

PLURAL ENDINGS

The rules for forming plural words from singular words are listed below.

SINGULAR FORM	PLURAL FORM	RULE	EXAMPLE Singular	Plural
a	ae	Retain the a and add e	pleura	pleurae
ax	aces	Drop the x and add ces	thorax	thoraces
en	ina	Drop en and add ina	lumen	lumina
is	es	Drop the is and add es	diagnosis	diagnoses
ix } ex }	ices	Drop the ix or ex and add ices	appendix apex	appendices apices
on	a	Drop on and add a	ganglion	ganglia
um	a	Drop um and add a	bacterium	bacteria
us	i	Drop us and add i	bronchus	bronchi
y	ies	Drop y and add ies	deformity	deformities
ma	mata	Retain the ma and add ta	carcinoma	carcinomata

30 WORKSHEET 1

Using the following word roots, *add an adjective ending* that means "pertaining to." Use the dictionary as a reference.

	WORD ROOT	MEANING		EXAMPLE
1.	narc	numbness	1.	narcotic
2.	gastr	stomach	2.	gastric
3.	hepat	liver	3.	hepatic
4.	duoden	duodenum (first part of the small intestine)	4.	duodenal
5.	bacteri	bacteria	5.	bacterial
6.	aque	watery	6.	aqueous
7.	cili	hairlike processes, especially eyelashes	7.	ciliary
8.	necr	death	8.	necroptic
9.	nephrocardi	nephro = kidney cardi = heart	9.	nephrocardiac
10.	fibr	fiber	10.	fibrous
11.	ossifer	os = bone fer = to bear	11.	ossiferous
12.	thorac	thorax, chest	12.	thoracic
13.	meningi	meninges	13.	meningieal
14.	membran	membrane	14.	membranous
15.	prophylac	guarding	15.	prophylactic
16.	muc	mucus	16.	mucous

WORKSHEET 2

Using the following word roots/combining forms, form medical words that have a *noun ending*. Use the dictionary as a reference. Underline the noun ending.

WR/CF	NOUN ENDING	MEANING
1. intern	1. intern<u>ist</u>	one who specializes in internal disease
2. leuk/em	2. leukemia	progressive, malignant disease of the blood-forming organs
3. sigmoid/oscop/	3. sigmoidoscopy	inspection of the sigmoid colon with a sigmoidoscope
4. alcohol	4. alcoholism	excessive consumption of alcohol
5. allerg	5. allergist	one who specializes in allergies
6. pub	6. pubis	pubic bone
7. senil	7. senilism	mental and physical weakness often associated with aging
8. man	8. mania	madness
9. ortho/ped	9. orthopedist	a specialist in orthopedics
10. pelv	10. pelvis	hip

32 WORKSHEET 3

Write the *plural form* for each word and briefly state the rule. Use the dictionary as a reference.

SINGULAR	PLURAL	RULE
1. enema	enemata	Retain the <u>ma</u> and add <u>ta</u>
2. aqua	aquae	a e
3. fornix	fornices	drop x ces
4. apex	apices	
5. bursa	bursae	a e
6. vertebra	vertebrae	a e
7. calcaneum	calcanea	drop um a
8. keratosis	keratoses	is es
9. bronchus	bronchi	us i
10. urinalysis	urinalyses	is es
11. speculum	specula	um a
12. uterus	uteri	us i
13. delivery	deliveries	y ies
14. spermatozoon	spermatozoa	on a
15. adenoma	adenomata	ma ta

WORKSHEET 4

Write the *plural form* for each word and briefly state the rule. Use the dictionary as a reference.

SINGULAR	PLURAL	RULE
1. medium	media	Drop <u>um</u> and add <u>a</u>
2. septum	septa	
3. coccus	cocci	
4. bursa	bursae	
5. ganglion	ganglia	
6. prognosis	prognoses	
7. thrombus	thrombi	
8. appendix	appendices	
9. bacterium	bacteria	
10. radius	radii	
11. conjunctiva	conjunctivae	
12. phenomenon	phenomena	
13. testis	testes	
14. apex	apices	
15. nevus	nevi	

CHAPTER 3

Prefixes

STUDENT OBJECTIVES

Upon completion of this chapter, you will be able to do the following:

Define prefix.

Identify prefixes of position and color, and apply this knowledge by completing Worksheets 1 and 2.

Identify prefixes of number, measurement, and direction, and apply this knowledge by completing Worksheets 3 and 4.

Identify miscellaneous prefixes, and apply this knowledge by completing Worksheet 5.

The major suffixes were presented in Chapters 1 and 2. This chapter emphasizes the major prefixes used in building a medical vocabulary. The first three chapters present the basic foundation for building medical words and should be used when studying the individual body systems chapters.

In order to learn medical terminology, it is easiest if you recognize the importance of breaking down medical words into components. This is achieved by developing the ability to recognize suffixes, prefixes, and combining forms.

Once you have learned the components in Chapters 1–3, you will experience no difficulty in defining the majority of medical terms in this textbook.

A prefix is a word element of one or more syllables and is always located at the beginning of a word. It is placed before a word root or with a suffix in order to change the meaning. In some words, a prefix can also serve as a combining form.

Example of a prefix with a word root is:

multi / par / ous = to bear many offspring

prefix   WR   suffix

Example of a prefix with a suffix is:

dia / rrhea = to flow

prefix   suffix

Example of a prefix that is also a combining form is:

leuk/o/cyte = white blood cell

CF   suffix

prefix

This chapter includes the major prefixes used in building medical terminology. The prefixes are grouped in sections in order to facilitate memorization.

PREFIXES OF POSITION

PREFIX	MEANING	EXAMPLE	PRONUNCIATION
ambi-	both, both sides	ambi/later/al side pertaining to	ăm - bĭ - LĂT - ěr - ăl
amphi-	on both sides	amphi/theatre	ăm - fē - THĒ - ă - těr
ante-	before, in front of	ante/cubit/al elbow pertaining to	ăn - tē - KŪ - bĭ - tăl
anter/o-		anter/o/posterior behind	ăn - těr - ō - pŏs - TĒ - rē - or
pre-		pre/operative operation	prē - ŎP - ěr - ā - tiv
pro-		pro/ot/ic ear pertaining to	prō - ŎT - ĭk

Continued on following page

PREFIX	MEANING	EXAMPLE		PRONUNCIATION
dextr/o-	to the right of	dextr/o/card/	ia	děks - trō - KĂR - dē - ăh
		heart	noun ending, condition (of)	
dors/o-	back	dors/o/sacr/	al	dor - sō - SĀ - krăl
		sacrum	pertaining to	
epi-	upon	epi/gastri/	um	ěp - ĭ - GĂS - trē - ŭm
		stomach	noun ending	
hypo-	under, below, beneath	hypo/derm/ic		hĭ - pō - DĔR - mĭk
		skin	relating to	
infra-		infra/pub/	ic	ĭn - fră - PŪ - bĭk
		pubis	relating to	
sub-		sub/nas/	al	sŭb - NĀ - zăl
		nose	pertaining to	
inter-	between	inter/cost/	al	ĭn - těr - KŌS - tăl
		ribs	pertaining to, adjective ending	
later/o-	side	later/ad*		LĂT - ěr - ăd
		toward		
mid-	middle	mid/stern/	um	mĭd - STĔR - nŭm
		chest	noun ending	
mes/o-		mes/o/derm		MĔS - ō - děrm
		skin		
medi-		medi/ad		MĒ - dē - ăd
		toward		
retro-	after, backward, behind	retro/spect		RĔT - rō - spěkt
		to look		
post-		post/nat/	al	pōst - NĀ - tăl
		birth	relating to	
postero-		postero/later/	al	pŏs - těr - ō - LĂT - ěr - ăl
		side	pertaining to side of	
sinistro-	left	sinistr/o/card/	ia	sĭn - ĭs - trō - KĂR - dē - ăh
		heart	noun ending, condition (of)	

*ad is also a prefix. See chart on Prefixes of Direction.

PREFIXES OF COLOR

PREFIX	MEANING	EXAMPLE	PRONUNCIATION
alb- albumin/o-	white protein	albumin/oid	ăl - BŪ - mĭ - noid
		resemble	

Continued on following page

PREFIXES OF COLOR—*Continued*

PREFIX	MEANING	EXAMPLE		PRONUNCIATION
leuc/o- ⎱ leuk/o- ⎰	white	leuk/em/	ia	loo - KĒ - mē - ăh
		blood	condition (of), noun ending	
chlor/o-	green	chlor/em/	ia	klō - RĒ - mē - ăh
		blood	condition (of), noun ending	
glauc/o- ⎱	gray	glauc/oma		glăw - KŌ - măh
		swelling		
polio- ⎰		polio/myel/	itis	pō - lē - ō - mĭ - ĕ - LĪ - tĭs
		spinal cord	inflammation	
cirrh/o- ⎱	yellow	cirrh/osis		sĭr - RŌ - sĭs
		abnormal condition (of)		
xanth/o- ⎰		xanth/em/	ia	zăn - THĒ - mē - ăh
		blood	condition (of), noun ending	
cyan/o-	blue	cyan/osis		sī - ă - NŌ - sĭs
		abnormal condition (of)		
melan/o-	black	melan/oma		mĕl - ăh - NŌ - măh
		tumor		
erythr/o- ⎱	red	erythr/o/cyte		ĕ - RĬTH - rō - sīt
		cell		
rube/o- ⎰		rube/osis		roo - bē - Ō - sĭs
		abnormal condition (of)		
purpur/o	purple	purpur/a		PŬR - pū - ră
		noun ending		

PREFIXES OF NUMBER AND MEASUREMENT

PREFIX	MEANING	EXAMPLE		PRONUNCIATION
primi-	first	primi/para*		prī - MĬP - ăh - răh
		to bear (offspring) to bring forth		
uni- ⎱	one	uni/para		ū - NĬP - ă - ră
		to bear (offspring) to bring forth		
mono- ⎰		mono/nucle/	us	mŏn - ō - NŪ - klē - ŭs
		nucleus	singular	
bi- ⎱	two	bi/later/	al	bī - LĂT - ĕr - ăl
di- ⎰		side	relating to	

Continued on following page

PREFIX	MEANING	EXAMPLE	PRONUNCIATION
diplo-	double	dipl/opia vision	dĭp - LŌ - pē - ăh
hemi- } semi- }	half, partial	hemi/pleg/ ia paralysis condition (of) semi/circul/ ar circle pertaining to	hĕm - ē - PLĒ - jē - ăh sĕm - ē - SŬR - kū - lăr
hyper-	over, above, excessive	hyper/active	hī - pĕr - ĂK - tĭv
hypo-	under, below	hypo/therm/ia heat condition (of), noun ending	hī - pō - THĚR - mē - ăh
multi- } poly- }	many, much	multi/para to bear (offspring) to bring forth poly/phob/ia fear condition (of)	mŭl - TĬP - ăh - răh pŏl - ē - FŌ - bē - ăh
tri-	three	tri/angul/ ar angle relating to	trī - ĂNG - gū - lĕr
quad- } quadri- }	four	quadri/pleg/ ia paralysis noun ending, condition (of)	kwŏd - rĭ - PLĒ - jē - ăh
macro-	large	macro/cephal/y head noun ending	măk - rō - SĔF - ăh - lē
micro-	small	micro/gastr/ ia stomach noun ending, condition (of)	mī - krō - GĂS - trē - ăh

*para is also a prefix. See chart on Prefixes of Direction.

PREFIXES OF NEGATION

PREFIX	MEANING	EXAMPLE	PRONUNCIATION
a- (usually used before a consonant) an- (usually used before a vowel) ar-	without, not, lack of	a/mast/ ia breast condition (of) an/esthes/ ia sensation condition (of) ar/rhythm/ ia rhythm noun ending, condition (of)	ă - MĂS - tē - ăh ăn - ĕs - THĒ - zē - ăh ăh - RĬTH - mē - ăh
im- } in- }	not	im/mature in/sane sound	ĭm - ăh - TŬR ĭn - SĀN

40 PREFIXES OF DIRECTION

PREFIX	MEANING	EXAMPLE	PRONUNCIATION
ab-	from, away from	ab/norm/ al regular, pertaining to usual	ăb - NŎR - măl
ad-	to, toward, near	ad/stern/ al breast relating to plate	ăd - STĔR - năl
circum-	around	circum/or/ al mouth pertaining to	sĕr - kŭm - Ō - răl
peri-	around	peri/oste/ um bone singular	pĕr - ē - ŎS - tē - ŭm
ec-	out, out from	ec/top/ ia place condition (of)	ĕk - TŌ - pē - ăh
ex-	out, out from	ex/cise to cut	ĕk - SĪZ
dia-	through, across	dia/rrhea flow	dī - ăh - RĒ - ăh
trans-	through, across	trans/fusion a pouring	trăns - FŪ - zhŭn
ecto-	outside	ecto/derm skin	ĔK - tō - dĕrm
exo-	outside	exo/trop/ ia turning condition (of)	ĕks - ō - TRŌ - pē - ăh
extra-	outside	extra/dur/ al hard pertaining to	ĕks - tră - DŪ - răl
endo-	in, within	endo/cardi/ um heart noun ending	ĕn - dō - KĂR - dē - ŭm
intra-	in, within	intra/muscul/ ar muscle relating to	ĭn - trăh - MŬS - kū - lăr
para-*	near, beside, beyond, abnormal	para/nas/ al nose pertaining to	păr - ă - NĀ - săl
super-	above	super/sensitive readily affected	soo - pĕr - SĔNS - ĭ - tĭv
supra-	above	supra/ren/ al kidney adjective ending	soo - pră - RĒ - năl
ultra-	beyond, excess	ultra/son/ ic sound adjective ending	ŭl - trăh - SŎN - ĭk

*para is also a suffix. When used as a suffix, it takes on the meaning "to bear." See chart on Prefixes of Number and Measurement.

MISCELLANEOUS PREFIXES

PREFIX	MEANING	EXAMPLE	PRONUNCIATION

anti- }
contra- }
	against	anti/bacteri/ al
		       bacteria pertaining to
		contra/ception
		          conceiving
			ăn - tĭ - băk - TĒ - rē - ăl
			
			kŏn - tră - SĔP - shŭn

brady-	slow	brady/card/ ia
		       heart noun ending,
		                condition (of)
			brād - ē - KĂR - dē - ăh

dys-	bad,
	painful,
	difficult
		dys/peps/ ia
		       digestion noun ending,
		                condition (of)
			dĭs - PĔP - sē - ăh

eu-	good, easy	eu/pnea breathing	ūp - NĒ - ăh
heter/o-	different	hetero/sex/ual pertaining to	hĕt - ĕr - ō - SĔK - shū - ăl
hidr/o	sweat	hidr/osis abnormal condition (of)	hĭ - DRŌ - sĭs
homo-	same	homo/sex/ual pertaining to	hō - mō - SĔK - shū - ăl
hydr/o-	water	hydro/phob/ia fear condition (of)	hĭ - drō - FŌ - bē - ăh
mal-	ill, bad, poor	mal/nutrition food substances	măl - nū - TRĬSH - ŭn
meta-	after, beyond, over, change	meta/carp/ al wrist pertaining to	mĕt - ăh - KĂR - păl
pan-	all	pan/hyster/ ectomy uterus excision	păn - hĭs - tĕr - ĔK - tō - mē
pseudo-	false	pseudo/pod foot	SOO - dō - pŏd
scler/o-	hard	scler/o/derma skin	sklē - rō - DĔR - mă
sym- } syn- }	union, together	syn/drome to run	SĬN - drōm
tachy-	rapid	tachy/pnea breathing	tăk - ĭp - NĒ - ăh

42

WORKSHEET 1

Place a slash after each prefix, then define the prefix.

WORD	DEFINE THE PREFIX
1. inter/dental	between
2. hypo/dermic	under
3. sinistro/cardia	left
4. epi/gastrium	upon
5. dors/algia	back
6. retro/active	after
7. lat/eral	side
8. postero/lateral	after
9. dextro/cardia	to right
10. sub/nasal	under
11. pro/thrombin	before
12. media/stinum	middle
13. infra/patellar	below
14. cyan/osis	blue
15. leuko/cyte	white
16. albumin/uria	white protein
17. xanth/oma	yellow
18. cirrh/otic	
19. glauc/oma	gray
20. melan/oma	black

WORKSHEET 2

Fill in the correct word from the right hand column that matches the definition in the statements below. Use only one word for each statement.

1. _____sinistropedal_____ left-footed

2. _____Acrocyanosis_____ abnormal condition of blueness of the extremities, including the lips and nailbeds

3. _____posteromedial_____ located behind and at the inner side of a part

4. _____leukorrhea_____ white or yellowish mucus discharge from the cervical canal or the vagina

5. _____retrocolic_____ back of the colon

6. _____erythema_____ abnormal redness of skin

7. _____ambilateral_____ pertaining to both sides

8. _____prenatal_____ before birth

9. _____infra-axillary_____ below the axilla

10. _____dorsodynia_____ pain in the back

11. _____melanoma_____ black tumor

12. _____intercostal_____ between the ribs

13. _____median_____ near the middle

14. _____midsternum_____ in the middle of the sternum

15. _____epigastric_____ pertaining to the region above the stomach

Ambilateral

Acrocyanosis

Dorsodynia

Epigastric

Erythema

Infra-axillary

Intercostal

Leukorrhea

Melanoma

Median

Midsternum

Anteroposterior

Posteromedial

Prenatal

Retrocolic

Sinistropedal

44 WORKSHEET 3

Place a slash after each prefix, then define the prefix.

WORD	DEFINE THE PREFIX
1. post/natal	after
2. quadri/plegia	four
3. hyper/lipidemia	above
4. primi/para	first
5. micro/gastria	small
6. tri/ceps	three
7. poly/dipsia	many
8. uni/sex	one
9. im/potent	not
10. an/aerobic	without
11. macro/cephaly	large
12. ultra/violet	beyond
13. ab/sorbent	from
14. extra/cellular	outside
15. intra/muscular	within
16. supra/renal (glands)	above
17. dia/rrhea	through
18. circum/ference	around
19. ad/hesion	near
20. peri/renal	around

WORKSHEET 4

Fill in the correct word from the right hand column that matches the definition in the statements below. Use only one word for each statement.

1. _quadriplegia_ paralysis affecting all four limbs   Circumoral

2. _macrocephal_ abnormally large head   Intracranial

3. _Unilateral_ affecting or occurring on only one side   Hemiparesis

4. _multiglandular_ concerning several or many glands   Hyperglycemia

5. _polyphobia_ many fears   Intramuscular

6. _hyperglycemia_ excessive sugar in the blood   Macrocephaly

7. _hemiparesis_ paralysis affecting only one side of the body   Microbe

8. _superlactation_ excessive or oversecretion of milk   Multiglandular

9. _intramuscular_ within a muscle   Primigravida

10. _intracranial_ within the cranium   Polyphobia

11. _suprasternal_ above the breast plate   Quadriplegia

12. _microbe_ a minute one-celled form of life   Superlactation

13. _transverse_ lying across, crosswise   Suprasternal

14. _circumoral_ around the mouth   Transverse

15. _primigravida_ a woman during her first pregnancy   Unilateral

46

WORKSHEET 5

Place a slash after each prefix, then define the prefix.

WORD	MEANING
1. brady/cardia	slow
2. tachy/pnea	fast
3. dys/pnea	difficult
4. eu/pnea	good
5. cyan/osis	blue
6. hidr/adenitis	sweat
7. hydro/phobia	water
8. mal/function	bad
9. peri/osteum	around
10. scler/oma	hardening

WORKSHEET 6

Fill in the correct word from the right hand column that matches the definitions in the statements below.

1. _____hydrophobia_____ fear of water   Bradypnea

2. _____bradypnea_____ abnormally slow breathing   Dyspnea

3. _____tachypnea_____ rapid breathing   Eupnea

4. _____dyspnea_____ difficult or bad breathing   Hidrosis

5. _____sclerosis_____ a condition of hardening   Hydrophobia

6. _____malnutrition_____ poor or bad nutrition   Malnutrition

7. _____panophobia_____ morbid fear of everything in   Panophobia
general

8. _____ a false encephalitis   Pseudoencephalitis

9. _____ condition of sweating   Sclerosis

10. _____ good, easy breathing   Tachypnea

C H A P T E R 4

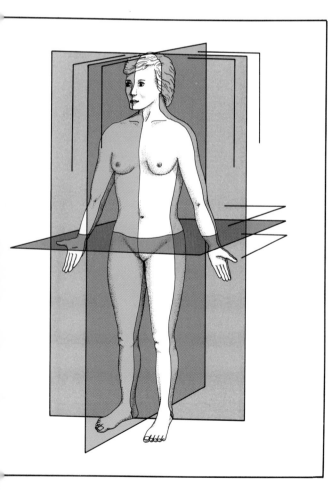

CHAPTER OUTLINE

The Body as a Whole

STUDENT OBJECTIVES

Upon completion of this chapter, you will be able to do the following:

List the levels of organization from the cellular level to the organism as a whole.

Define and identify three planes of the body.

List two dorsal cavities and two ventral cavities, and identify at least one organ within each cavity.

List and locate nine abdominopelvic regions and the four quadrants of this same area.

Define 16 directional terms and be able to use each term correctly.

Identify the word roots/combining forms related to the body as a whole.

Demonstrate an understanding of the chapter by completing the worksheets.

This chapter considers the terms that relate to the body as a whole rather than to any specific body system. Since this material is basic to an understanding of subsequent chapters, it is important that the information be understood by students attempting to master medical terminology.

LEVELS OF ORGANIZATION

The **cell** is the fundamental unit of life. As such, it must carry on all of the functions associated with life. Among these functions are reproduction, respiration, excretion, and adaptation to the environment. In highly complex organisms, cells are modified to carry on a specific activity, in addition to all of the other basic life functions. Muscle cells are designed for contraction; nerve cells transmit electrical impulses; and red blood cells carry oxygen to body tissues.

Groups of cells that perform the same basic activity are called **tissues.** Tissue types include epithelial (covering), connective (supporting and protecting), muscular (contracting), and nervous (conducting impulses) tissues. In addition, a variety of cell types compose the specialized tissue of blood.

Groups of tissues that work in close association and perform a special function are called **organs.** In addition to performing a specialized function, organs also have a more or less definite shape. For example, the shape of the stomach somewhat resembles a sac. The stomach is composed primarily of muscle tissue and epithelial tissue. The muscle tissue provides for the mixing of ingested food with gastric juices. These juices are secreted from the epithelial tissue in order to aid in the digestive process.

The next higher level of organization is a system. A **system** is composed of a group of organs that work together to perform a common function. For example, the mouth, pharynx, esophagus, stomach, small intestine, and colon, along with accessory organs, constitute the gastrointestinal system. Each of these organs performs one or more activities associated with digestion. Other body systems are as follows: integumentary, gastrointestinal, respiratory, cardiovascular, hematic and lymphatic, musculoskeletal, urogenital, reproductive, endocrine, nervous, and special senses.

The highest level of organization is the **organism,** which is a living entity composed of all of the body systems. These systems provide for all of the processes associated with life. They are responsible for its autonomous existence.

The levels of organization can be represented as follows:

Cells → Tissues → Organs → Systems → Organism

ANATOMICAL POSITION

The **anatomical position** places the body in a stance that is accepted by all anatomists throughout the world. In this position, the body is erect and the eyes are looking straight to the front. The upper limbs hang to the sides, with palms facing forward. The lower limbs are parallel, with the toes pointing forward. Whether the body lies face upward or downward, or whether the limbs are placed in any fashion, the positions and relationships of a structure are always described as if the body were in the anatomical position.

PLANES OF THE BODY

A **plane** of the body is an imaginary flat surface that passes through the body at different places in order to divide it for anatomical purposes. Several of the commonly used anatomical planes are illustrated in Figure 4-1. These planes include a midsagittal (median) plane, dividing the body into a right and left half; a sagittal plane, dividing the body into an unequal right and left side; a coronal (frontal) plane, dividing the body into an anterior (ventral) and posterior (dorsal) portion; and a transverse (horizontal) plane, running parallel to the ground, dividing the body or organs into superior (upper) and inferior (lower) portions.

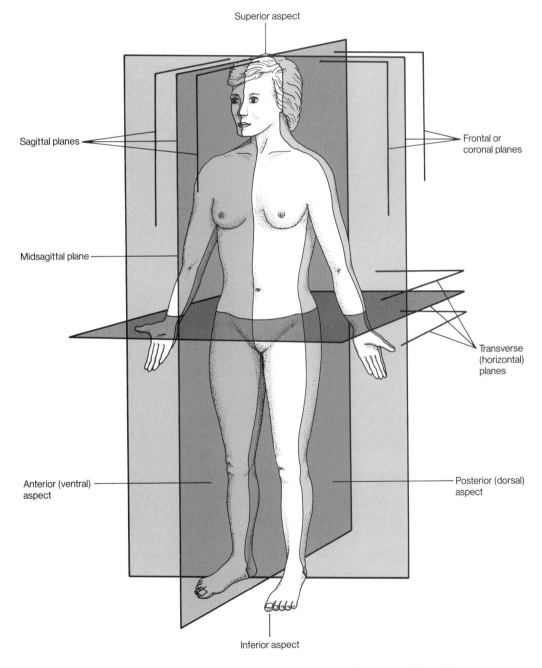

Figure 4-1. Body planes. (Note that the body is in the anatomical position.)

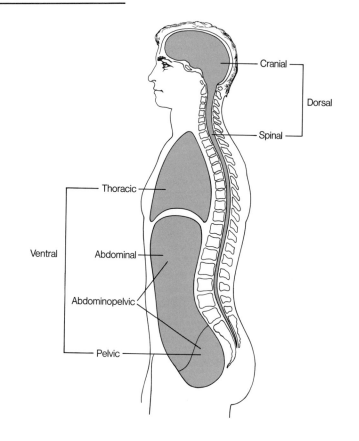

Figure 4-2. Body cavities.

BODY CAVITIES

The body is divided into four major cavities. A coronal plane divides these four cavities into two dorsal cavities and two ventral cavities (Fig. 4-2).

The **dorsal cavities** include the **cranial cavity**, which contains the brain, and the **spinal cavity**, which contains the spinal cord.

The **ventral cavities** include the **thoracic cavity**, which contains the heart, lungs, and associated structures, and the **abdominopelvic cavity**, which contains the digestive, excretory, and reproductive organs. The thoracic cavity is separated from the abdominopelvic cavity by a muscular wall, the diaphragm.

THE ABDOMINOPELVIC REGION

The abdominopelvic region may be divided into nine major sections by constructing an imaginary "tic-tac-toe" over this region. This provides anatomists with divisions to locate the placement of visceral organs. Detailed operative reports sometimes reference these divisions. The nine regions, from left to right and top to bottom, are as follows (Fig. 4-3):

Right hypochondriac. Upper right region beneath the ribs.
Epigastric. Region of the stomach.
Left hypochondriac. Upper left region beneath the ribs.
Right lumbar. Right middle lateral region.
Umbilical. Region of the navel.
Left lumbar. Left middle lateral region.
Right inguinal (iliac). Right lower lateral region.
Hypogastric. Lower middle region beneath the navel.
Left inguinal (iliac). Left lower lateral region.

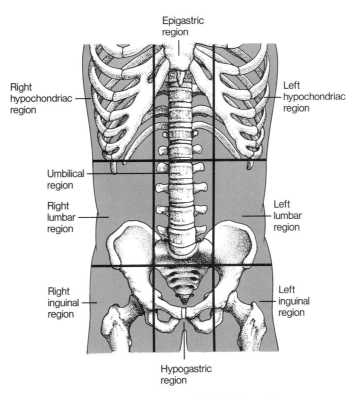

Epigastric region

Right hypochondriac region

Left hypochondriac region

Umbilical region

Right lumbar region

Left lumbar region

Right inguinal region

Left inguinal region

Hypogastric region

Figure 4–3. Anatomical divisions of the abdominopelvic region.

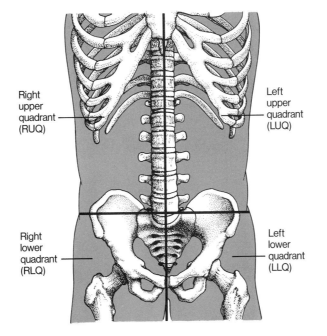

Right upper quadrant (RUQ)

Left upper quadrant (LUQ)

Right lower quadrant (RLQ)

Left lower quadrant (LLQ)

Figure 4–4. Abdominal quadrants.

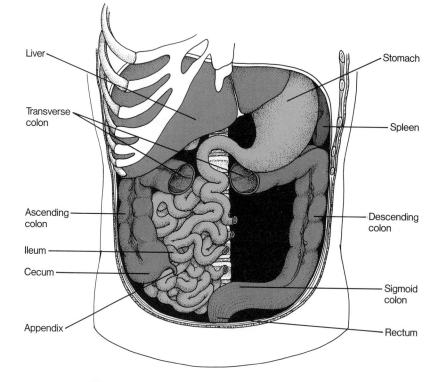

Liver

Transverse colon

Ascending colon

Ileum

Cecum

Appendix

Stomach

Spleen

Descending colon

Sigmoid colon

Rectum

Figure 4–5. *Organs of the abdominopelvic region.*

For purposes of clinical evaluation, the abdominopelvic region may be divided into four qudrants (sections) by an imaginary cross (Fig. 4-4):

Right upper quadrant (RUQ)   Left upper quadrant (LUQ)

Right lower quadrant (RLQ)   Left lower quadrant (LLQ)

Some organs of the abdominopelvic region are identified in Figure 4-5.

THE BACK

The back is divided into sections corresponding to the vertebrae, which are located in the spinal column. (For a more complete discussion, refer to Chapter 10, Musculoskeletal System.) These divisions are as follows:

Cervical (neck)

Thoracic (chest)

Lumbar (loin)

Sacral (lower back)

Coccyx (tailbone)

DIRECTIONAL TERMS

In order to explain where a structure is located in relation to one that is already known, anatomists use directional terms. These terms avoid confusion by expressing in only one word a specific position relative to another. In learning the following list, you should consider opposing terms for ease in memorization. The following directional terms are presented in such a fashion:

Superficial. Toward the surface of the body.
Deep (Internal). Away from the surface of the body.

Abduction. Movement away from the median plane of the body or one of its parts.
Adduction. Movement toward the median plane of the body.

Medial. Pertaining to the midline of the body or structure.
Lateral. Pertaining to a side.

Superior (Cephalad or Cranial). Toward the head or upper portion of a structure.
Inferior (Caudal or Caudad). Away from the head, or toward the tail or lower part of a structure.

Proximal. Near the attachment of an extremity to the trunk or a structure.
Distal. Farther from the attachment of an extremity to the trunk or a structure.

Anterior (Ventral). Near the front of the body.
Posterior (Dorsal). Near the back of the body.

Parietal. Pertaining to the outer wall of the body cavity.
Visceral. Pertaining to the covering of an organ.

Prone. Lying horizontal with the face downward, or denoting the hand with palms turned downward.
Supine. Lying on the back with the face upward, or denoting the position of the hand or foot with the palm or foot facing upward.

Inversion. Turning inward or inside out.
Eversion. Turning outward.

WORD ROOTS/COMBINING FORMS AND PREFIXES

WORD ROOTS/ COMBINING FORMS AND PREFIXES	MEANING	EXAMPLE		PRONUNCIATION
anter/o	anterior, front, before	<u>anter</u>/o/later/ side	al pertain- ing to	ăn - tĕr - ō - LĂT - ĕr - ăl
cyt/o	cell	<u>cyt</u>/o/logy study of		sī - TŎL - ō - jē
dist/o	distant	<u>dist</u>/al relating to		DĬS - tăl
dors/o	back	<u>dors</u>/o/dynia pain		dŏr - sō - DĬN - ē - ăh
epi-	upon, over, in addition to	<u>epi</u>/cardi/ heart	um noun ending	ĕp - ĭ - KĂRD - ē - ŭm

Continued on following page

WORD ROOTS/ COMBINING FORMS AND PREFIXES	MEANING	EXAMPLE	PRONUNCIATION
extern/o	outside	extern/al pertaining to	ĕks - TĔR - năl
hist/o	tissue	hist/o/logy study of	hĭs - TŎL - ō - jē
hyper-	above, excessive, beyond	hyper/tension pressure	hī - pĕr - TĔN - shŭn
hypo-	less, below, under	hypo/derm/ic skin pertaining to	hī - pō - DĔR - mĭk
infra-	below, under, after, beneath	infra/cost/al rib pertaining to	ĭn - fră - KŎS - tăl
later/o	side	later/al pertaining to	LĂT - ĕr - ăl

medi/o	middle	medi/o/stern/ al
		     ster- pertain-
		     num ing to
			mē - dē - ō - STĔR - năl

nucle/o	nucleus	nucle/ar pertaining to	NŪ - klē - ăr

peri-	around	peri/chondr/ al
		     cartilage pertain-
		     ing to
			pĕr - ĭ - KŎN - drăl

poster/o	posterior, behind, back	poster/o/later/al
		     side pertain-
		     ing to
			pŏs - tĕr - ō - LĂT - ĕr - ăl

proxim/o	near	proxim/al pertaining to	PRŎK - sĭm - ăl

supra-	above	supra/ren/ al
		     kidney pertain-
		     ing to
			soo - pră - RĒ - năl

trans-	across	trans/port carry	trăns - PŎRT
ventr/o	belly, belly-side	ventr/al pertaining to	VĔN - trăl
viscer/o	organ	viscer/al pertaining to	VĬS - ĕr - ăl

ABBREVIATIONS RELATED TO THE BODY AS A WHOLE

ABBREVIATION	TERM
AP	anterior-posterior
CNS	central nervous system
CV	cardiovascular
GI	gastrointestinal
GU	genitourinary
lat	lateral
LLQ	Left lower quadrant
LUQ	Left upper quadrant
MS	musculoskeletal
PA	posterior-anterior
RLQ	Right lower quadrant
ROM	range of motion
RUQ	Right upper quadrant
UGI	upper gastrointestinal
ULQ	upper left quadrant
URQ	upper right quadrant

58   ## WORKSHEET 1

From the list below, place each word in order from the most complex to the least complex in structure.

1. _Organism_   Cell

2. _System_   Organ

3. _Organ_   Organism

4. _tissue_   System

5. _Cell_   Tissue

Indicate if the following statements are true or false.

6. _T_ Groups of like cells that carry on the same function are called tissues.

7. _F_ Muscle cells transmit impulses.

8. _T_ Organs make up systems.

9. _F_ The specialized function of epithelial tissue is contraction.

10. _T_ The stomach is an organ.

11. _T_ All cells carry on life processes; that is, cells are living entities.

WORKSHEET 2

Label the body cavities on the diagram below, and compare your answers with Figure 4-2.

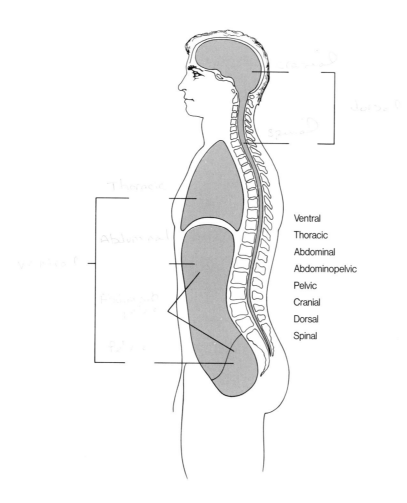

Ventral
Thoracic
Abdominal
Abdominopelvic
Pelvic
Cranial
Dorsal
Spinal

60   WORKSHEET 3

Using the diagrams provided in this chapter, complete the following sections of this worksheet.

List the body cavity (abdominopelvic, cranial, spinal, or thoracic) in which each of the following organs is located.

ORGAN	BODY CAVITY
1. brain	1. cranial
2. heart	2. thoracic
3. intestine	3. abdominopelvic
4. lungs	4. thoracic
5. spinal cord	5. spinal
6. stomach	6. abdominopelvic
7. urinary bladder	7. pelvic
8. ureters	8. abdominopelvic

In each of the following, underline the correct response.

9. The wrist is (proximal, distal) to the elbow.

10. The head is (superior, inferior) to the neck.

11. The ears are located on the (medial, lateral) aspect of the head.

12. The breast bone is (dorsal, ventral) to the spinal cord.

13. The breast bone is (anterior, posterior) to the spinal cord.

14. The muscles of the abdominal wall are (superficial, deep) to the organs of digestion.

15. Two membranes cover the lungs. The one closest to the lung is the (visceral, parietal) membrane.

16. The fingers are (proximal, distal) to the wrist.

17. A slight scratch on the skin is said to be a (deep, superficial) wound.

WORKSHEET 4

Label the abdominopelvic regions indicated on the diagram, and compare your answers with Figure 4-3.

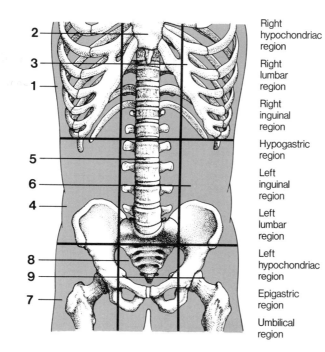

Right
hypochondriac
region

Right
lumbar
region

Right
inguinal
region

Hypogastric
region

Left
inguinal
region

Left
lumbar
region

Left
hypochondriac
region

Epigastric
region

Umbilical
region

62   WORKSHEET 5

On the diagram below, label the body planes indicated, and compare your answers with Figure 4-1.

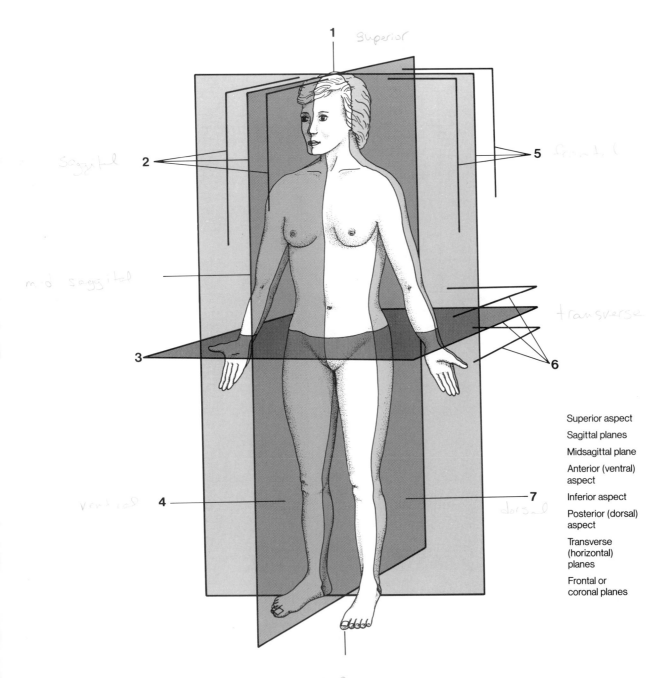

Superior aspect

Sagittal planes

Midsagittal plane

Anterior (ventral) aspect

Inferior aspect

Posterior (dorsal) aspect

Transverse (horizontal) planes

Frontal or coronal planes

WORKSHEET 6

On the diagram below, label the quadrant indicated, give the abbreviation, and name one organ found in that quadrant. Compare your answers with Figures 4-4 and 4-5.

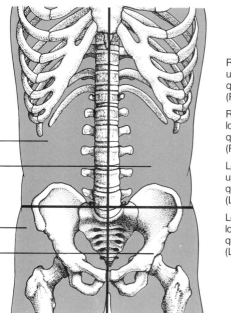

Right
upper
quadrant
(RUQ)

Right
lower
quadrant
(RLQ)

Left
upper
quadrant
(LUQ)

Left
lower
quadrant
(LLQ)

CHAPTER 5

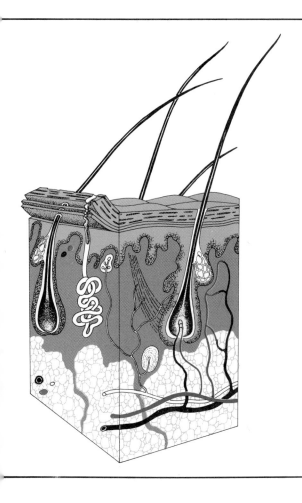

Integumentary System

STUDENT OBJECTIVES

Upon completion of this chapter, you will be able to do the following:

List the appendages of the integumentary system.

Define the main functions of the integumentary system, including its appendages.

Identify the word roots/combining forms and suffixes of the integumentary system and its appendages.

Identify five primary and secondary skin lesions.

Explain and identify some of the major skin problems caused by exposure.

Identify surgical, radiographic, clinical, and laboratory procedures and abbreviations related to the integumentary system.

Explain the pharmacology related to the treatment of integumentary disorders.

Build and analyze diagnostic, symptomatic, and surgical terms related to the integumentary system by completing the worksheets.

66 ANATOMY AND PHYSIOLOGY OF THE INTEGUMENTARY SYSTEM

All outer surfaces of the body are covered by the skin. The word **integument** is derived from the Latin term meaning a covering. Thus, the entire integumentary system consists not only of the skin but also of its appendages—hair, nails, sebaceous glands, sweat glands, and breasts.

The skin performs many important functions. It provides protection against injuries and invasion of bacteria and aids in the regulation of body temperature and the prevention of dehydration. It also functions as a reservoir for food and water, works as a sensory receptor, and is responsible for the synthesis of vitamin D.

The skin consists of two layers (strata) (Fig. 5-1):

1. The (1) **epidermis**, which is a layer of tissue with no blood or nerve supply, is the outermost layer of skin. It is in a state of continuous shedding. Cells that are formed in the innermost part of the epidermis mature and are pushed to the outermost layer. These cells are finally sloughed off and replaced by new cells.

2. The (2) **corium**, or **dermis**, is the layer of skin lying immediately under the epidermis. It is composed of living tissue that consists of numerous capillaries, lymphatics, and nerve endings. Hair follicles, sebaceous glands, and sweat glands are also located in the dermis.

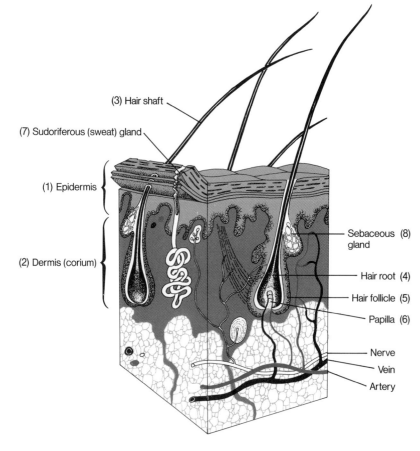

Figure 5-1. *Cross-section of the skin.*

Appendages of the Skin

HAIR

The visible part of the hair is referred to as the (3) **hair shaft** (see Fig. 5-1), while that which is embedded in the dermis is called the (4) **hair root**. The root, together with its coverings, forms the (5) **hair follicle**. At the bottom of the follicle is a loop of capillaries enclosed in a covering called the (6) **papilla**. The cluster of epithelial cells lying over the papilla reproduces and is responsible for the eventual formation of the hair shaft. As long as these cells remain alive, hair will regenerate even though it is cut or plucked or otherwise removed. Baldness **(alopecia)** is evident when the hairs of the scalp are not replaced. Men rather than women are more susceptible to this condition, which is due to hereditary factors.

NAILS

The nail bed covers the dorsal surface of the terminal phalanges, the most distal bones of each finger and toe. Most of the nail body is pink because of the underlying vascular tissue. The crescent-shaped white area near the root of the nail bed is the lunula. It has a whitish appearance because the vascular tissue underneath does not show through. The lunula is the area in which new growth occurs. The average growth rate is approximately 1 mm per week for fingernails, and somewhat slower for toenails. The major function of the nails is to protect the tips of the fingers and toes from bruises and other kinds of injuries.

GLANDS

Three kinds of microscopic glands are found within the skin (see Fig. 5-1).
1. The (7) **sudoriferous glands**, or **sweat glands**, are small structures that open as pores on the surface of the skin. They are found on the palms, soles, forehead, and armpits (axillae). On the palms of the hands, there are approximately 3000 sweat glands per square inch of skin. The main functions of the sudoriferous glands are to cool the body by evaporation, to excrete waste products through the pores of the skin, and to moisturize surface cells.
2. The (8) **sebaceous glands** are the oil-secreting glands of the skin. These glands are filled with cells, the centers of which are saturated with fatty droplets. As these cells disintegrate, they yield an oily secretion called **sebum**. The acidic nature of sebum helps to destroy harmful organisms on the surface of the skin and, thus, prevents infections. Sebaceous glands are present over the entire body except the soles of the feet and the palms of the hands. They are especially prevalent on the scalp and face, and around openings such as the nose, mouth, external ear, and anus, as well as the upper back and scrotum.
3. The **ceruminous glands** are modified sweat glands located in the skin that lines the external auditory canal. Instead of sweat, they secrete wax **(cerumen)**.

BREASTS

The breasts (Fig. 5-2), or mammary glands, are located in the upper anterior aspect of the chest. During puberty, girl's breasts begin to develop because they are exposed to periodic stimulation of two ovarian hormones, estrogen and progesterone. Estrogen is responsible for the fatty growth (1) **(adipose tissue)** and increased size of the breasts as they reach full maturity. The size of the breast is basically determined by the amount of fat around the

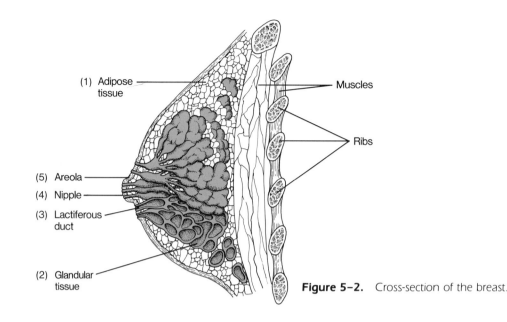

(1) Adipose tissue

Muscles

Ribs

(5) Areola
(4) Nipple
(3) Lactiferous duct

(2) Glandular tissue

Figure 5–2. *Cross-section of the breast.*

glandular tissue and is not indicative of functional ability. The other ovarian hormone, progesterone, forms the lobules that are present in the breast. Each breast has approximately 20 lobes of (2) **glandular tissue**. These lobes are drained by a (3) **lactiferous duct** (which carries milk) that opens on the tip of the raised (4) **nipple**. Circling the nipple, there is a border of slightly darker skin referred to as the (5) **areola**.

In females, full development of the breasts is achieved by the age of 16. The main purpose of the breasts is secretion of milk for the nourishment of newborn infants. Thus, pregnancy causes the breasts to enlarge for this function. At menopause, breast tissue begins to atrophy.

WORD ROOTS/COMBINING FORMS RELATED TO THE INTEGUMENTARY SYSTEM

WORD ROOT/ COMBINING FORM	MEANING	EXAMPLE	PRONUNCIATION
aden/o	gland	aden/o/pathy disease	ăd - ĕ - NŎP - ăh - thē
adip/o } lip/o	fat	lip/oid resemble	LĬP - oid

crypt/o	hidden	onych/o/crypt/osis
		nail abnormal
		             condition
		             (of)
			ŏn - ĭ - kō - krĭp - TŎ - sĭs

cutane/o }	skin	sub/cutane/ous under pertaining to	sŭb - kū - TĀ - nē - ŭs

Continued on following page

WORD ROOTS/COMBINING FORMS RELATED TO THE INTEGUMENTARY SYSTEM—*Continued*

WORD ROOT/ COMBINING FORM	MEANING	EXAMPLE	PRONUNCIATION

dermat/o	skin	dermat/o/tome
		                instrument
		                to cut
			DĔR - măh - tō - tōm

derm/o		derm/oid resemble	DĔR - moid
erythem/o	red	erythem/a noun ending	ĕr - ĭ - THĒ - mă
erythr/o		erythr/o/cyte cell	ĕ - RĬTH - rō - sīt

hidr/o	sweat	hidr/aden/ itis
		        gland inflamma-
		                    tion
			hī - drăd - ĕ - NĪ - tĭs

hist/o	tissue	hist/o/cyte cell	HĬS - tō - sīt

ichthy/o	dry, scaly	ichthy/osis
		            abnormal
		            condition (of)
			ĭk - thē - Ō - sĭs

kerat/o	horny substance	kerat/osis
		            abnormal
		            condition of
			kĕr - ă - TŌ - sĭs

lact/o	milk	lact/ation act of secreting	lăk - TĀ - shŭn
mamm/o	breast	mamm/ary relating to	MĂM - ă - rē
mast/o		mast/ectomy excision	măs - TĔK - tŏ - mē
melan/o	black	melan/oma tumor	mĕl - ă - NŌ - mă

myc/o	fungus	myc/o/log/ y
		        study noun
		        of ending
			mī - KŎL - ō - jē

onych/o	nail	onych/o/malacia softening	ŏn - ĭ - kō - mă - LĀ - sē - āh
pachy/o	thick, heavy	pachy/derma skin	păk - ē - DĔR - mă

pil/o	hair	pil/o/nid/ al
		        nest adjective
		              ending
			pī - lō - NĪ - dăl

Continued on following page

**WORD ROOTS/COMBINING FORMS RELATED TO THE
INTEGUMENTARY SYSTEM**—*Continued*

WORD ROOT/ COMBINING FORM	MEANING	EXAMPLE		PRONUNCIATION
scler/o	hard	scler/o/derma skin		sklē - rō - DĚR - mă
seb/o	sebum	seb/o/rrhea discharge, flow		sĕb - ō - RĒ - ăh
squam/o	scale	squam/ous composed of		SKWĀ - mŭs
steat/o	fat, fatty	steat/orrhea discharge		stē - ă - tō - RĒ - ăh
thel/o	nipple	thel/itis inflammation		thē - LĪ - tĭs
trich/o	hair	trich/o/myc/ osis fun- abnormal gus condition (of)		trĭk - ō - mĭ - KŌ - sĭs
ungu/o	nail	sub/ungu/al under adjective ending		sŭb - ŬNG - gwăl
xanth/o	yellow	xanth/oma tumor		zăn - THŌ - mă
xer/o	dry	xer/o/derma skin		zē - rō - DĚR - mă

SUFFIXES RELATED TO THE INTEGUMENTARY SYSTEM

SUFFIX	MEANING	EXAMPLE		PRONUNCIATION
-graph	instrument used for recording	mamm/o/graph breast		MĂM - ō - grăf
-graphy	process of recording	mamm/o/graph/y breast noun ending		măm - ŎG - ră - fē
-gram	record	mamm/o/gram breast		MĂM - ō - grăm
-therapy	treatment	dermat/o/therapy skin		dĕr - măh - tō - THĚR - ăh - pē

PATHOLOGY OF THE INTEGUMENTARY SYSTEM

Primary Skin Lesions

A skin lesion is an area of pathologically altered tissue (Fig. 5-3). When the skin tissue alteration is a direct result of an injury, wound, or infection, it is referred to as a primary lesion. Diagnoses are often dependent upon the visual appearance of a primary lesion. Measles rash, for example, appears as nonpalpable, discolored spots or patches **(macules)**. Warts, moles, and pimples, on the other hand, are seen as small, solid, circumscribed, raised areas of skin **(papules)**. When a papule measures more than 5 mm in diameter, it is referred to as a **nodule**.

A tumor is any new and abnormal growth **(neoplasm)** and must be examined in order to determine if it is cancerous **(malignant)** or noncancerous **(benign)**. In some individuals, benign tumors that are composed of a local proliferation of blood vessels **(hemangiomas)** are noted at birth **(congenital)**. These usually disappear shortly after birth. Hemangiomas are also called birthmarks or strawberry marks. Moles **(nevi)** are common skin tumors.

Hives **(urticaria)** are a vascular reaction of the skin characterized by the eruption of pale, slightly elevated patches **(wheals)**. They are white in the center, with a pale red periphery, and are accompanied by severe itching **(pruritus)**. Urticaria may be caused by foods, insect bites, pollens, drugs, or emotional stress, among other things.

Dermatitis, burns, chickenpox, and scabies produce skin lesions that appear as blisterlike elevations containing serous fluid **(vesicles)**. Vesicles larger than 1 cm are known as **bullae**. In some instances, especially in cases of dermatitis, the vesicles also contain pus **(pustules)**. Pimples associated with acne **(acne vulgaris)** are examples of pustules.

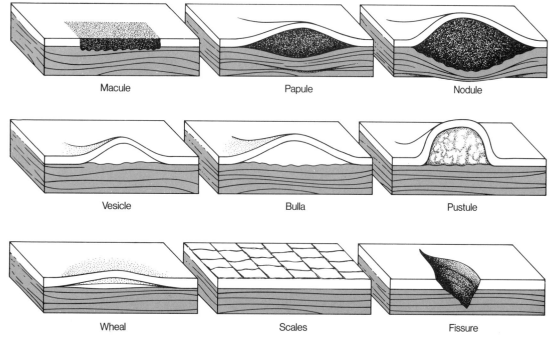

Macule   Papule   Nodule

Vesicle   Bulla   Pustule

Wheal   Scales   Fissure

Figure 5–3. *Lesions of the skin.*

Secondary Skin Lesions

Secondary skin lesions are pathological skin alterations that are a result of a primary skin lesion. Scabs **(crustations)** form over sores or wounds during the healing process. The crusts are composed of dry pus, lymph, or blood, and they may vary in color and thickness.

When trauma, chemicals, or burns cause a superficial loss of tissue, the resulting skin lesion is called an **excoriation**. Excoriation is often caused by a scraping away **(abrasion)** of epidermal tissue. In this condition, the skin is not broken **(contusion)**. A more serious injury results when an irregular tear occurs in the flesh **(laceration)**.

An open sore or lesion **(ulcer)** can be caused by traumas, caustics, intense heat or cold, hemostasis, or bacterial infection. Some ulcers form deep grooves in the skin **(fissures)** (see Fig. 5-3), with sloughing of dead **(necrotic)** tissues. As ulcers heal, a scar **(cicatrix)** is often evident. Scar tissue or a new growth of the skin consisting of dense tissue **(keloid)** may develop. The tissue response is out of proportion to the amount of scar tissue required for normal repair and healing. The result is a raised, firm, thickened **(hypertrophied)** scar that may grow for a prolonged period of time. A predisposition to keloid formation is thought to be hereditary and occurs more often in dark-skinned people. Although these complications can have serious cosmetic implications, they are not life-threatening.

Skin Problems Due to Exposure

Burns are thermal injuries to the outer surfaces of the body. They can be classified into three major categories, depending upon the degree of severity.

First-degree burns are superficial burns. The skin damage is limited to the top layers of the epidermis. These burns are distinguished by redness of the skin **(erythema)** and extreme sensitivity to sensory stimuli **(hyperesthesia)**, especially to touch.

Second-degree burns are characterized by the formation of blisters **(vesicles)**, which are caused by deeper penetration of heat. This condition causes body fluids to accumulate beneath the skin, which eventually rises, forming the vesicles. Normally, the second-degree burn will not result in the formation of scar tissue.

Third-degree burns penetrate both the epidermis and the dermis, which results in complete destruction of the skin tissue. This is the most serious type of burn. When more than two-thirds of the body's skin is destroyed, death usually results due to excessive loss of body fluids. Without the proper amount of body fluids, the brain, heart, and other organs cannot perform their normal functions. These types of burns usually result in scar formations, which can be altered only by the process of skin grafting **(dermatoplasty)**.

Other Skin Problems

Bedridden patients, especially those in nursing homes and hospitals, may develop bedsores **(decubitus ulcers)** as a result of impaired circulation.

Some of the other more common inflammations of the skin **(dermatitis)** are evidenced by itching, redness, and various skin lesions. A few selected inflammatory skin diseases are as follows:

Eczema. An acute or chronic cutaneous inflammatory condition with erythema, papules, vesicles, pustules, scales, crusts, or scabs alone or in combination. Eczema is more the description of a symptom than of a disease. It is a common allergic reaction in children, but can also occur in adults. This word has become synonymous with dermatitis caused by a number of external or internal factors acting singly or in combination.

Pemphigus. An acute or chronic disease of adults characterized by the occurrence of successive crops of vesicles **(bullae)** that appear suddenly on apparently normal skin and then disappear, leaving pigmented spots.

Psoriasis. A discrete pink or dull red lesion covered by characteristic silvery scaling. This condition may begin at any age as flat-topped papules covered with thin, grayish-white scales. Removal of scales often produces bleeding points.

OTHER TERMS RELATED TO THE INTEGUMENTARY SYSTEM AND ITS APPENDAGES

TERM	MEANING	PRONUNCIATION
acne	a chronic inflammatory disease of the sebaceous glands and hair follicles of the skin characterized by pustules, papules, and comedones (blackheads)	ĂK - nē
albinism	congenital nonpathological partial or total absence of pigment in skin, hair, and eyes	ĂL - bĭ - nĭzm
alopecia	natural or abnormal baldness or deficiency of hair, partial or complete, localized or generalized	ăl - ō - PĒ - shē - ăh
chloasma	an abnormal brown pigmentation of skin	klō - ĂZ - măh
comedo	blackhead; discolored dry sebum plugging an excretory duct of the skin	KŎM - ē - dō
ecchymosis, ecchymoses (pl.)	a form of macula appearing in large, irregularly formed hemorrhagic areas of the skin. The color is blue-black changing to greenish brown or yellow	ĕk - ĭ - MŌ - sĭs
fibrocystic disease of the breast	a common benign disease of the breast characterized by small, fluid-filled sacs of tissue. A surgical biopsy or mammography is often performed to differentiate this disease from carcinoma of the breast	fĭ - brō - SĬS - tĭk
gangrene	a necrosis, or death, of tissue usually due to deficient or absent blood supply	GĂNG - grēn
hirsutism	condition characterized by excessive growth of hair or the presence of hair in unusual places, especially in women	HĔR - soot - ĭzm

Continued on following page

OTHER TERMS RELATED TO THE INTEGUMENTARY SYSTEM AND ITS APPENDAGES—*Continued*

TERM	MEANING	PRONUNCIATION
impetigo	inflammatory skin disease marked by pustules that become crusted and rupture	ĭm - pĕ - TĪ - gŏ
melanoderma	a patchy or generalized skin discoloration caused by either an increase in the production of melanin by the normal number of melanocytes or an increase in the number of melanocytes	mĕl - ăh - nō - DĔR - măh
melanoma	a tumor made up of melanin-pigmented cells. When used alone, the term refers to malignant melanoma	mĕl - ă - NŌ - măh
systemic lupus erythematosus (SLE)	a chronic disease of unknown origin commonly marked by an erythematous rash on the face and other areas exposed to sunlight. It involves the vascular and connective tissues of many organs, resulting in a multiplicity of local and systemic manifestations. Etiology is unknown, but incidence is highest in females between puberty and menopause	sĭs - TĔM - ĭk LOO - pŭs ĕr - ĭ - them - ăh - TŌ - sŭs
onychia	inflammation of the nail bed, frequently with loss of the nail	ō - NĬK - ē - ăh
petechia, petechiae (pl.)	pin-sized hemorrhagic spots in the skin	pē - TĒ - kē - ăh
scabies	a contagious, parasitic skin disorder caused by mites	SKĀ - bēz
tinea	any fungal skin disease, commonly called ringworm, occurring in various parts of the body; the name indicates the part affected, for example: tinea barbae (beard), tinea corporis (body), tinea pedis (foot)	TĬN - ē - ăh
topical	pertaining to a particular surface area, as a topical anti-infective applied to a certain area of the skin and affecting only the area to which it is applied	TŎP - ĭ - kăl
vitiligo	an acquired cutaneous affection characterized by milk-white patches surrounded by areas of normal pigmentation. More common in the tropics and in blacks. Synonym: leukoderma	vĭt - ĭl - Ī - gō

TERMS RELATED TO THE BREASTS

TERM	MEANING	PRONUNCIATION
amastia	congenital absence of a breast; lack of breast development	ăh - MĂS - tē - ăh
athelia	absence of a nipple	ăh - THĒ - lē - ăh
gynecomastia	abnormally large mammary gland in the male; sometimes may secrete milk	jĭ - nĕ - kō - MĂS - tē - ăh
hypermastia	abnormally large breast	hĭ - pĕr - MĂS - tē - ăh
mastitis	inflammation of the breast	măs - TĪ - tĭs
peau d'orange	dimpled skin condition, resembling the skin of an orange, seen in lymphatic edema; it may also be present over the area of carcinoma of the breast	pō - dō - RAHNJ
thelitis	inflammation of the nipple	thē - LĪ - tĭs

SPECIAL PROCEDURES RELATED TO THE INTEGUMENTARY SYSTEM

RADIOGRAPHIC AND CLINICAL PROCEDURES

TERM	DESCRIPTION
intradermal tests	substance that is being tested is injected between the skin layers. Positive reaction results in red and inflamed area at the site of the injection within a given period of time (e.g., Mantoux test for tuberculosis; Schick test for diphtheria)
mammography	radiographic imaging or study of breast tissue, using photographic film, that does not require injection of a contrast medium. Used primarily in the assessment of breast masses and/or nipple discharge to detect the presence of malignancy.
patch tests	small square of gauze is impregnated with a suspected allergy-causing substance and is applied to the skin of the forearm. Swollen or reddened skin at the site of the patch after a given period of time indicates a positive reaction
scratch tests	scratches are made in rows on a patient's back or forearm. Extremely small quantities of allergens are introduced into these scratches. If no reaction occurs, the test is considered negative
thermography	a technique used to detect and record the heat present in very small areas of the body part being studied. Higher temperatures corre-

Continued on following page

RADIOGRAPHIC AND CLINICAL PROCEDURES—*Continued*

TERM	DESCRIPTION
	spond to an increased blood supply, which generally indicates the existence of pathology. This test is used as a means of diagnosing underlying pathological conditions, such as breast tumors. More accurate procedures have replaced thermography as a diagnostic method for breast cancer
xerography xeromammography	similar to mammography except image recordings are made on Xerox paper rather than x-ray film

SURGICAL PROCEDURES

TERM	DESCRIPTION	PRONUNCIATION
autograft	surgical transplantation of any tissue from one part of the body to another location in the same individual. Autografts are commonly used to replace skin lost in severe burns	ĂW - tō - grăft
biopsy of the breast	excision of a small piece of living tissue for microscopic exam usually performed to establish a diagnosis	BĪ - ŏp - sē
dermabrasion	planing of skin done by mechanical means (e.g., sandpaper) and mechanical methods on the frozen epidermis	DĔRM - ă - brā - zhŭn
electrodessication	destruction of tissue by dehydration performed by means of a high-frequency electric current	ē - lĕk - trō - dĕs - ĭ - KĀ - shŭn
electrolysis	the decomposition of a substance by passage of an electrical current through it. Hair follicles may be destroyed by use of this method	ē - lĕk - TRŎL - ĭ - sĭs
fulguration	destruction of tissue by means of long, high-frequency electric sparks	fŭl - gū - RĀ - shŭn
homograft	transplant tissue obtained from the same species	HŎ - mō - graft
lumpectomy	excision of a small primary breast tumor with the remainder of the breast left intact	lŭm - PĔK - tō - mē

Continued on following page

SURGICAL PROCEDURES—*Continued*

TERM	DESCRIPTION	PRONUNCIATION
mammoplasty, mastoplasty	surgical reconstruction of the breasts, sometimes augmented (added or increased) by substances such as fat tissue or silicone to alter the size and shape	MĂM - ăh - plăs - tē MĂS - tō - plăs - tē
mastectomy	surgical removal or excision of a breast	măs - TĔK - tō - mē
mastopexy	surgical fixation of a pendulous breast	MĂS - tō - pĕk - sē
mastotomy	incision and drainage of a breast abscess	măs - TŎT - ō - mē
radical mastectomy	the entire breast and neighboring lymph nodes are removed along with a significant margin of skin around the nipple and areola and around the tumor. The pectoralis major and minor muscles are removed. Depending on the amount of skin removed, skin grafting may be necessary	
skin grafting	using the skin from another part of the body, or from a donor, to repair a defect or trauma of the skin	GRĂFT - ĭng

PHARMACOLOGY RELATED TO THE INTEGUMENTARY SYSTEM

MEDICATION	ACTION
anti-infectives (antibacterials and antifungals)	eliminate epidermal infections. They can be administered either topically or systemically. Topical medications create a skin environment that is lethal to microbes. Generally, a specific fungicide must be prescribed for a given fungus strain, while one antibiotic effectively eliminates several types of bacteria
anti-inflammatory drugs (topical corticosteroids)	these topically applied drugs relieve three common symptoms of skin disorders: pruritus (itching), vasodilation, and inflammation
antipruritics	agents that prevent or relieve itching
antiseptics	topically applied compounds or agents that destroy bacteria, thus preventing the development of infections in cuts, scratches, and surgical incisions

Continued on following page

PHARMACOLOGY RELATED TO THE INTEGUMENTARY SYSTEM—Cont.

MEDICATION	ACTION
keratolytics	destroy and soften the outer layer of skin so that it is sloughed off (shed). The strong keratolytics are effective for removing warts and corns. Milder preparations are used to promote the shedding of scales and crusts in eczema, psoriasis, and seborrheic dermatitis. Very weak keratolytics irritate inflamed skin, acting as tonics that speed up the healing process
parasiticides	kill insect parasites that infest the skin. Scabicides kill the mites that cause scabies. Pediculicides kill the lice that cause pediculosis
protectives and astringents	function by covering, cooling, drying, or soothing inflamed skin. Protectives do not penetrate the skin or soften it, but form a long-lasting film. This protects the skin from air, water, and clothing during the natural healing process. Astringents shrink the blood vessels locally, dry up secretions from seepy lesions, and lessen the sensitivity of the skin
topical anesthetics	prescribed for pain on skin surfaces or mucous membranes that is caused by wounds, hemorrhoids, or sunburns. These topical anesthetics relieve pain and itching by numbing the skin layers and mucous membranes. They are applied directly to the painful areas by means of sprays, creams, gargles, suppositories, and other preparations

ABBREVIATIONS RELATED TO THE INTEGUMENTARY SYSTEM

ABBREVIATION	TERM
bx	biopsy
Derm.	dermatology
FS	frozen section
H	hypodermic
ID	intradermal
SLE	systemic lupus erythematosus
STD	skin test dose
Subcu.	subcutaneous
ung.	ointment

WORKSHEET 1

A. Using the word root/combining form mast/o (breast), build medical words to mean:

1. _____ pain in the breast

2. _____ inflammation of a breast

3. _____ any disease of the breast

4. _____ hemorrhage from the breast

5. _____ drooping or pendulous breast

6. _____ without or lack of breast (development)

B. Using the word root/combining form mamm/o (breast), build medical words to mean:

1. _____ inflammation of the breast

2. _____ pertaining to the breast

3. _____ pain in the breast

C. Using the word root/combining form adip/o or lip/o (fat), build medical words to mean:

1. _____ tumor consisting of fat

2. _____ hernia containing fat or fatty tissue

3. _____ resembling fat

4. _____ beginning or formation of fat

D. Using the word root/combining form derm/o, dermat/o (skin), build medical words to mean:

1. _____ inflammation of the skin

2. _____ pain in the skin

3. _____ one who specializes in studying skin diseases

4. _____ resembling the skin

5. _____ pertaining to skin repair or skin grafting

E. Using the word root/combining form erythem/o, erythr/o (redness), build medical words to mean:

1. _____ redness of the skin

2. _____ pertaining to (adjective ending) erythema

F. Using the word root/combining form hidr/o (sweat), build medical words to mean:

1. _____ condition of sweating

2. _____ adenoma of a sweat gland

3. _____ without or absence of sweat

G. Using the word root/combining form onych/o (nail), build medical words to mean:

1. _____ inflammation of the nail bed

2. _____ tumor of the nail or nail bed

3. _____ pain in the nails

4. _____ nourishment of the nails

5. _____ resembling or similar to a nail

6. _____ any disease of the nail

7. _____ condition or disease of the nails caused by a fungus

8. _____ softening of the nails

9. _____ dropping off of the nails

10. _____ condition of a hidden (ingrown) toenail

H. Using the word root/combining form trich/o (hair, hair bulb), build medical words to mean:

1. _____ resembling hair, or hairlike

2. _____ study of the hair (care and treatment)

3. _____ any disease of the hair

4. _____ abnormal fear of hair or of touching it

5. _____ inflammation of hair bulbs

6. _____ condition or disease of the hair caused by a fungus

WORKSHEET 2

Fill in the correct word from the right hand column that matches the definition in the statements below.

1. _____ infestation with lice

Alopecia

2. _____ inflammation of the nail bed frequently resulting in loss of the nail

Chloasma

3. _____ any fungal skin disease, especially ringworm

Ecchymosis

4. _____ a contagious skin disease transmitted by the itch mite

Impetigo

5. _____ a skin infection marked by vesicles that become pustular and crusted, and rupture

Onychia

6. _____ severe itching of the skin, also known as hives

Pediculosis

7. _____ hyperpigmentation in certain areas of the skin, occurs in yellowish-brown patches or spots

Petechiae

8. _____ hemorrhagic spot or bruise, larger than a petechia

Scabies

9. _____ minute or small hemorrhagic spots on the skin

Tinea

10. _____ loss or absence of hair

Urticaria

82   WORKSHEET 3

Build a surgical term for the following:

1. _____mastectomy or mammectomy_____ excision or removal of a breast

2. _____ surgical incision of a breast

3. _____ surgical fixation or suspension of a pendulous breast

4. _____ surgical repair or reconstruction of a breast

5. _____ excision of fat or adipose tissue

6. _____ surgical removal of the nail

7. _____ surgical incision of a nail

8. _____ skin graft taken from other individuals

9. _____ skin graft taken from one's self

10. _____ excision of a small piece of mammary tissue (for microscopic examination)

WORKSHEET 4

Define the following diagnostic and symptomatic terms. Use your dictionary as a reference.

1. acne _____

2. eczema _____

3. athelia _____

4. thelitis _____

5. gynecomastia _____

6. peau d'orange _____

7. comedo _____

8. cicatrix of skin _____

9. albinism _____

10. decubitus ulcer _____

WORKSHEET 5

Grammar Review—Integumentary System

Write the plural form for the following words.

SINGULAR	PLURAL
1. keratosis	1. ______________
2. milium	2. ______________
3. capillus	3. ______________
4. bacillus	4. ______________
5. mamma	5. ______________

Build words with adjective endings that mean "pertaining to" for the following.

NOUN	ADJECTIVE
6. allergy	6. ______________
7. epithelium	7. ______________
8. cerumen	8. ______________
9. keratosis	9. ______________
10. pilonid	10. ______________

Form words with noun endings for the following.

WORD ROOT	NOUN
11. albin	11. ______________
12. alopec	12. ______________
13. dermatolog	13. ______________
14. derm	14. ______________
15. dermatopath	15. ______________

WORKSHEET 6

Identify the following skin lesions, and compare your answers with Figure 5-3.

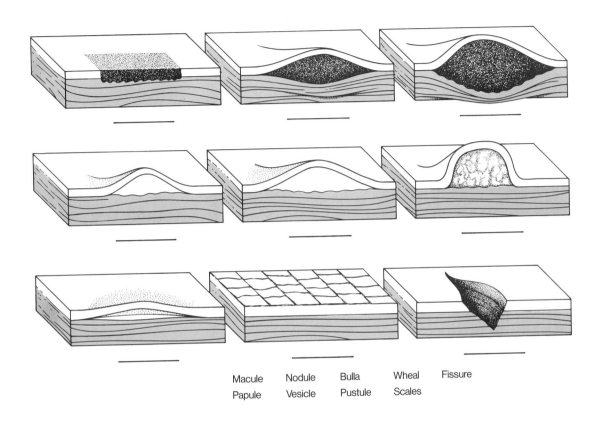

Macule   Nodule   Bulla   Wheal   Fissure

Papule   Vesicle   Pustule   Scales

86   WORKSHEET 7

Radiographic and Clinical Procedures

Choose the word(s) that best describes the following statements:

intradermal tests   positive
mammography   scratch tests
negative   thermography
patch tests   xerography

1. The Mantoux test for tuberculosis and the Schick test are known as _____ _____ .

2. _____ is a radiographic image of breast tissue, using photographic film, that does not require injection of a contrast medium.

3. Extremely small quantities of allergens are introduced into rows of scratches on a patient's back or forearm. If no reaction occurs, the test is considered to be _____ .

4. The tests are known as _____ _____ .

5. Radiographic image of breast tissue is made on Xerox paper rather than x-ray film using _____ .

6. Small square of gauze is impregnated with a suspected allergy-causing substance and is applied to the skin of the forearm. These tests are known as _____ _____ .

7. When performing patch tests, the swollen or reddened skin at the site of the patch after a given period of time indicates a _____ reaction.

8. When performing an intradermal test, a red and inflamed area at the site of the injection within a given period of time indicates a _____ reaction.

WORKSHEET 8

Pharmacology

Choose the medication or term that best describes the following statements:

anti-infectives
anti-inflammatory drugs
antipruritics
antiseptics
astringents
corticosteroids

keratolytics
parasiticides
protectives
topical anesthetics
vasodilation

1. _____ - _____ _____
   relieve three common symptoms of skin disorders: pruritus, vasodilation, and inflammation.

2. _____ are topically applied disinfectants that destroy bacteria.

3. _____ destroy and soften the outer layer of skin so that it is
   sloughed off.

4. _____ inhibit itching due to inflammation, thereby preventing
   infections resulting from excessive scratching.

5. _____ - _____ eliminate epidermal infec-
   tions. They can be administered either topically or systemically. Generally, a specific
   fungicide must be prescribed for a given fungus strain.

6. _____ kill insect parasites that infest the skin. Pediculicides kill
   the lice that cause pediculosis. Scabicides kill the mites that cause scabies.

7. _____ _____ are prescribed for pain on the
   skin surfaces or mucous membranes which is caused by wounds, hemorrhoids, or
   sunburns.

8. _____ do not penetrate the skin or soften it, but form a long-
   lasting film that protects the skin from air, water, and clothing during the healing
   process.

9. _____ shrink the blood vessels locally, dry up secretions from
   seepy lesions, and lessen the sensitivity of the skin.

10. Anti-inflammatory drugs are topically applied and relieve pruritus, inflammation,
    and _____ .

CHAPTER 6

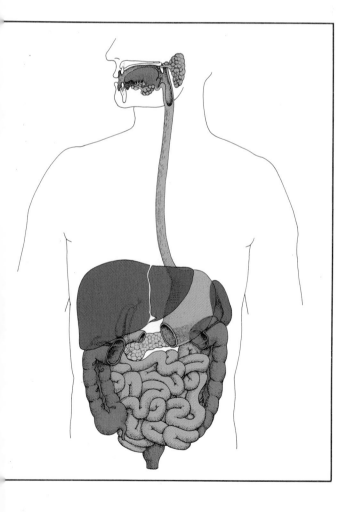

Gastrointestinal System

STUDENT OBJECTIVES

Upon completion of this chapter, you will be able to do the following:

Explain the main functions of the digestive system.

Identify the organs of the alimentary canal.

Identify the accessory organs of digestion.

Define the role of the liver and gallbladder in digestion.

Identify the word roots/combining forms and suffixes of the organs and structures of the digestive system.

Identify and discuss associated pathology related to the gastrointestinal system.

Identify radiographic, endoscopic, surgical, and laboratory procedures and abbreviations related to the gastrointestinal system.

Explain the pharmacology related to the treatment of gastrointestinal disorders.

Build and analyze diagnostic, symptomatic, and surgical terms related to the gastrointestinal system by completing the worksheets.

90 ANATOMY AND PHYSIOLOGY OF THE DIGESTIVE SYSTEM

The twofold purpose of the digestive system is to prepare the food that we eat for absorption by millions of body cells and to eliminate waste materials from the body.

When food is ingested, it is in a form that cannot reach the cells because of its inability to pass through the intestinal mucosa into the bloodstream. Therefore, the consumed food must be altered not only physically but also chemically. Thus, digestion can be defined as the complete process of changing the chemical and physical composition of food in order to facilitate assimilation of the nourishing ingredients of food by the cells of the body.

The organs of the gastrointestinal (GI) system form a tube that begins at the mouth and terminates at the anus. This tube is referred to as the alimentary canal or the digestive tract. It measures approximately 30 feet in adults.

As you read the following paragraphs, refer to Figure 6-1.

Mouth (Oral Cavity, Buccal Cavity)

The gastrointestinal (GI) tract is a continuous tubular passageway that begins at the (1) **oral cavity**, or mouth. The structures within the oral cavity are the cheeks, or **bucca**, and the (2)

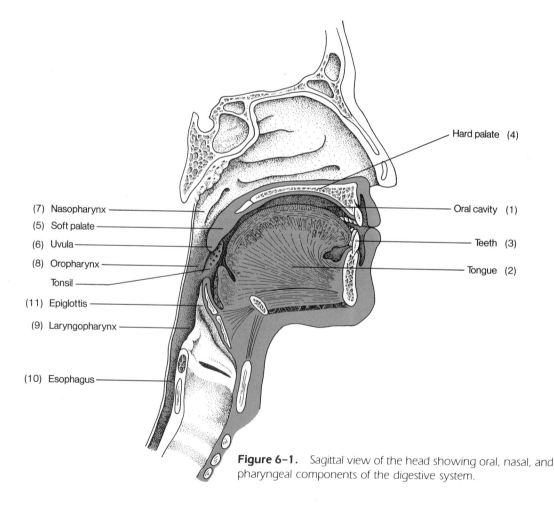

Hard palate (4)

Oral cavity (1)

Teeth (3)

Tongue (2)

(7) Nasopharynx

(5) Soft palate

(6) Uvula

(8) Oropharynx

Tonsil

(11) Epiglottis

(9) Laryngopharynx

(10) Esophagus

Figure 6–1. Sagittal view of the head showing oral, nasal, and pharyngeal components of the digestive system.

tongue and its muscles, which extend across the floor of the mouth. The main functions of the tongue are manipulation of food during the chewing process, deglutition (swallowing), speech production, and determination of taste. The surface of the tongue has rough elevations; these elevations are taste buds. These sense organs are called papillae and are capable of perceiving a variety of flavors found in our foods, such as bitterness, sweetness, saltiness, and sourness.

The (3) **teeth** are also found in the oral cavity and play an important role in the initial stages of digestion. The teeth that are located in the front of the oral cavity, the incisors and cuspids, cut and tear the food into small pieces. The teeth located in the rear of the oral cavity are called molars. They further crush and grind the food into finer particles. Teeth are covered by hard enamel, which gives them a white and smooth appearance. Beneath the enamel is the main structure of the tooth, the dentin. Dentin is surrounded by a thin layer of modified bone called cementum. In the innermost part of the tooth is the pulp, which stores the nerves and blood vessels of the tooth. The teeth are imbedded in pink fleshy tissue known as gums, or gingiva.

Two of the other structures located within the mouth are the hard and soft palates. The (4) **hard palate** lies in the anterior portion of the roof of the oral cavity, while the (5) **soft palate** lies in its posterior portion. The soft palate forms a partition between the mouth and the nasopharynx and is continuous with the hard palate. The entire oral cavity, like the rest of the digestive tract, is lined with mucous membrane.

After the food is chewed, it is formed into a round, sticky mass called a bolus. The bolus is pushed by the tongue from the mouth into the **pharynx** (also called the throat). Its downward movement is guided into the pharynx by the soft, fleshy V-shaped tissue called the (6) **uvula**. The uvula hangs from the superior roof of the oral cavity. The pharynx is a muscular tube. It is divided into three major sections:

1. The (7) **nasopharynx** (the part of the throat behind the nose).
2. The (8) **oropharynx** (the part of the throat behind the mouth).
3. The (9) **laryngopharynx** (the part of the throat above the larynx). The laryngopharynx is further divided into two tubes: one that leads to the lungs, called the trachea; and one that leads to the stomach, called the (10) **esophagus**.

A small flap of tissue, the (11) **epiglottis**, covers the trachea. The main function of the epiglottis is to prevent food from entering the trachea, thus allowing all food to be channeled to the stomach through the esophagus.

Stomach

The (1) **stomach** is a saclike structure located in the abdominal cavity directly below the diaphragm (Fig. 6-2). It is continuous with the (2) **esophagus**. Thus, food continues its descent down the stomach. The stomach mixes the undigested food with gastric juices to further break it down for digestion. Within the stomach, there are a considerable number of folds called rugae. The rugae appear only when the stomach is empty. As the stomach fills, the interior walls become smooth. The interior lining of the stomach is composed of mucous membranes and contains the glands that secrete hydrochloric acid (HCl) and gastric juices. Once the food, or bolus, is mixed with gastric juices and HCl, it forms a semi-creamy fluid called chyme.

There are two valves in the stomach. The first valve is called the (3) **cardiac valve**, or **cardiac sphincter**, and is located at the top of the stomach. It connects the esophagus to the stomach. The second valve is called the (4) **pyloric valve**, or **pyloric sphincter**, and is located at the base of the stomach. It connects the stomach to the small intestine. Both valves are composed of a round band of muscles called sphincters, which contract and expand to allow food to enter and leave the stomach.

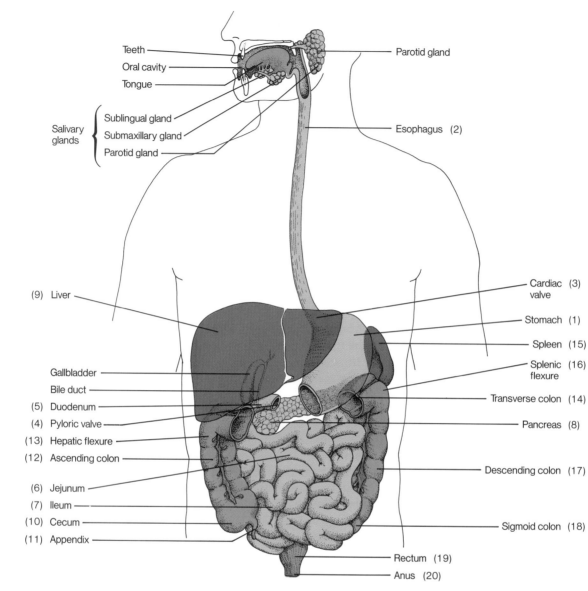

Teeth
Oral cavity
Tongue

Parotid gland

Salivary glands
{
Sublingual gland
Submaxillary gland
Parotid gland
}

Esophagus   (2)

(9) Liver

Cardiac   (3) valve

Stomach   (1)

Spleen   (15)

Splenic   (16) flexure

Gallbladder
Bile duct
(5) Duodenum
(4) Pyloric valve
(13) Hepatic flexure
(12) Ascending colon

Transverse colon   (14)

Pancreas   (8)

Descending colon   (17)

(6) Jejunum
(7) Ileum
(10) Cecum
(11) Appendix

Sigmoid colon   (18)

Rectum   (19)
Anus   (20)

Figure 6–2. *The human digestive system.*

Small Intestine

The small intestine is approximately 1 inch in diameter and is a continuation of the gastro-intestinal tube (see Fig. 6-2). The small intestine consists of three parts:

1. The (5) **duodenum**, the uppermost division, which is about 10 inches long.
2. The (6) **jejunum**, which is approximately 8 feet long.
3. The (7) **ileum**, which is about 12 feet long. Most of the absorption of food takes place in the ileum by tiny fingerlike projections called villi. Inside the villi is a network of fine capillaries, veins, and arteries. This network allows the absorption of food into the bloodstream.

There are also many other intestinal digestive glands located in the mucous membrane lining of the small intestine. These microscopic glands secrete additional digestive juices.

The (8) **pancreas** and (9) **liver** produce digestive secretions, and these secretions are added to the chyme at the beginning of the small intestine. With the exception of some forms of fat, water, and waste products, all of the food ingested into the body is absorbed through the walls of the small intestine.

Colon

The colon (see Fig. 6-2) is a continuation of the gastrointestinal tube and is attached to the ileum by the ileocecal valve. This valve is composed of sphincter muscles that serve to close the ileum at the point at which the small intestine is connected to the colon.

The large intestine has an average diameter of $2\frac{1}{2}$ inches and is approximately 5 feet long. It is divided into two major divisions: the cecum and the colon.

The (10) **cecum** is the first 2 or 3 inches of the large intestine. Attached to the cecum is a wormlike projection, the (11) **vermiform appendix**, which performs no function in the digestive system.

The colon consists of the following parts:
1. The (12) **ascending colon**, which extends from the cecum to the lower border of the liver (13) **(hepatic flexure)**.
2. The (14) **transverse colon**, which passes horizontally across the abdomen to the left toward the (15) **spleen** (16) **(splenic flexure)**.
3. The (17) **descending colon**, which continues down to form the (18) **sigmoid colon**.
4. The (19) **rectum**, which serves as a storage area for the waste products of digestion, leads to the orifice called the (20) **anus**. The anus is kept closed by internal and external **sphincters**, or muscles, except during the process of defecation (elimination of feces).

ACCESSORY ORGANS OF DIGESTION

Liver

The (1) **liver** is the largest glandular organ in the body and weighs approximately 3 to 4 pounds (Fig. 6-3). It is located beneath the diaphragm in the right upper quadrant (RUQ) of the abdominal cavity. The liver performs so many vital functions that people cannot survive without it. Some important functions of the liver include the following:
1. Produces bile, which is used in the small intestines to emulsify and absorb fats.
2. Removes glucose (sugar) from blood, which it synthesizes and stores as glycogen (starch).
3. Stores vitamins, such as B_{12}, A, D, E, and K.
4. Breaks down or transforms some toxic products into less harmful compounds.
5. Maintains normal levels of glucose in the blood.
6. Destroys old erythrocytes and releases bilirubin.
7. Produces various blood proteins, such as prothrombin and fibrinogen, which aid in the clotting of blood.

Pancreas

The (2) **pancreas** is an elongated, somewhat flattened organ that lies posterior and slightly inferior to the stomach (see Fig. 6-3). The pancreas acts as both an endocrine gland and an

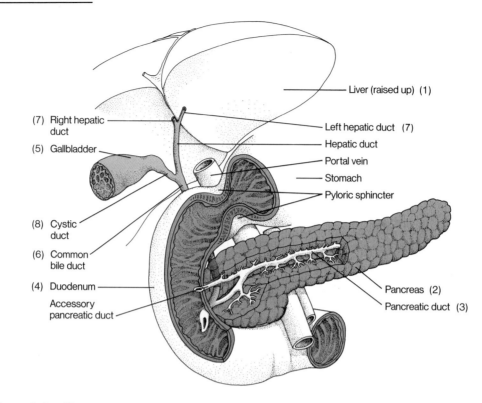

Liver (raised up) (1)

(7) Right hepatic duct

Left hepatic duct (7)

Hepatic duct

(5) Gallbladder

Portal vein

Stomach

Pyloric sphincter

(8) Cystic duct

(6) Common bile duct

(4) Duodenum

Accessory pancreatic duct

Pancreas (2)

Pancreatic duct (3)

Figure 6–3. *The liver, gallbladder, pancreas, and duodenum, with associated blood vessels and ducts.*

exocrine gland. In the digestive system, it provides digestive juices that pass through the (3) **pancreatic duct**, thereby giving it its exocrine function. These enzymatic juices aid in the digestive process. The pancreatic duct extends along the gland and enters the (4) **duodenum** in the company of the bile duct from the liver. By secreting digestive juices through a duct, the pancreas functions as an exocrine gland in the GI system. But in the endocrine system, the pancreas releases hormones directly into the bloodstream and functions as an endocrine, or ductless, gland. The endocrine function of the pancreas is related to the islets of Langerhans, whose beta cells secrete the hormone insulin and alpha cells secrete the hormone glucagon, which regulate blood sugar levels. A more detailed discussion of the pancreatic endocrine functions is found in Chapter 13.

Gallbladder

The (5) **gallbladder** (see Fig. 6-3) serves as a storage area for bile. During the process of digestion, when there is a need for some bile, the gallbladder releases it into the duodenum through the (6) **common bile duct**. Bile is also drained from the liver through the (7) **hepatic ducts**. The hepatic ducts connect with the (8) **cystic duct** from the gallbladder, forming the **common bile duct**.

WORD ROOTS/COMBINING FORMS RELATED TO THE MOUTH

WORD ROOT/ COMBINING FORM	MEANING	EXAMPLE	PRONUNCIATION

or/o
stomat/o
	mouth	or/al
		  pertaining to
		stomat/itis
		  inflammation
			ŎR - ăl
			
			stō - mă - TĪ - tǐs

gloss/o
lingu/o
	tongue	gloss/ectomy
		  excision
		lingu/al
		  pertaining to
			glŏs - ĔK - tō - mē
			
			LĬNG - gwăl

bucc/o	cheek	bucc/al pertaining to	BŬK - ăl

cheil/o
labi/o
	lip	cheil/o/plasty
		  surgical repair
		labi/al
		  pertaining to
			KĪ - lō - plăs - tē
			
			LĀ - bē - ăl

dent/o
 	
odont/o
	tooth	dent/al
		  pertaining
		  to
		ortho/dont/ist
		straight one who
		       specializes
			DĔNT - ăl
			
			ŏr - thō - DŎN - tǐst

gingiv/o	gum	gingiv/ectomy excision	jǐn - jǐ - VĔK - tō - mē

sial/o	saliva, salivary gland	sial/o/lith/ iasis
		    stone presence
		       of
			sī - ăh - lō - lǐ - THĪ - ăh - sǐs

WORD ROOTS/COMBINING FORMS RELATED TO THE PHARYNX AND ESOPHAGUS

WORD ROOT/ COMBINING FORM	MEANING	EXAMPLE	PRONUNCIATION
pharyng/o	pharynx	pharyng/itis inflammation	făr - ǐn - JĪ - tǐs
tonsill/o	tonsil	tonsill/itis inflammation	tŏn - sǐl - Ī - tǐs
esophag/o	esophagus	esophag/ectomy excision	ē - sǒf - ăh - JĔK - tō - mē

WORD ROOTS/COMBINING FORMS RELATED TO THE
STOMACH AND ABDOMEN

WORD ROOT/ COMBINING FORM	MEANING	EXAMPLE	PRONUNCIATION
celi/o	belly, abdomen	celi/ac relating to	SĒ - lē - ăk
gastr/o	stomach	gastr/itis inflammation	găs - TRĪ - tĭs
lapar/o	abdominal wall, abdomen	lapar/o/scopy visual examination	lăp - ăr - ŎS - kō - pē
pylor/o	pylorus	pylor/o/my/o/ tomy mus- cut cle into	pī - lō - rō - mī - ŎT - ō - mē
sphincter/o	sphincter	sphincter/o/tomy cut into	sfĭnk - tĕr - ŎT - ō - mē

WORD ROOTS/COMBINING FORMS RELATED TO THE
SMALL INTESTINE AND COLON (LARGE INTESTINE)

WORD ROOT/ COMBINING FORM	MEANING	EXAMPLE	PRONUNCIATION
duoden/o	duodenum	duoden/al pertaining to	dū - ō - DĒ - năl
enter/o	intestines (usually small intestine)	enter/o/stomy forming a new opening	ĕn - tĕr - ŎS - tō - mē
jejun/o	jejunum	jejun/o/rrhaphy suture	jĕ - joo - NŎR - ăh - fē
ile/o	ileum	ile/o/stomy forming a new opening	ĭl - ē - ŎS - tō - mē
col/o	colon	col/o/stomy forming a new opening	kō - LŎS - tō - mē
proct/o	anus, rectum	proct/o/log/ ist study one of who special- izes	prŏk - TŎL - ō - jĭst

Continued on following page

WORD ROOTS/COMBINING FORMS RELATED TO THE
SMALL INTESTINE AND COLON (LARGE INTESTINE)—*Continued*

WORD ROOT/ COMBINING FORM	MEANING	EXAMPLE	PRONUNCIATION
rect/o	rectum	rect/o/cele swelling, hernia	RĔK - tō - sēl
an/o	anus, opening of the rectum	an/o/rect/ al rec- relating tum to	ā - nō - RĔK - tăl
sigmoid/o	sigmoid colon	sigmoid/o/scopy visual examination	sĭg - moi - DŎS - kō - pē

WORD ROOTS/COMBINING FORMS RELATED TO THE
ACCESSORY ORGANS OF DIGESTION: LIVER, PANCREAS,
AND BILIARY SYSTEM

WORD ROOT/ COMBINING FORM	MEANING	EXAMPLE	PRONUNCIATION
bil/i	biliary system	bil/i/ary pertaining to	BĬL - ē - ā - rē
cirrh/o	yellow, tawny	cirrh/osis abnormal condition (of)	sĭr - RŌ - sĭs
cholangi/o	bile vessel	cholangi/oma tumor	kō - lăn - jē - Ō - mă
chol/e	bile, gall	chol/em/ ia blood noun ending, condition of	kō - LĒ - mē - ăh
cholecyst/o	gallbladder	cholecyst/o/gram record	kō - lē - SĬS - tō - grăm
choledoch/o	bile duct	choledoch/o/lith/o/tomy cal- inci- cu- sion lus	kō - lĕd - ō - kō - lĭ - THŎT - ō - mē
hepat/o	liver	hepat/o/megaly enlargement	hĕp - ăh - tō - MĔG - ăh - lē
pancreat/o	pancreas	pancreat/ectomy excision	păn - krē - ăt - ĔK - tō - mē

Continued on following page

**WORD ROOTS/COMBINING FORMS RELATED TO THE
ACCESSORY ORGANS OF DIGESTION: LIVER, PANCREAS,
AND BILIARY SYSTEM**—*Continued*

WORD ROOT/ COMBINING FORM	MEANING	EXAMPLE	PRONUNCIATION
peritone/o	peritoneum	peritone/al relating to	pĕr - ĭ - tō - NĒ - ăl
splen/o	spleen	splen/ectomy excision	splē - NĔK - tō - mē

SUFFIXES RELATED TO THE GASTROINTESTINAL SYSTEM

SUFFIX	MEANING	EXAMPLE	PRONUNCIATION
-chlorhydria	hydrochloric acid	a/chlorhydr/ia with- condition out (of)	ă - klōr - HĪ - drē - ăh
-crine	to secrete	ex/o/crine out- side	ĔKS - ō - krĭn
-emesis	vomit	hemat/emesis blood	hĕm - ăt - ĔM - ĕs - sĭs
-iasis	abnormal condition, formation of, presence of,	chole/lith/iasis gall stone, calcu- lus	kō - lē - lĭ - THĪ - ăh - sĭs
-lith	calculus, stone	chole/lith gall	KŌ - lē - lĭth
-phagia	ingesting, swallowing, eating	dys/phag/ia diffi- noun ending cult	dĭs - FĀ - jē - ăh
-prandial	pertaining to a meal	post/prandi/al after adjective ending	pōst - PRĂN - dē - ăl
-rrhea	discharge, flow	dia/rrhea flow	dī - ăh - RĒ - ăh

PATHOLOGY OF THE GASTROINTESTINAL SYSTEM

Ulcers

An ulcer is an open sore or lesion of the skin or mucous membrane. It is not uncommon for ulcers to be accompanied by formation of pus. Most ulcers occur in the stomach or duodenal lining of the intestine. Digestive acids break down the mucous membranes so that the underlying tissue is exposed and destroyed. If left untreated, the tissue destruction eventually leads to perforation. When this occurs, a hole **(perforated ulcer)** permits food and enzymes to enter the abdominal cavity and results in contamination of other organs.

Generally, an ulcer may develop any place in which gastric juice and acid digest damaged mucous membrane. These ulcers develop most commonly in the first portion of the duodenum, next most frequently in the stomach, and rarely in the lower portion of the esophagus. They may be of long duration **(chronic)** or arise suddenly **(acute)**. Chronic ulcers are more common in the duodenum, while acute ulcers are usually found in the stomach.

Inflammation of the colon with formation of ulcers in the lining of the intestine **(ulcerative colitis)** can occur at any age but is most common in young adults. Anxiety and nervous tension may be etiological factors. The chief symptom is severe diarrhea, which is often accompanied by blood and mucus in the stool. The patients may feel very weak, lose weight, and sometimes experience anemia. They may also suffer from pain in the joints **(arthralgia)**. In severe cases, it might be necessary to perform an ileostomy to drain the intestinal contents to the outside of the body.

Hernias

A hernia is an abnormal protrusion or projection of an organ or tissue through the structures that normally contain it (Fig. 6-4). They may be abdominal, inguinal, or umbilical.

Hernias are found most commonly in the abdominal region, but they may develop in the diaphragm **(diaphragmatic hernia)** or in the form of a hiatus **(hiatal hernia)**. With this

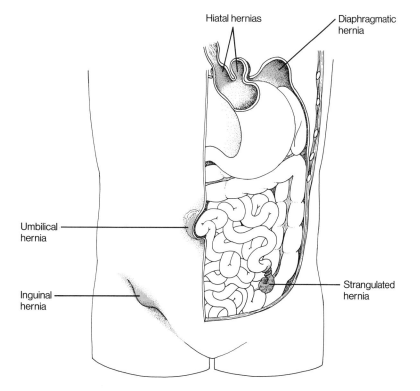

Figure 6–4. Types of hernias.

condition, the lower end of the esophagus and the adjacent part of the stomach herniate into the thorax **(gastroesophageal hernia)**. This results in a gastroesophageal reflux causing stomach acids to back up into the esophagus.

The **inguinal hernia** occurs in the groin where the abdominal folds of flesh meet the thighs. Inguinal hernias account for about 80 percent of all hernias. In the initial stages, such a hernia may hardly be noticeable and appears as a soft lump under the skin, no larger than a marble. In the early stages, an inguinal hernia is usually reducible—it can be pushed gently back into its normal place. With this type of hernia, there may be little pain. As time passes, the pressure of the contents of the abdomen against the weak abdominal wall may increase the size of the opening as well as the size of the hernia lump. The **strangulated hernia** cuts off circulation, and the herniated blood vessel is likely to become gangrenous. This is also known as an incarcerated hernia, as it results in complete bowel obstruction.

The protrusion of part of the intestine at the navel **(umbilical hernia)** is more frequent in women than men and is treated surgically.

Hernias may also be found in newborns **(congenital)** or they may be acquired at an early age. The term rupture is sometimes used to describe a hernia.

Bowel Obstructions

One of the disorders that are prevalent in the elderly is an intestinal obstruction, when the bowel twists on itself **(volvulus)**. Volvulus may be evident when there is an absence of the rumbling noise caused by the propulsion of gas through the intestines **(borborygmus)**. Surgery is required to untwist the bowel.

Telescoping of the bowel within itself **(intussusception)** is a rare type of intestinal obstruction that occurs in children, usually before the age of 3. If the condition is not corrected within 4 days, death can result. Sometimes the barium enema administered to diagnose this abnormality may even correct it, but surgery is usually necessary.

Hemorrhoids

The enlargement of the veins in the mucous membrane of the anal canal causes hemorrhoids, or piles. These may be either internal (found inside the rectal area) or external (found just outside the rectal area).

Hemorrhoids are usually caused by straining to evacuate a fecal concretion **(fecalith)**. They sometimes develop during pregnancy because of pressure on the veins from the enlarged uterus. They may also result from pressure on the veins caused by a disorder of the liver or the heart or may be symptomatic of a tumor that exerts pressure against the veins.

Temporary relief from hemorrhoids can usually be obtained by cold compresses, sitz baths, fecal softeners, or an analgesic ointment. Treatment of an advanced hemorrhoidal condition is by surgical removal **(hemorrhoidectomy)**.

Liver Disorders

One of the symptoms of many liver disorders is a yellowing of the skin **(jaundice)**. This condition is also known as icterus and may result when the bile duct is blocked, causing bile to enter the bloodstream. Jaundice is noted in patients who suffer from cirrhosis of the liver and is believed to be related to poor nutrition and drinking too much alcohol. Icterus may also be exhibited in patients who suffer from an infection of the liver **(hepatitis)**.

Two of the forms of hepatitis include hepatitis A (infectious hepatitis, caused by A virus) and hepatitis B (serum hepatitis, caused by B virus). Type A virus is highly contagious and usually enters by the oral route through ingestion of food, milk, water, and seafood obtained from contaminated water. Type B virus is usually transmitted by the parenteral (other than the mouth) route (e.g., blood transfusions, semen, and so forth). Health care personnel are especially prone to hepatitis B, but there is now a vaccine that provides immunity to type B hepatitis.

Diverticulosis

Diverticulosis is a condition in which small, blisterlike pockets develop in the walls of the large intestine. These pouch-like areas may balloon out from the large intestine. The small pockets usually do not cause any problems unless they become inflamed (**diverticulitis**). Pain (usually in the left lower part of the abdomen), extreme constipation (**obstipation**) or diarrhea, fever, swelling of the abdomen, and occasional blood in the bowel movement are some of the symptoms of diverticulitis. The usual treatment for diverticulitis consists of bed rest, antibiotics, and a soft diet.

OTHER TERMS RELATED TO THE GASTROINTESTINAL SYSTEM

TERM	MEANING	PRONUNCIATION
absorption	the passing of simple nutrients into the bloodstream	ăb - SORP - shŭn
aerophagia	swallowing of air	ā - ĕr - ō - FĀ - jē - ăh
anorexia	loss of appetite	ăn - ō - RĔK - sē - ăh
ascites	accumulation of serous fluid in the peritoneal cavity	ăh - SĪ - tēz
borborygmus	gurgling, splashing sound heard over the large intestine; caused by passage of flatus through the intestine	bŏr - bō - RĬG - mŭs
bulimia	an eating disorder characterized by binge eating followed by purging	bū - LĬM - ē - ăh
cirrhosis	a chronic disease of the liver	sĭr - RŌ - sĭs
cleft lip	harelip; a congenital cleft or separation of the upper lip. May be associated with cleft palate	
cleft palate	congenital fissure or split in the roof of the mouth	klĕft/PĂL - ăt
colic	spasm in any hollow or tubular soft organ accompanied by pain	KŎL - ĭk
deglutition	swallowing	dĕg - loo - TĬSH - ŭn
diarrhea	frequent passage of unformed watery bowel movements. It is a frequent	dī - ăh - RĒ - ăh

Continued on following page

OTHER TERMS RELATED TO THE GASTROINTESTINAL SYSTEM—*Cont.*

TERM	MEANING	PRONUNCIATION
	symptom of gastrointestinal disturbances	
digestant	an agent capable of aiding digestion	dĭ - JĔS - tănt
dyspepsia	poor digestion	dĭs - PĔP - sē - ăh
dysphagia	inability or difficulty in swallowing	dĭs - FĀ - jē - ăh
emesis	vomiting	ĔM - ĕ - sĭs
emulsification	the breaking down of large fat globules in the intestine to smaller, uniformly distributed particles; accomplished largely through the action of bile acids, which lower surface tension	ē - mŭl - sĭ - fĭ - KĀ - shun
enteritis	inflammation of the small intestine	ĕn - tĕr - Ī - tĭs
eructation	producing gas from the stomach, usually with a characteristic sound; belching	ĕ - rŭk - TĀ - shŭn
fecalith	fecal concretion	FĒ - kăh - lĭth
flatus	gas in the digestive tract	FLĀ - tŭs
halitosis	offensive breath	hăl - ĭ - TŌ - sĭs
hematemesis	vomiting blood	hĕm - ăh - TĔM - ĕ - sĭs
intussusception	the slipping of one part of an intestine into another part just below it; telescoping	ĭn - tŭs - sŭs - SĔP - shŭn
jaundice	yellowness of skin and whites of eyes, mucous membranes, and body fluids due to deposition of bile pigment resulting from excess bilirubin in the blood	JĂWN - dĭs
leukoplakia	formation of white spots or patches on the mucous membrane of the tongue or cheek. They tend to grow into larger patches or take the form of ulcers	loo - kō - PLĀ - kē - ăh
obstipation	extreme constipation, often due to obstruction	ŏb - stĭ - PĀ - shŭn
peristalsis	a progressive wavelike movement that occurs involuntarily in hollow tubes of the body, especially the alimentary canal	pĕr - ĭ - STĂL - sĭs

Continued on following page

OTHER TERMS RELATED TO THE GASTROINTESTINAL SYSTEM—*Cont.*

TERM	MEANING	PRONUNCIATION
pilonidal cyst	a dermoid cyst containing hairs that is found in the sacrococcygeal region	pī - lō - NĪ - dăl/sǐst
polyphagia	excessive food intake	pŏl - ē - FĀ - jē - ăh
pyloric stenosis	narrowing of the pyloric orifice; may be due to excessive thickening of the circular muscle of the pylorus	pī - LŎR - ĭk/stĕ - NŌ - sĭs
regurgitation	return of solids or fluids to the mouth from the stomach	rē - gŭr - jǐ - TĀ - shŭn
steatorrhea	excessive amount of fat in the feces, as in the malabsorption syndromes	stē - ăh - tō - RĒ - ăh
visceroptosis	prolapse or downward displacement of the viscera (internal organs enclosed within a cavity), especially the abdominal organs	vǐs - ěr - ŏp - TŌ - sǐs

SPECIAL PROCEDURES RELATED TO THE GASTROINTESTINAL SYSTEM

RADIOGRAPHIC AND CLINICAL PROCEDURES

TERM	DESCRIPTION
barium enema (lower GI)	radiographic examination of the colon (large bowel or large intestine). An enema using a barium solution is administered while a series of radiographs is taken. After the barium is expelled, another radiograph of the abdomen is taken
barium swallow (upper GI)	barium solution is swallowed for a radiographic examination of the upper gastrointestinal tract in order to visualize the esophagus, stomach, and duodenum
esophagram (barium swallow)	a diagnostic series of radiographs of the esophagus. While the patient is drinking a barium solution, the radiologist uses a TV monitor to follow the progress of the solution from the mouth to the stomach. A series of radiographs is taken throughout the procedure
intravenous cholangiography	injection of dye into a vein in order to take radiographs of bile vessels
oral cholecystography	radiographs are taken of the gallbladder following an oral administration of dye
liver scan	radioactive substance is injected intravenously (IV). This media is absorbed by the liver cells in order to visualize the liver. Some of

Continued on following page

RADIOGRAPHIC AND CLINICAL PROCEDURES—*Continued*

TERM	DESCRIPTION
	the abnormalities that can be diagnosed with liver scanning are tumors, cysts, hepatomegaly, hepatitis, ruptures, and abscesses
percutaneous transhepatic cholangiography	a needle is inserted through the skin into the liver. A contrast media is injected to visualize the bile ducts
spleen scan	radioactive material is injected intravenously. This media is absorbed by the spleen cells in order to visualize the spleen. Abnormalities such as cysts, abscesses, tumors, splenomegaly, and ruptures can be diagnosed

ENDOSCOPIC PROCEDURES

TERM	DESCRIPTION
colonoscopy, colonofiberoscopy	method of examining the colon by using a colonic fiberscope with a four-way controlled tip to facilitate its passage through the flexures of the sigmoid colon and transverse colon under fluoroscopic guidance. This procedure permits the removal of polyps in the ascending colon
esophagoscopy with biopsy	visualization of the esophagus with removal of tissue. This is usually performed to establish or confirm a diagnosis
peritoneoscopy, laparoscopy	the scope is inserted into the abdominal cavity through a small incision in the abdominal wall. It is used to inspect the abdominal cavity for tumors or other abnormalities
proctosigmoidoscopy	endoscopic procedure for visualization of benign and malignant lesions of the rectosigmoid. It permits excisional biopsy of small lesions such as polyps and segmental biopsy of large lesions for diagnosis. This procedure is also used to determine such abnormalities as tumors, polyps, cancer, and diverticulitis
gastrointestinal endoscopy	a flexible fiberoptic tube is placed through the mouth or anus to visualize parts of the gastrointestinal tract

SURGICAL PROCEDURES

TERM	DESCRIPTION	PRONUNCIATION
adenoidectomy	removal of adenoids	ăd - ĕ - noid - ĔK - tō - mē
anastomosis	surgical formation of a passage or opening between two hollow viscera or vessels	ăh - năs - tō - MŌ - sĭs

Continued on following page

SURGICAL PROCEDURES—*Continued*

TERM	DESCRIPTION	PRONUNCIATION
appendectomy	excision of appendix	ăp - ĕn - DĔK - tō - mē
cecectomy	removal of cecum	sē - SĔK - tō - mē
cheiloplasty	surgical reconstruction of the lip	KĪ - lō - plăs - tē
cholecystectomy	excision of the gallbladder	kō - lē - sĭs - TĔK - tō - mē
choledocholithotomy	incision into bile duct for removal of gallstones	kō - lĕd - ō - kō - lĭ - THŎT - ō - mē
choledochoplasty	surgical reconstruction of a bile duct	kō - lĕd - ō - kō - PLĂS - tē
colostomy	surgical creation of an opening between the colon and the surface of the abdomen	kō - LŎS - tō - mē
diverticulectomy	excision of diverticulum and closure of the resulting defect	dī - vĕr - tĭk - ū - LĔK - tō - mē
esophagojejunostomy	formation of a communication between the esophagus and jejunum	ĕ - sŏf - ăh - gō - jē - jū - NŎS - tō - mē
exploratory laparotomy	incision of the abdomen that allows the physician to explore the abdominal cavity to determine the extent of disease	lăp - ăr - ŎT - ō - mē
glossectomy	partial or complete excision of the tongue	glŏs - SĔK - tō - mē
hemorrhoidectomy	excision of hemorrhoids	hĕm - ō - roid - ĔK - tō - mē
hepatic lobectomy	removal of a lobe of the liver	hĕ - PĂT - ĭk/lō - BĔK - tō - mē
hernioplasty, herniorrhaphy	surgical repair of a hernia	HĔR - nē - ō - plăs - tē hĕr - nē - OR - ă - fē
ileostomy	creation of a surgical passage through the abdominal wall into the ileum	ĭl - ē - ŎS - tō - mē
liver biopsy	excision of a small piece of liver tissue for microscopic examination in order to establish or confirm a diagnosis	BĪ - ŏp - sē
proctoplasty	surgical reconstruction of the rectum or colon	PRŎK - tō - plăs - tē

Continued on following page

SURGICAL PROCEDURES—*Continued*

TERM	DESCRIPTION	PRONUNCIATION
pyloromyotomy	incision of the longitudinal and circular muscles of the pylorus	pĭ - lō - rō - mĭ - ŎT - ō - mē
stomatoplasty	surgical reconstruction of the mouth	STŌ - măh - tō - plăs - tē

LABORATORY PROCEDURES

TERM	DESCRIPTION
fasting blood sugar (FBS)	used to detect abnormalities of glucose metabolism. The level of glucose in the blood is determined after the patient has fasted for 8 hours
glucose tolerance test (GTT)	determines the ability to metabolize glucose. After an overnight fast, the patient ingests a measured amount of glucose. Blood and urine samples are usually obtained at intervals of 30 minutes, 1, 2, and 3 hours after ingestion of the glucose. In a healthy individual, the blood sugar level peaks in 30 to 60 minutes and then returns to normal
serum bilirubin	may indicate excessive hemolysis, hepatic disorders, or obstructive conditions of the bile ducts. Serum bilirubin is formed from the breakdown of hemoglobin. In the liver, bilirubin is secreted into the bile and then excreted into the intestinal tract through the bile ducts
occult blood	determines bleeding in gastrointestinal disorders. Because this test is so sensitive, the patient is instructed to have a meat-free diet for 3 days before the test. The presence of undigested meat can give a false-positive reading

PHARMACOLOGY RELATED TO THE GASTROINTESTINAL SYSTEM

MEDICATION	ACTION
antacids	neutralize excess acid in the stomach and help relieve gastritis and ulcer pain. Antacids are also used to relieve indigestion and reflux esophagitis (heartburn)
antiflatulents	reduce the feelings of gassiness and bloating (flatulence) that accompany indigestion. They facilitate the passing of gas by breaking down gas bubbles to smaller size and by mildly stimulating intestinal motility
antiemetics (antinauseants)	suppress nausea and vomiting, mainly by acting on the brain control to stop the nerve impulses. There are many uses for these

Continued on following page

PHARMACOLOGY RELATED TO THE GASTROINTESTINAL SYSTEM—*Cont.*

MEDICATION	ACTION
	drugs, including motion sickness and dizziness associated with inner ear infections. Some antihistamines and tranquilizers have antiemetic properties
antidiarrheals	relieve diarrhea either by absorbing excess fluids and bacteria that cause diarrhea, or by lessening intestinal motility (slowing the movement of fecal material through the intestine). This then allows more time for absorption of water
antispasmodics	act on the autonomic nervous system to slow peristalsis, thereby relieving intestinal cramping
cathartics (laxatives and purgatives)	promote bowel movement and/or defecation. When used in smaller doses, they relieve constipation and are called laxatives. When used in larger doses, they evacuate the entire GI tract and are called purgatives. Purgatives are used prior to surgery or intestinal radiological examinations
emetics	used to induce vomiting, especially in cases of poisoning

ABBREVIATIONS RELATED TO THE GASTROINTESTINAL SYSTEM

ABBREVIATION	MEANING
A.C., a.c.	before meals
BaE	barium enema
B.I.D., b.i.d.	twice a day
BM	bowel movement
FBS	fasting blood sugar
GI	gastrointestinal
GTT	glucose tolerance test
HCl	hydrochloric acid
h.s.	at bedtime
IVC	intravenous cholangiography
NPO	nothing by mouth
P.C., p.c.	after meals
PD	postprandial (after meals)
P.O.	orally
p.r.n.	as required

Continued on following page

ABBREVIATIONS RELATED TO THE GASTROINTESTINAL SYSTEM—*Cont.*

ABBREVIATION	MEANING
q.d.	every day
Q.I.D., q.i.d.	four times a day
Stat.	immediately
T.I.D., t.i.d.	three times a day
TPN	total parenteral nutrition

NOTE: Many of these abbreviations deal with pharmacology and the administration of medication. They are not unique to the gastrointestinal system.

WORKSHEET 1

A. Using the word root/combining form esophag/o (esophagus), build medical words to mean:

1. ___esophagitis___ inflammation of the esophagus

2. _____ pain in the esophagus

3. _____ surgical repair of the esophagus

4. _____ endoscope for examination of the esophagus

5. _____ excision of (part of) the esophagus

B. Using the word root/combining form gastr/o (stomach), build medical words to mean:

1. _____ excision or removal of the stomach

2. _____ inflammation of the stomach

3. _____ pain in the stomach

4. _____ any disease of the stomach

5. _____ paralysis of the stomach

6. _____ enlargement of the stomach

7. _____ downward displacement or dropping of the stomach

8. _____ suture of the stomach

9. _____ study of the stomach and intestines

10. _____ narrowing (or shrinkage) of the stomach

C. Using the word root/combining form duoden/o, jejun/o, or ile/o, build medical words to mean:

1. _____ pertaining to the duodenum

2. _____ inflammation of the duodenum

3. _____ inflammation of the jejunum

4. _____ inflammation of the jejunum and ileum

5. _____ pertaining to the ileum and cecum

110

D. Using the word root/combining form enter/o (small intestine), build medical words to mean:

1. _____ pertaining to the small intestine

2. _____ inflammation of the small intestine

3. _____ any disease of the small intestine

4. _____ surgical fixation of the small intestine (to the abdominal wall)

5. _____ surgical repair of the small intestine

E. Using the word root/combining form col/o, (colon), build medical words to mean:

1. _____ inflammation of the colon

2. _____ visual examination of the colon

3. _____ any disease or disorder of the colon

4. _____ inflammation of the colon and rectum

5. _____ a downward displacement of the colon

F. Using the word root/combining form proct/o or rect/o (rectum), build medical words to mean:

1. _____ pain in the rectum

2. _____ inflammation of the rectum

3. _____ narrowing or constriction of the rectum

4. _____ prolapse of the rectum

5. _____ paralysis of the anus (anal muscles)

G. Using the word root/combining form chole (bile, gall), build medical words to mean:

1. _____ the gallbladder

2. _____ calculus or stone in the gallbladder

3. _____ presence of or formation of a calculus in the gallbladder

4. _____ crushing of a gallstone

5. _____ vomiting of bile

6. _____ pertaining to the bile duct

7. _____ presence of or formation of a calculus in the common bile duct

8. _____ inflammation of the common bile duct

9. _____ excision of a portion of the common bile duct

10. _____ suture of the common bile duct

H. Using the word root/combining form hepat/o (liver) or pancreat/o (pancreas), build medical words to mean:

1. _____ any tumor of the liver

2. _____ pain in the liver

3. _____ enlargement of the liver

4. _____ cirrhosis of the liver

5. _____ inflammation of the pancreas

6. _____ pertaining to the pancreas (adj. ending)

7. _____ removal of all or part of the pancreas

112   WORKSHEET 2

Fill in the correct word from the right hand column that matches the definition in the statements below.

1. _____hematemesis_____   vomiting blood   Anorexia

2. _____   difficulty or inability to swallow   Bulimia

3. _____   intestinal concretion formed around a   Cirrhosis
                           center of fecal matter

4. _____   bad breath   Dyspepsia

5. _____   loss of appetite   Dysphagia

6. _____   poor digestion   Fecalith

7. _____   black stool   Halitosis

8. _____   chronic liver disease   Hematemesis

9. _____   intractable constipation   Melena

10. _____   binging and purging   Obstipation

WORKSHEET 3

Build a surgical term for the following:

1. _____gingivectomy_____ excision of gum tissue (in pyorrhea)

2. _____ partial or complete excision of the tongue

3. _____ surgical repair of the esophagus

4. _____ surgical removal of part or all of the stomach

5. _____ establishment of a permanent passage between the stomach and jejunum

6. _____ visual examination of the rectum and sigmoid colon

7. _____ creation of a passage between the stomach, small intestine, and colon

8. _____ surgical repair of the intestines

9. _____ fixation of the intestine (to the abdominal wall)

10. _____ surgical creation of a permanent opening into the jejunum

11. _____ surgical creation of a permanent opening into the colon

12. _____ fixation of a movable liver (to the abdominal wall)

13. _____ surgical repair of the anus or rectum

14. _____ removal of the gallbladder

15. _____ surgical repair of a bile duct

114   WORKSHEET 4

Define the following diagnostic and symptomatic terms. Use the dictionary as a reference.

1. leukoplakia _____

2. gastrectasis _____

3. cheilitis
    chilitis } _____

4. enterospasm _____

5. aerophagia _____

6. ptyalism _____

7. regurgitation _____

8. stenosis _____

9. diverticulum _____

10. volvulus _____

WORKSHEET 5

Grammar Review—Gastrointestinal System

Use the dictionary and refer to Chapter 2 in order to complete this exercise.

1. Using the WR duoden (duodenum), form a word with an adjective ending that means pertaining to. _____duodenal_____

2. Using the WR hepat (liver), form a word with an adjective ending that means pertaining to. _____

3. Using the CF/WR gastroentero (stomach and intestines), form a word with a noun ending that means one who specializes in stomach disorders. _____

4. Using the WR rect (anus), form a word with an adjective ending that means pertaining to. _____

5. Using the WR bulim (hunger), form a word with a noun ending. _____
_____

6. Using the CF/WR proctolog (study of rectal disease), form a word with a noun ending that means one who specializes in rectal diseases. _____

Write the plural form for the following words.

SINGULAR	PLURAL
7. ruga	_____
8. omentum	_____
9. stoma	_____
10. diverticulum	_____

116   WORKSHEET 6

Label the figure below, and compare your answers with Figure 6-1.

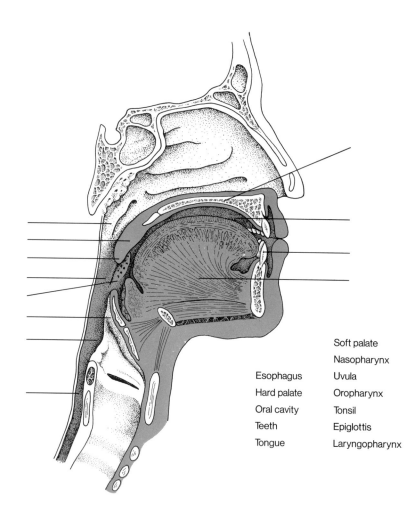

Esophagus   Soft palate

Hard palate   Nasopharynx

Oral cavity   Uvula

Teeth   Oropharynx

Tongue   Tonsil

                 Epiglottis

                 Laryngopharynx

WORKSHEET 7

Label the figure below, and compare your answers with Figure 6-2.

Appendix

Parotid gland

Esophagus

Cardiac
valve

Stomach

Spleen

Splenic
flexure

Pancreas

Transverse colon

Descending colon

Sigmoid colon

Rectum

Anus

Ileum

Cecum

Tongue

Salivary
glands

Sublingual gland

Submaxillary gland

Parotid gland

Liver

Gallbladder

Bile duct

Duodenum

Pyloric valve

Hepatic flexure

Ascending colon

Jejunum

Teeth

Oral cavity

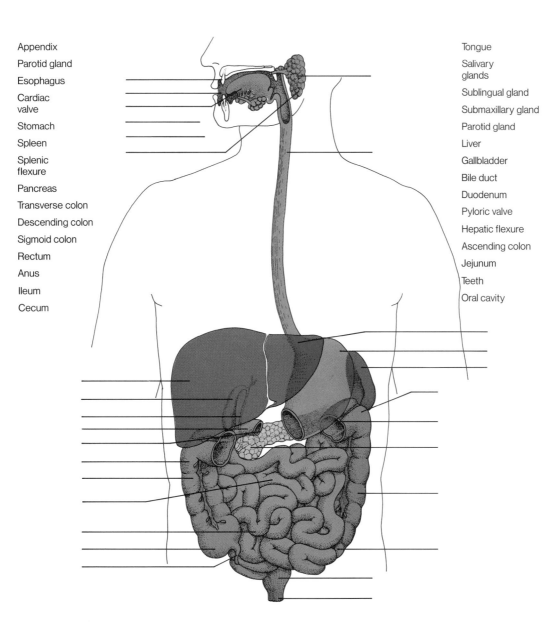

WORKSHEET 8

Special Procedures, Pharmacology, and Abbreviations

Choose the term that best describes the following statements:

anastomosis
antacids
antidiarrheals
antiflatulents
b.i.d.
cathartics
choledochoplasty
emetics
FBS
intravenous cholangiography
laparoscopy

lower GI
occult blood
oral cholecystography
p.c.
proctosigmoidoscopy
pyloromyotomy
q.i.d.
spleen scan
Stat.
stomatoplasty
upper GI

1. _____ after meals

2. _____ used to determine bleeding in gastrointestinal disorders

3. _____ used to induce vomiting, especially in cases of poisoning

4. _____ twice a day

5. _____ surgical reconstruction of a bile duct

6. _____ an enema with a barium solution is administered while a series of radiographs are taken of the large intestine

7. _____ the scope is inserted into the abdominal cavity through a small incision in the abdominal wall in order to diagnose tumors or other abnormalities

8. _____ surgical reconstruction of the mouth

9. _____ promote bowel movement and/or defecation

10. _____ surgical formation of a passage or opening between two hollow viscera or vessels

11. _____ oral administration of dye is taken prior to radiographs of the gallbladder

12. _____ radioactive material is injected intravenously in order to visualize the spleen

13. _____ reduce the feelings of gassiness and bloating that accompany indigestion

14. _____ neutralize excess acid in the stomach and help relieve gastritis and ulcer pain

15. _____ used to detect abnormalities of glucose metabolism

16. _____ injection of dye into a vein in order to take radiographs of bile vessels

17. _____ four times a day

18. _____ immediately

19. _____ endoscopic procedure for visualization of benign and malignant lesions of the rectosigmoid colon

20. _____ barium solution is swallowed for a radiographic examination of the esophagus, stomach, and duodenum

CHAPTER 7

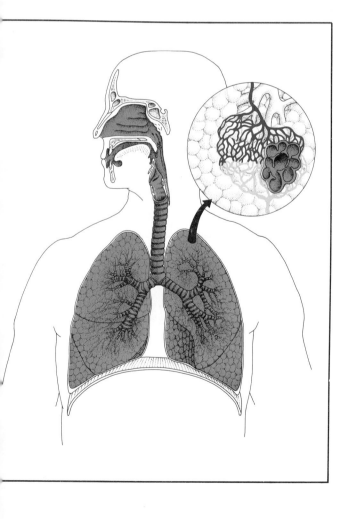

Respiratory System

STUDENT OBJECTIVES

Upon completion of this chapter, you will be able to do the following:

List the major structures of the respiratory system, and briefly describe the function of each.

Differentiate external and internal respiration.

Describe the function of the diaphragm in the breathing process.

Identify the word roots/combining forms and suffixes associated with the respiratory system.

Identify and discuss associated pathology related to the respiratory system.

Identify radiographic, clinical, surgical, and laboratory procedures and abbreviations related to the respiratory system.

Explain the pharmacology related to the treatment of respiratory disorders.

Build and analyze diagnostic, symptomatic, and surgical terms related to the respiratory system by completing the worksheets.

122 ANATOMY AND PHYSIOLOGY OF THE RESPIRATORY SYSTEM

Respiratory activity consists of two separate, simultaneous operations that involve the exchange of oxygen (O_2) and carbon dioxide (CO_2).

External Respiration

The first operation, **external respiration**, refers to the exchange of O_2 and CO_2 between the organism and the external environment. In this operation, oxygen-rich air from the environment is brought into the lungs during inspiration (inhalation), and CO_2 is removed from the body during expiration (exhalation). More familiarly, external respiration is called **lung breathing**.

Internal Respiration

The second operation, **internal respiration**, refers to the exchange of O_2 and CO_2 at the cellular level. Oxygen contained in the red blood cells is exchanged for the waste carbon dioxide in the tissues. This exchange is also called **tissue breathing**. Just as the organism as a whole requires the exchange of gases to maintain life, each individual cell must also exchange gases for the metabolic process. Ultimately, CO_2 will be transferred to the lungs to be expelled.

Structures Associated with Breathing

As you read the following paragraphs, refer to Figure 7-1. This will provide a better understanding of the anatomy and physiology of the respiratory system.

During the breathing process, air from the environment is drawn into the nose and passes through the (1) **nasal cavity (turbinates)** to the **pharynx (throat)**. The pharynx is a muscular tube that constitutes the first major section of the air passages to the lungs. It is about 5 inches long and consists of three sections:

1. The (2) **nasopharynx**, posterior to the nose.
2. The (3) **oropharynx**, posterior to the mouth.
3. The (4) **laryngopharynx**, above the larynx.

Within the nasopharynx is a collection of lymphatic tissue known as (5) **adenoids**, or **pharyngeal tonsils**. Another collection of lymphatic tissue called (6) **palatine tonsils**, or more commonly, **tonsils**, is located in the oropharynx.

Beneath the laryngopharynx is the (7) **larynx** (voice box). This structure is responsible for sound production, or **phonation**. A leaf-shaped flap on top of the larynx, the (8) **epiglottis**, seals off the air passage to the lungs during swallowing to ensure that food or liquids do not obstruct the flow of air to the lungs.

The extension of the air passage tube beneath the larynx is the (9) **trachea**. It is composed of smooth muscle embedded with C-shaped cartilage rings. These rings provide the necessary rigidity to keep the air passage open at all times. The trachea divides into two branches called (10) **bronchi** (singular form, **bronchus**). One bronchus leads to the right lung and the other to the left lung. Like the trachea, the bronchi contain C-shaped cartilage rings. Without them, the trachea or bronchi may possibly collapse and endanger life.

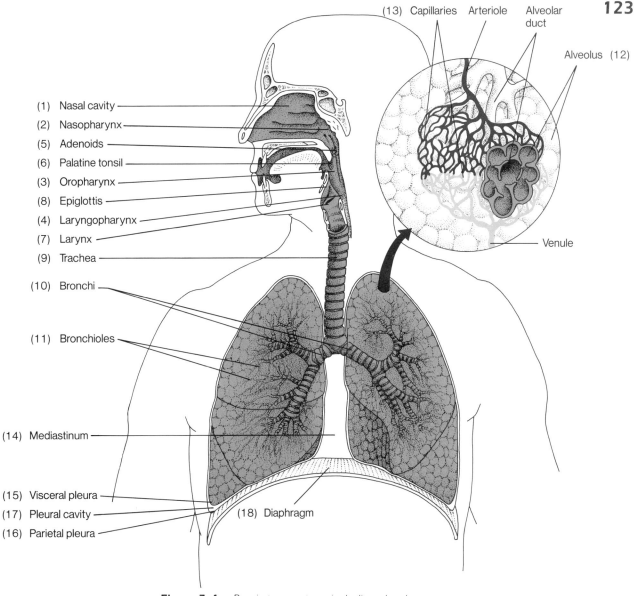

(13) Capillaries   Arteriole   Alveolar duct

Alveolus (12)

(1) Nasal cavity
(2) Nasopharynx
(5) Adenoids
(6) Palatine tonsil
(3) Oropharynx
(8) Epiglottis
(4) Laryngopharynx
(7) Larynx
(9) Trachea
(10) Bronchi
(11) Bronchioles
(14) Mediastinum
(15) Visceral pleura
(17) Pleural cavity
(16) Parietal pleura

(18) Diaphragm

Venule

Figure 7–1. *Respiratory system, including alveolus.*

Each bronchus divides into small branches called (11) **bronchioles** (little bronchi), which terminate in air sacs called (12) **alveoli** (singular form, **alveolus**). An alveolus resembles a small balloon because it expands and contracts with inflow and outflow of air (see Fig. 7-1). (13) **Capillary beds** of the circulatory system lie adjacent to the thin tissue membranes of the alveoli. Carbon dioxide passes from the blood within the pulmonary capillaries into the alveolar spaces, while oxygen from the alveoli passes into the blood. After the blood becomes oxygenated, it returns to the heart where it is pumped to all body tissues. At the tissue level, O_2 from the blood is exchanged for tissue CO_2. This exchange of gases is called internal respiration.

The lungs are divided into lobes: three lobes in the right lung and two lobes in the left lung. The space between the right and left lungs is called the (14) **mediastinum**. It contains the heart, aorta, esophagus, and the bronchi.

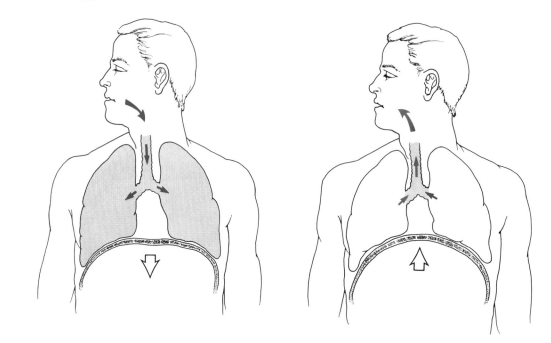

Figure 7–2. *Diaphragm contracts and flattens during inhalation, then relaxes during exhalation.*

A double fold of serous membrane, the pleura, surrounds the lungs. The innermost layer lying next to the lung is the (15) **visceral pleura**; the outermost layer is the (16) **parietal pleura**. These two membranes provide for a potential space, the (17) **pleural cavity**. This cavity contains a small amount of lubricating fluid that permits the visceral pleura to glide smoothly over the parietal pleura during respiration.

The ability of the lungs to fill with air and to expel air depends on a pressure differential between the atmosphere and the chest cavity. A large muscular partition, the (18) **diaphragm**, lies between the chest cavity and abdominal cavity. By contracting and relaxing, the diaphragm produces the needed pressure differential for respiration. When the diaphragm contracts, it partially descends into the abdominal cavity, decreasing the pressure within the chest (Fig. 7-2). This allows air to enter the lungs. When the diaphragm relaxes, it slowly re-enters the thoracic cavity. This increases the pressure within, and air slowly passes from the lungs. The intercostal muscles assist the diaphragm in changing the volume of the thoracic cavity. As the diaphragm contracts, the intercostal muscles elevate the rib cage. Both of these activities result in enlarging the thoracic cavity. Consequently, air from the environment passes into the lungs. The reverse activity causes the air to pass from the lungs into the environment.

WORD ROOTS/COMBINING FORMS RELATED TO THE RESPIRATORY SYSTEM

WORD ROOT/ COMBINING FORM	MEANING	EXAMPLE	PRONUNCIATION
nas/o	nose	nas/al pertaining to	NĀ - zl

Continued on following page

WORD ROOTS/COMBINING FORMS RELATED TO THE
RESPIRATORY SYSTEM —*Continued*

WORD ROOT/ COMBINING FORM	MEANING	EXAMPLE	PRONUNCIATION
rhin/o	nose	rhin/o/plasty surgical repair	RĪ - nō - plăs - tē
adenoid/o	adenoid	adenoid/ectomy excision	ăd - ĕ - noid - ĔK - tō - mē
tonsill/o	tonsils	tonsill/o/tome instrument to cut	tŏn - SĬL - ō - tōm
sinus/o	sinus, cavity	sinus/itis inflammation	sī - nŭs - Ī - tĭs
pharyng/o	pharynx, throat	pharyng/o/scope instrument to view	făr - ĬN - gō - skōp
epiglott/o	epiglottis	epiglott/itis inflammation	ĕp - ĭ - glŏt - TĪ - tĭs
laryng/o	larynx	laryng/o/scopy visual examination	lăr - ĭn - GŎS - kō - pē
trache/o	trachea	trache/o/tomy incision	trā - kē - ŎT - ō - mē
bronchi/o bronch/o	bronchus, bronchi (pl.)	bronchi/ectasis dilation bronch/o/scope instrument to view	brŏng - kē - ĔK - tă - sĭs BRŎNG - kă - skōp
pneumat/o	air, breath	pneumat/ic pertaining to	nū - MĂT - ĭk
pulmon/o	lung	pulmon/ary pertaining to	PŬL - mō - nĕ - rē
pneumon/o pneum/o	lung, air	pneumon/itis inflammation pneum/o/thorax chest	nū - mō - NĪ - tĭs nū - mō - THŌ - răks
lob/o	lobe	lob/ectomy excision	lō - BĔK - tō - mē
alveol/o	alveolus	alveol/ar pertaining to	ăl - VĒ - ō - lăr

Continued on following page

WORD ROOTS/COMBINING FORMS RELATED TO THE RESPIRATORY SYSTEM—*Continued*

WORD ROOT/ COMBINING FORM	MEANING	EXAMPLE	PRONUNCIATION
pleur/o	pleura	pleur/itis inflammation	ploo - RĪ - tĭs
phren/o	diaphragm, mind	phren/o/spasm twitching	FRĔN - ō - spăzm
pector/o		pector/algia pain	pĕk - tō - RĂL - jē - ăh

steth/o	chest	steth/o/scope
		          instrument
		          to view
			STĔTH - ō - skōp

thorac/o		thorac/ic pertaining to	thō - RĂS - ĭk

spir/o	breathe	spir/o/meter
		       instrument
		       for measuring
			spī - RŎM - ĕt - ĕr

coni/o	dust	pneum/o/coni/osis lung abnormal condition	nū - mō - kō - nē - Ō - sĭs

anthrac/o	coal	anthrac/osis
		       abnormal
		       condition
			ăn - thrăh - KŌ - sĭs

ox/o	oxygen, O_2	hyp/ox/emia de- blood ficient	hī - pŏk - SĒ - mē - ăh
orth/o	straight	orth/o/pnea breathing	ŏr - thŏp - NĒ - ăh
atel/o	incomplete, imperfect	atel/ectasis dilation	ăt - ē - LĔK - tăh - sĭs

SUFFIXES RELATED TO THE RESPIRATORY SYSTEM

SUFFIX	MEANING	EXAMPLE	PRONUNCIATION
-capnia	carbon dioxide, CO_2	hyper/capnia exces- sive	hī - pĕr - KĂP - nē - ăh
-osmia	smell	an/osmia lack	ăn - ŎZ - mē - ăh

Continued on following page

SUFFIXES RELATED TO THE RESPIRATORY SYSTEM—*Continued*

SUFFIX	MEANING	EXAMPLE	PRONUNCIATION
-phonia	voice	dys/phonia bad	dĭs - FŌ - nē - ăh
-pnea	breathing	a/pnea with- out	ăp - NĒ - ăh
-ptysis	spitting	hem/o/ptysis blood	hē - MŎP - tĭ - sĭs
-thorax	chest	hem/o/thorax blood	hē - mō - THŌ - răks

PATHOLOGY OF THE RESPIRATORY SYSTEM

Chronic Obstructive Pulmonary Disease (COPD)

Chronic obstructive pulmonary disease, also called chronic obstructive lung disease (COLD), includes respiratory disorders characterized by the lungs' decreased ability to perform their function of ventilation. Diagnostic criteria include a history of difficulty in breathing **(dyspnea)**, with or without a chronic cough. COPD includes bronchial asthma, chronic bronchitis, pulmonary emphysema, and bronchiectasis. An overdevelopment of tissue **(hyperplasia)** within the bronchial passages is characteristic of COPD.

Bronchial asthma often results as a response to an allergen. With this condition, there are spasms of the bronchi **(bronchospasms)** that cause a sudden or violent attack **(paroxysm)** of dyspnea. The asthmatic episode results in an increase in mucus secretion and, over a period of time, a thickening of the epithelium and muscle layers **(hyperplasia)**. Treatment includes the use of agents that loosen and break down mucus **(mucolytics)** in order to clear the obstructed air passages. In addition, medications that relax the smooth muscles of the bronchial passages **(bronchodilators)** provide relief.

Chronic bronchitis is an inflammation of the bronchi caused by the presence of infectious agents such as viruses or pathogenic bacteria. This disorder may also be caused by various physical and chemical agents, including dust and fumes. Due to its chronic nature, hyperplasia of the bronchial walls occurs. Associated with chronic bronchitis is a heavy, productive cough often accompanied by chest pain **(thoracodynia)**.

Pulmonary emphysema is a disease in which the alveoli lose elasticity. The air sacs expand **(dilate)** but are unable to contract to their initial form. Air becomes trapped in the alveoli, and the act of exhaling becomes very difficult for the emphysematous patient. This causes a characteristic "barrel chest" appearance.

Emphysema is often a secondary problem to some other respiratory disorder, including asthma, tuberculosis, or chronic bronchitis. It is also associated with long-term heavy smoking. Frequently, the patient experiences difficulty in breathing in any but the erect sitting or standing positions **(orthopnea)**.

In bronchiectasis there is a dilation of the bronchus or bronchi that usually leads to secondary infections involving the lower portions of the lungs. The patient produces copious amounts of sputum mixed with pus **(purulent sputum)**. Treatment of this condition includes the use of medications that relax the smooth muscles of the bronchi **(bronchodilators)** or medications that loosen and liquify sputum **(mucolytics)**. In addition, antibiotics and postural drainage are used in the treatment of this disorder.

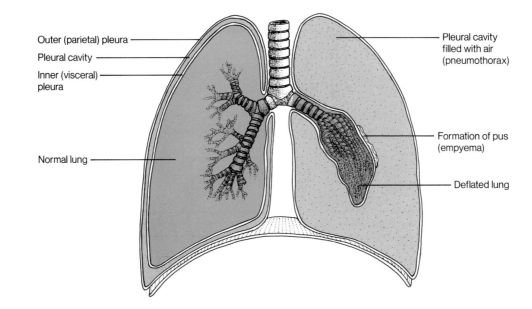

Outer (parietal) pleura

Pleural cavity

Inner (visceral) pleura

Normal lung

Pleural cavity filled with air (pneumothorax)

Formation of pus (empyema)

Deflated lung

Figure 7–3. Pneumothorax is air in the pleural cavity that can cause a lung to collapse. Empyema is a collection of pus in the cavity between the pleura and the lung tissue.

Pleural Effusions

An effusion is the passage of any fluid or gas into a cavity of the body. Some of the most common types of effusions are those that develop in the pleural cavity. Two techniques used in the diagnosis of pleural effusion are listening to the sounds of the chest cavity with a stethoscope **(auscultation)** and gently tapping the chest with the fingers to determine the position, size, or consistency of the underlying structures **(percussion)**. Different types of pleural effusions include the escape of pus **(pyothorax, empyema)**, serum **(hydrothorax)**, blood **(hemothorax)**, air **(pneumothorax)**, or a mixture of pus and air **(pyopneumothorax)** into the pleural cavity (Fig. 7-3).

Pneumoconiosis

Some employees are frequently exposed to environments that lead to lung disorders. These environments contain minute particles of substances, which are inhaled. After prolonged exposure, pathological changes are evident in the lungs. Such a condition is referred to as pneumoconiosis. The several different types of pneumoconioses derive their names from the types of dust particles that are found in the lung. These include asbestos **(asbestosis)**, coal dust **(anthracosis)**, limestone **(chalicosis)**, iron **(siderosis)**, or sand **(silicosis)**.

Atelectasis

Atelectasis is a condition in which a lung, lobe, or alveoli is in an airless state, or more simply, collapsed. It may occur at birth **(congenital)**, when the lungs fail to inflate properly in the newborn infant **(neonate)**. It also may be caused by the presence of disease, such as pneumonia. Other instances that result in atelectasis include situations in which retained secretions, foreign bodies (e.g., tumors), enlarged lymph nodes, or other obstructions press upon the lung, or portions of the lung, causing it to collapse.

Pneumonia

Pneumonia is an inflammatory disease of the lungs and may be caused by a variety of agents, including bacteria, viruses, diseases, chemicals, or other substances. Infectious

Table 7–1. PNEUMONIAS

SPECIFIC MICROBIAL CAUSES	DISEASES THAT MAY BE ACCOMPANIED BY PNEUMONIA	PNEUMONIA NOT CAUSED BY INFECTIONS
Viruses Adenoviruses influenza Rhinoviruses respirosyncytial Coxsackie Coronaviruses *Mycoplasmas* Mycoplasma pneumoniae *Cocci* Pneumococcus Staphylococcus Hemolytic streptococcus *Protozoon* (probable) Pneumocystis carinii *Bacilli* Hemophilus influenzae Mycobacterium tuberculosis Klebsiella pneumoniae (Friedländer's bacillus) Gram-negative bacilli *Chlamydiae* C. trachomatis C. psittaci *Fungi* Histoplasma capsulatum Coccidioides immitis *Rickettsiae* Rickettsia rickettsii Rickettsia burnetii	Tularemia Brucellosis Rheumatic fever Syphilis Typhus Typhoid Rocky Mountain fever Q fever Acute viral respiratory disease Infectious mononucleosis Trichiniasis Acquired immune deficiency syndrome Psittacosis Plague Legionnaire's disease Rickettsial diseases	Oil aspiration Radiation Chemicals Vegetable dusts Silo-filler's disease

From Thomas, CL (ed): *Taber's Cyclopedic Medical Dictionary*. FA Davis, Philadelphia, 1985, p 1325, with permission.

pneumonias are primarily attributed to bacteria or viruses. Some pneumonias occur as a secondary complication of another disease. Still other pneumonias develop because of food or liquid inhalation **(aspiration pneumonia)**, injury to the chest **(traumatic pneumonia)**, or inhalation of oily substances **(lipid** or **lipoid pneumonia)**. Some pneumonias affect only a lobe of the lung **(lobar pneumonia)**, while others affect both the right and left lungs **(bilateral** or **double pneumonia)**. Chest pain **(thoracodynia)**, purulent sputum, and spitting of blood **(hemoptysis)** are frequent symptoms of the disease. Solidification of the lungs may be due to a pathological engorgement of lung tissue **(consolidation)**. Table 7-1 lists some of the more common types of pneumonias.

Cystic Fibrosis

Cystic fibrosis is a hereditary disorder that affects the exocrine glands. The disease causes widespread **(systemic)** involvement, especially of the lungs, pancreas, and digestive tract. Mucus that is produced in an individual afflicted with cystic fibrosis is extremely thick **(viscid)** and causes a blockage of the bronchioles. Air becomes trapped in the lungs. The use of mists **(aerosols)** and postural drainage may provide relief. Improved diagnosis and treatment of this condition has extended life expectancy, and many children survive to young adulthood.

Respiratory Distress Syndrome (RDS, Hyaline Membrane Disease, HMD)

This condition is most frequently seen in premature infants or infants born to diabetic mothers. Prior to birth, lung tissue normally develops a phospholipid substance called surfactant. This substance aids in decreasing the surface tension of the alveoli. In order to expand **(compliance)**, lungs require surfactant. Lacking surfactant, the alveoli collapse and inhalation becomes extremely difficult. Radiography reveals a membrane that has a ground-glass appearance **(hyaline membrane)**. Clinical symptoms are noticeable immediately after birth and include cyanosis, tachypnea, flaring of the nostrils **(nares)**, intercostal retraction, and a characteristic grunt audible during exhalation. Although severe cases result in death, some forms of therapy are effective.

OTHER TERMS RELATED TO THE RESPIRATORY SYSTEM

TERM	MEANING	PRONUNCIATION
anosmia	absence of the sense of smell; hence the absence of the sense of taste	ăn - ŎZ - mē - ăh
anoxia, hypoxia	absence or deficiency of oxygen in the tissues	ăh - NŎK - sē - ăh hĭ - PŎK - sē - ăh
anoxemia, hypoxemia	absence or deficiency of oxygen in the blood	ăn - ŏk - SĒ - mē - ăh hĭ - pŏk - SĒ - mē - ăh
asphyxia	a condition in which there is insufficient oxygen; literally means without pulse	ăs - FĬK - sē - ăh

Continued on following page

OTHER TERMS RELATED TO THE RESPIRATORY SYSTEM—*Continued*

TERM	MEANING	PRONUNCIATION
compliance	the ease with which lung tissue can be stretched	kŏm - PLĪ - ăns
coryza	head cold; upper respiratory infection (URI)	kŏ - RĪ - zăh
croup	a condition resulting from an acute obstruction of the larynx caused by allergy, foreign body, infection, or new growth. The symptoms include a resonant, barking cough, suffocative and difficult breathing, laryngeal spasm, and sometimes the formation of a membrane	croop
Cheyne-Stokes respiration	breathing characterized by a fluctuation in the depth of respiration. The patient breathes deeply for a short time, then breathes very slightly, then not at all. This pattern occurs over and over again. Cheyne-Stokes respiration is usually caused by diseases that affect the respiratory centers, such as heart failure or brain damage	CHĀN - stōks rĕs - pĭ - RĀ - shŭn
epistaxis	nosebleed; nasal hemorrhage	ĕp - ĭ - STĂK - sĭs
intermittent positive-pressure breathing	a procedure that employs a mechanical device that causes the lungs to inflate when positive pressure is exerted, and deflate when the pressure is removed	
laryngeal stridor	abnormal sound caused by a spasm or swelling of the larynx	lăr - ĪN - jē - ăl/STRĪ - dŏr
mucus	viscous fluid secreted by mucous membranes that communicate with the air	MŪ - kŭs
naris, nares (pl.)	nostril	NĂ - rĭs
pleurisy, pleuritis	inflammation of the pleural membrane characterized by a stabbing pain that is intensified by coughing or deep breathing	PLOOR - ĭ - sē ploo - RĪ - tĭs
postural drainage	positioning a patient so that gravity aids in the drainage of secretions from the bronchi and lobes of the lungs	

Continued on following page

OTHER TERMS RELATED TO THE RESPIRATORY SYSTEM—*Continued*

TERM	MEANING	PRONUNCIATION
pulmonary edema	excessive fluid in the lungs that induces cough and dyspnea; common in left heart failure	PŬL - mō - nĕ - rē ĕ - DĒ - măh
rale, crackle	an abnormal respiratory sound heard on auscultation caused by exudates, spasms, hyperplasia, or when air enters moisture-filled alveoli	răl
sputum, sputa (pl.)	an abnormal viscous fluid formed in the lower respiratory tract that often contains blood, pus, and bacteria	SPŪ - tŭm
stenosis of the trachea, tracheostenosis	a constricture or narrowing of the trachea	stĕ - NŌ - sĭs/TRĀ - kē - ăh trā - kē - ō - stĕn - Ō - sĭs
tuberculosis	a disease caused by an acid-fast bacilli. It is acquired by inhaling viable tubercle bacilli into the lungs. Though primarily a lung disease, it might affect any organ of the body	tū - bĕr - kū - LŌ - sĭs

SPECIAL PROCEDURES RELATED TO THE RESPIRATORY SYSTEM

RADIOGRAPHIC AND CLINICAL PROCEDURES

TERM	DESCRIPTION
bronchography	examination of the bronchial tree following the intratracheal injection of an opaque solution
chest radiographs	series of radiographs designed to evaluate the chest, heart, lungs, and rib cage
computed tomography of the bronchial tree	a computerized visualization of the bronchi to determine pathology, especially tumors
pulmonary angiography	radiograph of the pulmonary vasculature after injection of a contrast medium into the pulmonary arteries in order to detect pulmonary embolisms and congenital or acquired defects
PA (posteroanterior) view	refers to the direction x-ray beams travel through the body. The beams travel from the back to the front. This is the preferred view for chest radiographs
pulmonary function studies	a series of tests designed to evaluate the volume and air-flow rate of the lungs. This is sometimes calculated by the use of a com-

Continued on following page

RADIOGRAPHIC AND CLINICAL PROCEDURES—*Continued*

TERM	DESCRIPTION
	puter attached to a sterile cylinder that the patient uses to perform various breathing exercises
tomography of the lung, laminography, planigraphy	a sequence of radiographs, each representing a "slice" of the lung at different depths. Tomography permits examination of a single layer or plane of an organ

ENDOSCOPIC PROCEDURES

TERM	DESCRIPTION
bronchoscopy	examination of the bronchial passageways. In this procedure, a flexible fiberoptic endoscope is passed into the bronchus for diagnosis, biopsy, specimen collection, or assessment of changes
laryngoscopy	visualization of the larynx using a laryngoscope. This procedure is important in diagnosing malignant neoplasms after biopsy

SURGICAL PROCEDURES

TERM	DESCRIPTION	PRONUNCIATION
bronchoplasty	surgical repair of the bronchus; surgical closure of a bronchial fistula	BRŎNG - kō - plăs - tē
bronchotomy	incision of the bronchus	brŏng - KŎT - ō - mē
laryngectomy	partial or total removal of the larynx, usually performed as a treatment for cancer	lăr - ĭn - JĔK - tō - mē
laryngoplasty	surgical repair of the larynx	lăh - RĬNG - gō - plăs - tē
pleurectomy, decortication	excision of part of the pleura	ploor - ĔK - tō - mē / dē - kŏr - tĭ - KĀ - shŭn
pneumonectomy	excision of a lung or lobe of the lung	nū - mō - NĔK - tō - mē
rhinoplasty	surgical repair or reconstruction of the nose	RĪ - nō - plăs - tē
thoracentesis	a surgical puncture and drainage of the pleural cavity	thō - răh - sĕn - TĒ - sĭs
tracheoplasty	surgical repair of the trachea	TRĀ - kē - ō - plăs - tē
tracheostomy	creation of an opening in the trachea during tracheal obstruction	trā - kē - ŎS - tō - mē

Continued on following page

SURGICAL PROCEDURES—*Continued*

TERM	DESCRIPTION	PRONUNCIATION
tracheotomy	incision of the trachea for exploration, for removal of a foreign body, or for obtaining a biopsy specimen	trā - kē - ŎT - ō - mē

LABORATORY PROCEDURES

TERM	DESCRIPTION
arterial blood gases (ABG)	among other things, this test assesses the O_2 and CO_2 levels in arterial blood. Since the concentration of these gases is greatly influenced by renal and respiratory functions, blood gas studies provide information for assessing and managing respiratory and renal disturbances
sputum culture and sensitivity (CS)	bacteriological procedure used to isolate the organism causing disease, especially pneumonia. When the causative organism is isolated, this test determines which antibiotic will be effective for treatment
throat culture	a bacteriological test used to identify throat pathogens, especially group A streptococci. Strep infections must be treated with appropriate antibiotics because they may cause serious secondary disorders

PHARMACOLOGY RELATED TO THE RESPIRATORY SYSTEM

MEDICATION	ACTION
antihistamine	opposes the action of histamine. Histamines are tissue substances that dilate blood vessels, thereby initiating the inflammatory response: local redness, heat, swelling, and pain. This medication is the primary agent used in treating allergic rhinitis (hay fever)
antitussive	prevents or relieves coughing, usually by acting on the medullary center of the brain to inhibit the cough reflex
bronchodilator	causes the smooth muscles of bronchi and bronchioles to relax, thereby increasing their lumen. Bronchodilators "open up" the air passages
decongestant	reduces congestion or swelling, especially in the nasal passages, or turbinates, by constricting blood vessels
expectorant	facilitates the removal of sputum, a pathological secretion of the bronchopulmonary membrane. Expectorants act either directly or reflexly on the bronchial glands to increase the volume of their secretions
mucolytic	liquifies tenacious, or "sticky," mucus so that it can be more readily coughed up

ABBREVIATIONS RELATED TO THE RESPIRATORY SYSTEM

ABBREVIATION	MEANING
ABG	arterial blood gases
AFB	acid-fast bacillus
AP view	anteroposterior view (radiology)
ARDS	adult respiratory distress syndrome
CO_2	carbon dioxide
COPD	chronic obstructive pulmonary disease
COLD	chronic obstructive lung disease
CPR	cardiopulmonary resuscitation
CXR	chest x-ray; chest radiograph
FEF	forced expiratory flow
FEV	forced expiratory volume
FVC	forced vital capacity
IPPB	intermittent positive-pressure breathing
O_2	oxygen
PND	paroxysmal nocturnal dyspnea
PA view	posteroanterior view (radiology)
RD	respiratory disease
SOB	short(ness) of breath
T&A	tonsillectomy and adenoidectomy
TB	tuberculosis
TPR	temperature, pulse, and respiration
URI	upper respiratory infection
VC	vital capacity

WORKSHEET 1

A. Using the word root/combining form rhin/o or nas/o (nose), build medical words to mean:

1. _____ nosebleed

2. _____ inflammation of the (mucous membranes) of the nose

3. _____ discharge from the nose

4. _____ pertaining to the nose

B. Using the word root/combining form laryng/o (larynx or voice box), build medical words to mean:

1. _____ inflammation of the larynx

2. _____ visual examination of the (interior) larynx

3. _____ spasm of the larynx

4. _____ stricture (narrowing) of the larynx

5. _____ pertaining to the larynx and the trachea

6. _____ disease of the larynx

C. Using the word root/combining form bronch/o or bronchi/o (bronchus), build medical words to mean:

1. _____ instrument to visually examine the bronchus

2. _____ inflammation of the bronchus

3. _____ dilation of the bronchus

4. _____ originating in the bronchus

5. _____ bronchial hemorrhage

6. _____ spasm of the bronchus

7. _____ pathological condition of bronchus

D. Using the word root/combining form pulmon/o, pneumon/o, or pneum/o (air, lung), build medical words to mean:

1. _____ inflammation of lungs

2. _____ air in the (pleural cavity) chest

3. _____ excision of a lung

4. _____ pertaining to the lung

E. Using the word root/combining form thoraclo (chest), build medical words to mean:

1. _____ surgical puncture of the chest

2. _____ pain in the chest

3. _____ pertaining to the chest

F. Using the suffix -pnea (breathing), build medical words to mean:

1. _____ good (normal) breathing

2. _____ rapid breathing

3. _____ breathing in an upright position

4. _____ temporary loss of breathing

5. _____ increased breathing

6. _____ slow breathing

7. _____ decreased breathing

8. _____ difficult (labored) breathing

138   WORKSHEET 2

Fill in the correct word from the right hand column that matches the definitions in the statements below.

1. _____ sputum _____ pathological fluid formed in the lungs or bronchi   Anosmia

2. _____ abnormal respiratory sounds heard in auscultation indicating pathology   Anoxemia

3. _____ spitting of blood   Apnea

4. _____ tapping of chest cavity   Atelectasis

5. _____ listening to chest sounds   Auscultation

6. _____ irregular breathing characterized by alteration in depth of respiration and apnea   Cheyne-Stokes respiration

7. _____ collapsed lung, lobe, or alveoli   Coryza

8. _____ pus in body cavity, especially the pleural cavity   Empyema

9. _____ lack of sense of smell   Epiglottis

10. _____ absence (decrease) of blood O_2 Epistaxis

11. _____ temporary absence of breathing   Hemoptysis

12. _____ head cold (upper respiratory infection)   Percussion

13. _____ structure to prevent choking   Rales/Crackles

14. _____ nosebleed   Sputum

WORKSHEET 3

Build surgical terms to mean:

1. _____laryngectomy_____ excision of the larynx

2. _____ excision of a lung

3. _____ excision of a single lobe from the lung

4. _____ surgical repair of the nose

5. _____ surgical puncture of the chest

6. _____ suture of the lungs

7. _____ fixation of the lung (to the thoracic wall)

8. _____ surgical repair of the bronchus

9. _____ formation of an artificial opening in the trachea

10. _____ incision of the larynx

11. _____ surgical repair of the larynx

12. _____ removal of a lung stone

140   **WORKSHEET 4**

Define each of the symptomatic or diagnostic terms. Use the dictionary, if necessary.

1. alveolitis _____

2. bronchomycosis _____

3. pneumoconiosis _____

4. silicosis _____

5. laryngoplegia _____

6. bronchiectasis _____

7. hemothorax _____

8. pleural effusion _____

9. auscultation _____

WORKSHEET 5

Special Procedures, Pharmacology, and Abbreviations

Choose the word(s) that best describes the following statements:

antihistamine
antitussive
AP
arterial blood gases
bronchodilator
bronchography
COLD
culture and sensitivity
decongestant

IPPB
laminography
laryngoscopy
mucolytic
PND
pulmonary angiography
pulmonary function studies
throat culture

1. _____ tests designed to evaluate volume and air-flow rate of the lungs

2. _____ radiography of the bronchial tree following the intratracheal injection of a contrast medium

3. _____ a sequence of radiographs, each representing a "slice" of the lung at different depths

4. _____ a bacteriological test used to identify throat pathogens, especially group A streptococci

5. _____ anteroposterior view (radiology)

6. _____ chronic obstructive lung disease

7. _____ prevents or relieves coughing

8. _____ primary agent used to relieve discomfort associated with allergic rhinitis by opposing the action of histamine

9. _____ reduces congestion and swelling of the nasal passages by constricting blood vessels

10. _____ helps to liquify "sticky" mucus so that it can be coughed up more readily

11. _____ relaxes smooth muscles of the bronchi in order to increase their lumen

12. _____ intermittent positive-pressure breathing

142

13. _____ assesses the O_2 and CO_2 levels of arterial blood in order to evaluate and manage respiratory and renal disturbances

14. _____ isolation of an organism and the determination of an effective antibiotic for treatment; used especially in pneumonia

WORKSHEET 6

Grammar Review—Respiratory System

A. Provide the noun for each of the adjectives listed below. Use the dictionary, if necessary.

1. hyperplastic _____ hyperplasia _____

2. orthopnic _____

3. paroxysmal _____

4. embolic _____

5. mucous _____

B. Provide the plural form for each of the singular forms listed below. Use the dictionary, if necessary.

6. lumen _____

7. sputum _____

8. thorax _____

9. bronchus _____

10. trachea _____

11. naris _____

WORKSHEET 7

Label the following, and check your answers with Figure 7-1.

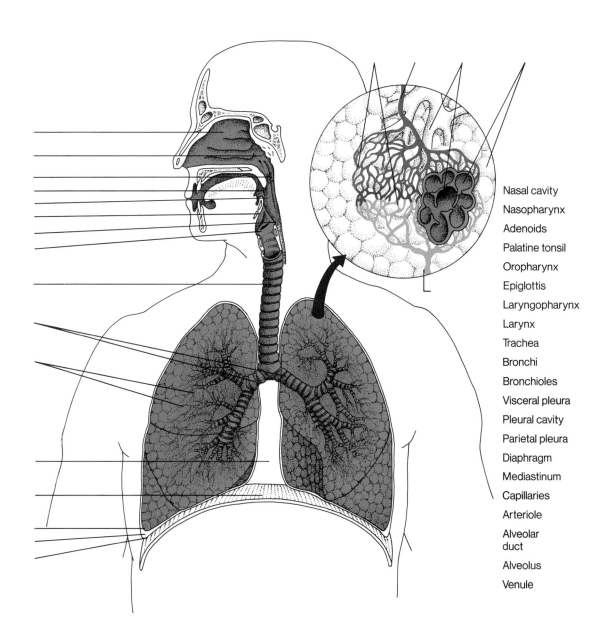

Nasal cavity

Nasopharynx

Adenoids

Palatine tonsil

Oropharynx

Epiglottis

Laryngopharynx

Larynx

Trachea

Bronchi

Bronchioles

Visceral pleura

Pleural cavity

Parietal pleura

Diaphragm

Mediastinum

Capillaries

Arteriole

Alveolar
duct

Alveolus

Venule

CHAPTER 8

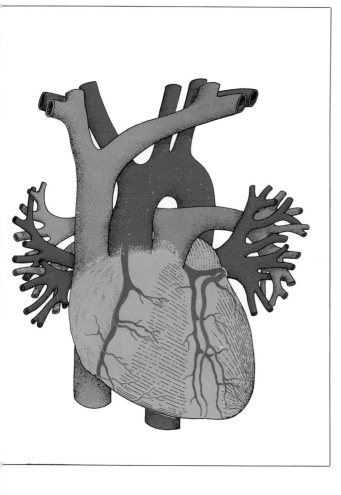

CHAPTER OUTLINE

Cardiovascular System

STUDENT OBJECTIVES

Upon completion of this chapter, you will be able to do the following:

List and describe the major difference in the walls of the three types of blood vessels.

Name the four chambers of the heart, and state the function of each chamber.

Differentiate systemic and pulmonary circulation.

Define systolic and diastolic blood pressures.

List the structures in sequential order through which the electrical current passes through the conduction system.

Identify the word roots/combining forms and suffixes associated with the cardiovascular system.

Identify and discuss associated pathology related to the cardiovascular system.

Identify radiographic, clinical, surgical, and laboratory procedures and abbreviations related to the cardiovascular system.

Explain the pharmacology related to the treatment of disorders of the cardiovascular system.

Build and analyze diagnostic, symptomatic, and surgical terms related to the cardiovascular system by completing the worksheets.

146 ANATOMY AND PHYSIOLOGY OF THE CARDIOVASCULAR SYSTEM

Discussions in earlier chapters addressed the anatomy and physiology of various body systems. Each of these systems, composed of millions of cells, requires a constant supply of food and vital products in order to function. In addition, each cell within these systems must be cleansed and purified of accumulated waste products. Since body cells are not always located near the source of the products they require and they are not always near the organs necessary for elimination of waste, a transportation system is required. Two distinct body systems, the cardiovascular system and the lymphatic system, are responsible for transportation of products to and from the cells of the body.

The cardiovascular system is composed of the heart, blood vessels, and blood. The lymphatic system is composed of lymph glands, lymph vessels, and lymph.

Only the heart and blood vessels are discussed in this chapter. Blood is considered with the lymphatic system because of the similarity between them (see Chapter 9).

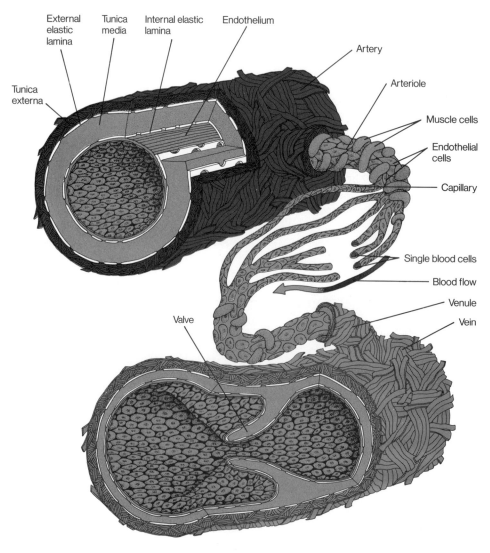

Figure 8-1. Diagram of an artery, a capillary, and a vein.

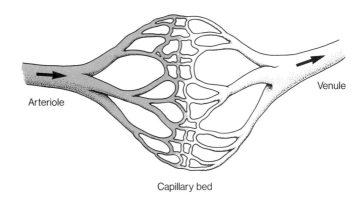

Figure 8–2. *Schematic representation of a capillary bed. The capillary system is the gateway for the return of blood to the heart. Blood flows from the heart through the arterial system to the capillaries. Transfer of products into and out of the blood vessels occurs at the capillary level.*

Arteriole

Venule

Capillary bed

Vascular System

Three types of vessels carry blood throughout the body. Each differs in structure, depending on its function. These vessels are the arteries, capillaries, and veins (Figs. 8-1 and 8-2).

ARTERIES

Arteries carry blood from the heart to body tissues and organs. The blood is propelled through the arteries by the pumping action of the heart. Consequently, arterial walls are thick and muscular and capable of expanding to accommodate the surge of blood that results when the heart contracts. The expansion of the arterial walls at each heartbeat is referred to as a pulse. Because of the pressure against the arterial walls associated with the pumping action of the heart, a cut or severed artery is a serious condition.

The blood in the arteries (except for the pulmonary artery) contains a high concentration of oxygen (O_2). Such blood is referred to as oxygenated blood. It is characterized by a bright red color.

Arteries branch to form smaller vessels called **arterioles** (little arteries). Arterioles further divide to form the smallest vessels of the circulatory system, the **capillaries**.

CAPILLARIES

Capillaries are microscopic vessels that join the arterial system with the venous system. Although seemingly the most insignificant of the three vessel types because of size (only one blood cell at a time is able to pass through the lumen), they are functionally the most important. The walls of the capillaries are composed of a single layer of endothelial cells. The thinness of these walls makes it possible for substances to pass quite readily into and out of the vessels. Consequently, the primary function of the vascular system—providing cells with vital products—is accomplished by the capillaries.

It is important to note that the vast number of capillaries makes their combined diameter so great that blood flows through them very slowly. This allows sufficient time for the exchange of materials to occur between blood and body cells. The pathway for this exchange is as follows:

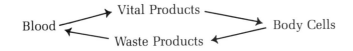

Blood → Vital Products → Body Cells
Body Cells → Waste Products → Blood

VEINS

Veins carry blood to the heart from body organs and tissues. Veins are formed from smaller vessels called venules (little veins), which develop from the union of capillaries. Capillaries connect arterioles to venules. This connection provides a gateway for the return of blood to the heart. Since the extensive network of capillaries throughout the body absorbs the propelling pressure exerted by the heart, the blood in veins now must rely on other methods of propulsion in order to return to the heart. These methods include skeletal muscle contraction (especially in the legs), gravity (in the upper areas of the body), and respiratory activity (in the thoracic area). In addition, valves aid in the return of blood to the heart. Valves are small structures within the vein that prevent the backflow of blood. Valves are especially important in the legs because blood must travel a long distance against the force of gravity in order to reach the heart.

Blood carried in the veins (except for the pulmonary vein) contains a high concentration of carbon dioxide (CO_2). This gas is a waste product of cell metabolism and is produced by all cells of the body. When CO_2 is present in blood, the blood takes on a characteristic purple color. Such blood is said to be deoxygenated. Deoxygenated blood is continuously transported to the lungs, where the CO_2 is expelled.

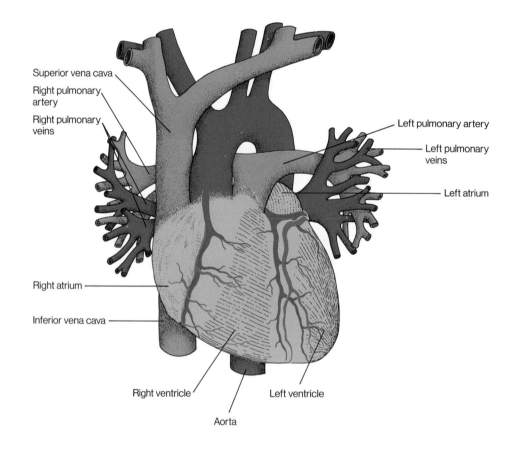

Figure 8–3. Diagram of the heart.

The Heart   149

The heart is a hollow, muscular organ that pumps blood through the arteries, capillaries, and veins. It is enclosed in a fibroserous sac called the pericardium. The heart has three distinct layers of tissue:

1. The **endocardium**, which is a serous membrane that lines the four chambers of the heart and its valves. It is continuous with the arteries and veins.
2. The **myocardium**, which is the muscular layer of the heart.
3. The **epicardium**, which is the outermost layer of the heart.

The heart is divided into four chambers (Fig. 8-3). These chambers are the **right atrium**, **right ventricle**, **left atrium**, and **left ventricle**. The two upper chambers, the atria, collect blood; the two lower chambers, the ventricles, pump blood from the heart. The right side of the heart provides for the oxygenation of blood (pulmonary circulation), and the left side is responsible for the transportation of blood to body cells, which compose all the systems of the body (systemic circulation). The muscular wall dividing the right side of the heart from the left is called the **septum**.

Refer to Figure 8-4 as you read the following paragraphs on blood flow through the heart and major blood vessels.

Body cells produce waste products during metabolism. These waste products include carbon dioxide (CO_2), a gas that must be removed or tissue death will occur. The thin-walled capillaries allow CO_2 to enter the blood, where it is transported to the heart by way of two large veins: the (1) **superior vena cava**, which collects and carries blood from the top portion of the body; and the (2) **inferior vena cava**, which collects and carries blood from the lower portion of the body. The superior and inferior vena cava deposit the deoxygenated blood into the right upper chamber of the heart, the (3) **right atrium**. From the right

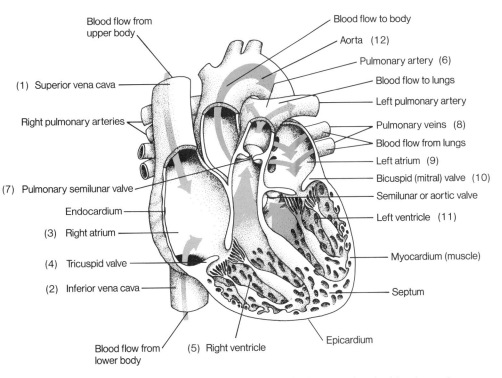

Figure 8-4. Diagram of the blood flow through the heart and major blood vessels.

150

atrium, blood passes through the (4) **tricuspid valve** to the (5) **right ventricle**. The tricuspid valve prevents blood from returning to the right atrium during contraction of the ventricle. When the heart contracts, blood leaves the right ventricle by way of the (6) **pulmonary artery**. The (7) **pulmonic semilunar valve (pulmonary valve)** in the pulmonary artery restrains blood from passing back into the right ventricle. In the lungs, this artery branches into millions of capillaries, each lying in close proximity to the alveoli. Here CO_2 in the blood is replaced by O_2 that has been drawn into the lungs during inhalation. The blood is now oxygenated and takes on a bright red appearance.

The pulmonary capillaries unite to form the (8) **pulmonary veins**, which carry blood back to the heart. The right and left pulmonary veins carry oxygenated blood into the (9) **left atrium** of the heart. The blood passes from the left atrium through the (10) **bicuspid valve** (also called the **mitral valve**) to the (11) **left ventricle**. Upon contraction of the heart, the oxygenated blood leaves the left ventricle through the largest artery of the body, the (12) **aorta**. Within the aorta is a valve called the aortic semilunar valve, or aortic valve. This valve permits blood to flow in only one direction—from the left ventricle to the aorta. The aorta branches into many smaller arteries that carry blood to all parts of the body. Some arteries derive their name from the organs or areas of the body that they vascularize. For example, the coronary arteries vascularize the heart muscle, the renal arteries vascularize the kidneys, and so forth.

It is important to recognize that the O_2 present in the blood passing through the chambers of the heart cannot be used by the myocardium. Instead, an arterial system, called the coronary arteries, branches from the aorta and provides the heart muscle with its own blood supply. If the flow of blood in the coronary arteries is diminished, myocardial damage may result. When severe damage occurs, necrosis of muscle tissue results. Refer to Figure 8-4 and trace the pathway that the blood follows as it passes through the heart.

Blood Pressure

Each heartbeat is composed of two phases: the contraction phase, or systole, when the blood is forced out of the heart; and a relaxation phase, or diastole. Blood pressure measures the force exerted by the blood against the arterial walls during these two phases. Systole indicates the maximum force exerted by the blood against the arterial walls; diastole, the weakest. These are recorded as two figures separated by a diagonal line; the systolic pressure is given first, followed by the diastolic pressure. For example, a blood pressure may be recorded as 120/80; 120 is the systolic pressure, and 80 is the diastolic pressure.

Several factors influence the blood pressure, including the resistance of blood flow in the blood vessels, the pumping action of the heart, the viscosity, or thickness, of the blood, the elasticity of the arteries, and the quantity of blood in the vascular system. Elevated blood pressure is called **hypertension**; decreased blood pressure is called **hypotension**.

Conduction System of the Heart

Within the heart is a specialized cardiac tissue known as conductive tissue. Its sole function is the initiation and propagation of contraction impulses.

The conductive tissue consists of four masses of highly specialized cells (Fig. 8-5):
- Sinoatrial node, or SA node.
- Atrioventricular node, or AV node.
- Bundle of His.
- Purkinje fibers.

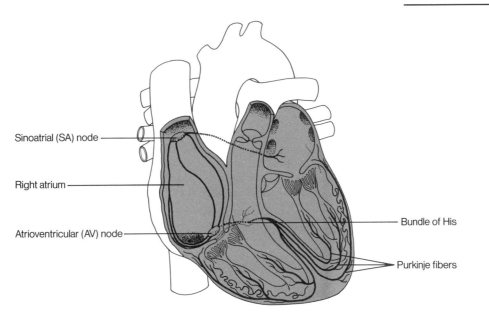

Figure 8-5. *The conduction system of the heart.*

The SA node, which is located in the upper portion of the right atrium, possesses its own intrinsic rhythm. Without being stimulated by external nerves, it has the ability to initiate and propagate each heartbeat, thereby setting the basic pace for the cardiac rate. For this reason, it is commonly known as the pacemaker. Cardiac rate may be altered by impulses from the autonomic nervous system. Such an arrangement allows outside influences to accelerate or decelerate the rate of the heartbeat. For example, during a period of physical exertion the heart beats faster, and during a restful interval the rate becomes slower.

Each electrical impulse discharged by the SA node is transmitted to the AV node, causing the atria to contract. The AV node is located at the base of the right atrium. From this point, a tract of conduction fibers called the bundle of His, composed of a right and left branch, relays the impulse to the Purkinje fibers. These fibers extend up the walls of the ventricles. The Purkinje fibers transmit the impulse to both the right and left ventricles, causing them to contract. The blood is now forced out of the heart through the pulmonary artery and the aorta.

In summary, the sequence of involvement of the four structures in the heart that are responsible for the conduction of a contraction impulse is as follows:

SA node → AV node → Bundle of His → Purkinje fibers

Impulse transmission through the conduction system generates weak electrical currents that can be detected on the surface of the body. These electrical impulses can be recorded on an instrument called an **electrocardiograph**. The deflection of the needle of the electrocardiograph produces waves or peaks designated by the letters P, Q, R, S, and T, each of which is associated with a specific electrical event. The P wave is the depolarization (contraction) of the atria, and the QRS complex is the depolarization (contraction) of the ventricles. The T wave, which appears a short time later, is the repolarization (recovery) of the ventricles (Fig. 8-6).

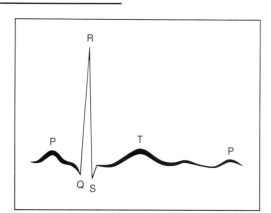

Figure 8-6. Normal ECG deflections. The ECG gives important information concerning the spread of excitation to the different parts of the heart, and it is of value in the diagnosis of abnormal cardiac rhythm and myocardial damage.

WORD ROOTS/COMBINING FORMS RELATED TO THE CARDIOVASCULAR SYSTEM

WORD ROOT/ COMBINING FORM	MEANING	EXAMPLE	PRONUNCIATION
angi/o ⎫ vas/o ⎭	vessel	angi/o/rrhaphy suture vas/o/spasm twitching	ăn - jē - ŎR - ăh - fē VĂS - ō - spăzm
aort/o	aorta	aort/o/stenosis narrowing	ā - ŏr - tō - stĕ - NŌ - sĭs
arteriol/o	little artery, arteriole	arteriol/itis inflammation	ăr - tĕr - ĭ - ō - LĪ - tĭs

ather/o	fatty deposit, fatty degeneration	ather/o/scler/ osis
		    hard- abnor-
		    en- mal
		    ing con-
		    dition
		    (of)
			ăth - ĕr - ō - sklē - RŌ - sĭs

atri/o	atrium	atri/al pertaining to	Ā - trē - ăl
cardi/o	heart	cardi/o/megaly enlargement	kăr - dē - ō - MĔG - ăh - lē
embol/o	embolus, plug	embol/ectomy excision	ĕm - bō - LĔK - tō - mē
hemangi/o	blood vessel	hemangi/oma tumor	hĕ - măn - jē - Ō - măh

oxy/o	oxygen, O_2	oxy/gen/ ic
		    to pertaining
		    pro- to
		    duce
			ŏk - sĭ - JĔN - ĭk

Continued on following page

WORD ROOTS/COMBINING FORMS RELATED TO THE
CARDIOVASCULAR SYSTEM—*Continued*

WORD ROOT/ COMBINING FORM	MEANING	EXAMPLE	PRONUNCIATION
phleb/o ⎱ ven/o ⎰	vein	phleb/itis inflammation ven/ous pertaining to	flĕ - BĪ - tĭs VĒ - nŭs
thromb/o	clot (of blood)	thromb/osis abnormal condition	thrŏm - BŌ - sĭs
sphygm/o	pulse	sphygm/o/manometer instrument for measuring pressure	sfĭg - mō - măn - ŎM - ĕt - ĕr
venul/o	venule	venul/itis inflammation	vĕn - ū - LĪ - tĭs

SUFFIXES RELATED TO THE CARDIOVASCULAR SYSTEM

SUFFIX	MEANING	EXAMPLE	PRONUNCIATION
-gram	record, a writing	angi/o/gram vessel	ĂN - jē - ō - grăm
-graph	instrument for recording	electr/o/cardi/o/graph elec- heart tricity	ē - lĕk - trō - KĂR - dē - ō - grăf
-manometer	instrument to measure pressure	sphygm/o/manometer pulse	sfĭg - mō - măn - ŎM - ĕt - ĕr
-stenosis	narrowing	aort/o/stenosis aorta	ā - ŏr - tō - stĕ - NŌ - sĭs
-tension	pressure	hyp/o/tension below	hĭ - pō - TĔN - shŭn

PATHOLOGY OF THE CARDIOVASCULAR SYSTEM

Atherosclerosis

Atherosclerosis is a vascular disorder that may lead to hardening of the arteries (arteriosclerosis). Loss of vascular elasticity and narrowing of the vascular channel are characteristic of

154   atherosclerosis. In this disorder, the innermost lining of the artery **(tunica intima)** becomes thickened with soft fatty deposits **(atheromatous plaques**, or **atheromas)**. As the atheromas increase in size, they impede the flow of blood to the tissues, become hardened, and may even rupture. In some cases, the circulation increases in the area of the atheroma because of the development of additional vessels, thus averting tissue injury. If additional circulation is not established, the tissues near the atheroma experience a deficiency in oxygen **(isch-emia)**, which may progress to tissue death **(necrosis)**. Atheromas may involve the abdomi-nal, coronary, or cerebral arteries, as well as the major arteries of the legs.

Coronary Artery Disease (CAD)

Any disease that alters the ability of the coronary arteries to deliver the amount of blood that is required by the heart muscle is referred to as coronary artery disease. Its usual cause, however, is arteriosclerosis (Fig. 8-7).

About 20 percent of the total coronary output is needed to supply the oxygen require-ments of the heart muscle. When the coronary arteries are not able to deliver this amount, localized areas of the heart experience ischemia. Myocardial ischemia causes a suffocating chest pain **(angina pectoris**, or **angina)** and difficulty in breathing **(dyspnea)**. When pain cannot be controlled with medication, bypass surgery, which is designed to circumvent the obstruction, may be required. In this surgery, the saphenous vein from the lower leg (or another vein) is used to bypass the obstruction. One end of the graft vessel is sewn to the

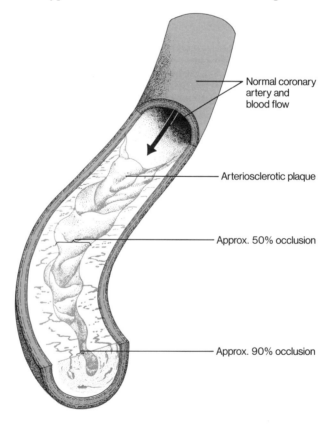

Normal coronary artery and blood flow

Arteriosclerotic plaque

Approx. 50% occlusion

Approx. 90% occlusion

Figure 8–7.   Arteriosclerosis.

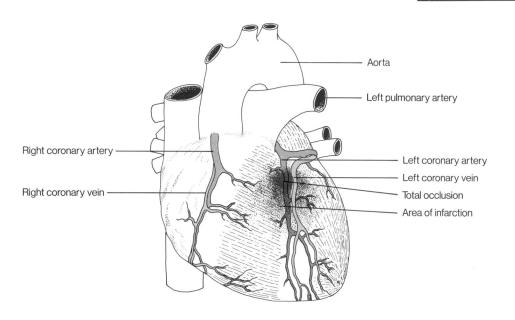

Figure 8-8. Myocardial infarction.

aorta, and the other end is sewn to the coronary artery below the blocked area **(anastomosis)**. This re-establishes the blood flow to the heart muscle.

Coronary artery disease may ultimately produce an acute myocardial infarction (MI). In this life-threatening condition, blood supply to part of the heart is totally suppressed, causing necrosis, or infarction, in a portion of the myocardium (Fig. 8-8). The clinical symptoms of an acute myocardial infarction include intense angina, profuse sweating **(diaphoresis)**, paleness **(pallor)**, and dyspnea. An arrhythmic heartbeat, accompanied by either a rapid heart action **(tachycardia)** or slow heart action **(bradycardia)**, may also accompany MI.

As the heart muscle undergoes necrotic changes, several enzymes are released, one of which is transaminase. The rapid elevation of the transaminase level in circulating blood helps differentiate MI from pericarditis, aortic aneurysm, and acute pulmonary embolism.

Valvular Heart Disease

The valves of the heart are generally thin, smooth structures that permit the flow of blood through the chambers of the heart. Birth defects or certain infections, especially those caused by scarlet fever or rheumatic fever, may produce scarring of the valves. When this occurs, there may be a narrowing of the valves **(stenosis)** or an inability of the valves to close properly **(insufficiency)**. Although medications may prove helpful, heart surgery frequently is the only recourse. Whenever possible, the original valve is repaired **(valvotomy, or commissurotomy)**, but more often it is replaced with an artificial device. (Fig. 8-9).

Patients who have had open heart surgery, rheumatic or scarlet fever, or valvular disease are often more susceptible to infections of the inner lining of the heart chambers **(bacterial endocarditis)** than are individuals who have not had these problems. Therefore, in order to ward off the threat of endocarditis, treatment with antibiotics is undertaken prior to certain procedures **(prophylactic treatment)**. These procedures include tooth removal, root canal, and other minor surgeries.

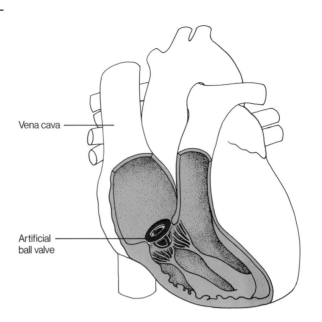

Vena cava

Artificial
ball valve

Figure 8–9. Replacement surgery may be performed to replace a damaged heart valve

Varicose Veins

Varicose veins develop when the valves of the veins are damaged. A backflow of blood, especially in the legs, causes the veins to enlarge, exerting excessive pressure on the valves. Blood accumulates in the flabby areas of the vein, and excess fluid eventually seeps from the vein, resulting in edema of the surrounding tissue.

Varicose veins can result from a congenital weakness of the valves, pregnancy, occupations that necessitate standing for long periods of time, and from a vascular condition called phlebitis.

In phlebitis, the walls of the vein become inflamed. There is usually pain and tenderness. A cordlike mass may develop under the skin, but as the disease subsides, this mass diminishes. If the infection occurs in a deep vein and involves the inner layer of vein tissue, clots may form **(thrombophlebitis)**. A more serious condition may subsequently develop when the thrombus breaks loose from the vein wall and begins to travel in the vascular system **(embolus)**. Death may result if the embolus lodges in a vital organ. Emboli may be removed directly by excision **(embolectomy)** or indirectly by means of a balloon catheter **(angioplasty)**. A deflated balloon catheter is inserted into the vein below the embolus and is passed beyond the place where the embolus is located. The balloon is then inflated. By withdrawing the catheter, the embolus is drawn to a small incision in the surface of the skin and removed.

Treatment of mild cases of varicose veins includes rest periods during which the legs are elevated. Elastic stockings may also bring relief. In extreme cases, the affected vein is tied **(ligated)** and removed **(stripped)**.

OTHER TERMS RELATED TO THE CARDIOVASCULAR SYSTEM

TERM	MEANING	PRONUNCIATION
aneurysm	a localized abnormal dilation of a blood vessel of the heart that may result in a rupture. This condition is due to a congenital defect or weakness in the wall of the heart or blood vessel	ĂN - ū - rĭzm
arrhythmia	irregularity in heart action	ăh - RĬTH - mē - ăh
cardiomyopathy	any disease of the heart muscle that is not caused by an impairment of coronary circulation and ischemia. Cardiomyopathies may be caused by viral infections, metabolic disorders, or general systemic diseases	kăr - dē - ō - mĭ - ŎP - ă - thē
cardioversion	conversion of a cardiac arrhythmia to a normal sinus rhythm by the use of a device called a cardioverter. This instrument produces countershocks to the heart through electrodes placed on the chest wall	KĂR - dē - ō - věr - zhŭn
coarctation	narrowing of a vessel, especially the aorta	kō - ărk - TĀ - shŭn
congenital septal defect	small hole(s) within the atrial septum or ventricular septum present at birth	kŏn - JĔN - ĭ - tăl SĔP - tăl/DĒ - fĕkt
congestive heart failure, cardiac decompensation	failure of the heart to pump required supplies of blood to the tissues and organs. The most common cause of heart failure is impaired coronary blood flow	kŏn - JĔS - tĭv hărt/făl - yer KĂR - dē - ăk dē - kŏm - pĕn - SĀ - shŭn
embolus, emboli (pl.)	a foreign object, a quantity of air or gas, a bit of tissue or tumor, or a piece of thrombus that circulates in the bloodstream or lymphatic channels until it becomes lodged in a vessel	ĔM - bō - lŭs
hypothermia	having a body temperature below normal; may be induced for certain surgical procedures, especially those involving the heart	hĭ - pō - THĔR - mē - ăh
fibrillation	quivering or spontaneous muscle contractions, especially in the heart, causing ineffectual cardiac contractions. These often may be corrected using a defibrillator	fĭ - brĭl - Ā - shŭn

Continued on following page

OTHER TERMS RELATED TO THE CARDIOVASCULAR SYSTEM—*Cont.*

TERM	MEANING	PRONUNCIATION
Holter monitor	a small, portable ECG monitor, about the size of a transistor radio, that assesses heart and pulse activity as a person engages in daily activity. This test is used for people who experience chest pain and palpitations only during exertion or while performing daily activities	
lipoproteins	conjugated proteins in which lipids form part of the molecule. They are classified into three groups: HDL (high-density lipoproteins), LDL (low-density lipoproteins), and VLDL (very-low-density lipoproteins). Their concentrations and proportions provide information on cardiovascular abnormalities, hypertension, atherosclerosis, and coronary artery disease	lĭp - ō - PRŌ - tēn
mitral stenosis	narrowing of the bicuspid valve, obstructing the flow of blood from atrium to ventricle, usually due to rheumatic heart disease	MĪ - trăl/stě - NŌ - sĭs
mitral valve prolapse (MVP)	a common and occasionally serious condition in which the cusp or cusps of the mitral valve prolapse into the left atrium during systole. In some patients, it causes non-anginal chest pain, palpitations, dyspnea, and fatigue	
murmur, bruit	a soft blowing sound heard on auscultation; may result from vibrations associated with the movement of blood and/or valvular action	MŬR - mŭr brwē or broot
pacemaker (artificial)	an electrical device that controls the beating of the heart by a rhythmic series of electrical discharges	
patent ductus arteriosus	abnormal persistence of an open lumen in the ductus arteriosus after birth. This small vessel connects the pulmonary artery to the aorta, causing the fetal blood to bypass the lungs	PĀ - tĕnt/DŬK - tŭs ăr - tē - rē - Ō - sŭs

Continued on following page

OTHER TERMS RELATED TO THE CARDIOVASCULAR SYSTEM—*Cont.*   **159**

TERM	MEANING	PRONUNCIATION
shunt	a passage between two blood vessels or between two sides of the heart	shŭnt
tetralogy of Fallot	a congenital cardiac anomaly consisting of four defects: narrowing of the pulmonary arteries, septal defects of the ventricles, malposition of the aorta causing it to receive blood from both right and left ventricles, and hypertrophy of the right ventricle	tĕ - TRĂL - ō - jē/făl - Ō

SPECIAL PROCEDURES RELATED TO THE CARDIOVASCULAR SYSTEM

RADIOGRAPHIC AND CLINICAL PROCEDURES

TERM	DESCRIPTION
cardiac catheterization, cardiac angiography, coronary arteriography, angiocardiography	helps the physician assess the heart, major coronary vessels, valves, and septum. Although the types of catheterization vary considerably, the usual technique involves the introduction of a cardiac catheter into the right side of the heart through an arm vein or leg vein. The catheter is advanced through the vena cava, right atrium, right ventricle, and pulmonary artery. On the left side, the catheter is introduced through an artery of the arm or leg. It is advanced through the ascending aorta, left ventricle, and sometimes to the left atrium. Through the catheters, pressures are recorded, radiopaque dye is injected for angiography, and cardiac output is determined
Doppler ultrasonography	assesses the velocity of blood flow through a vessel. Ultrahigh-frequency sound waves are transmitted through the skin to a vein or artery. These waves are reflected off of moving RBCs, determining the speed of blood through the vessels. This test is used to detect deep vein thromboses (DVTs), peripheral arterial aneurysms, and carotid arterial occlusive diseases. Doppler ultrasonography is an alternative to arteriography and venography
echocardiography	uses ultrasound to provide a method for assessing the structures of the heart. A small transducer is directed at different areas of the heart, and the high-frequency sound waves that are emitted are deflected from the structures of the heart, producing "echoes." These are viewed as lines and spaces on an oscilloscope, providing a representation of the heart and its structures. The test is noninvasive, and no particular preparation is required. Echocardiography can detect abnormal pericardial fluid, valvular disorders, aneurysms, tumors, chamber size, and blood output

Continued on following page

RADIOGRAPHIC AND CLINICAL PROCEDURES—*Continued*

TERM	DESCRIPTION
electrocardiography (ECG)	a graphic representation of the electrical impulses generated by the conduction system of the heart during the cardiac cycle. These impulses generate weak electrical currents that can be detected on the surface of the body by electrodes and can be recorded by an instrument called an electrocardiograph and recorded on graph paper known as "rhythm strips." The ECG is used mainly to diagnose coronary artery disease, myocardial infarction, abnormal rhythms, electrolyte imbalance, pericardial effusions, and pericarditis
impedance plethysmography (IPG)	graphic recording of changes in electrical resistance (impedance) caused by variations in blood volume. Electrodes are placed on the surface of the skin, and voltage changes are recorded. These changes correspond to the blood volume changes when deep vein thromboses are present. This test is used to diagnose and monitor deep vein thromboses
phonocardiography	provides a graphic display of the heart sounds during the cardiac cycle. It is used to identify, time, and differentiate heart sounds and murmurs. A specialized microphone is placed over the heart to detect sound, which is electronically amplified and graphically recorded on a monitor. An ECG is simultaneously recorded on the monitor to provide a reference point for each of the sounds and their duration. In this procedure, abnormal acoustic events can be permanently recorded in order to evaluate treatment
stress/exercise testing	measures the efficiency of the heart during a period when it is subjected to predetermined exercise (treadmill or bicycle). Recording electrodes (ECG) are placed on the patient's chest and attached to a monitor. Exercise is initiated. At different times during the test, the ECG, heart rate, and blood pressure are recorded. The test is clinically significant when the ECG is abnormal, extreme fatigue or weakness occurs, or abnormal blood pressure changes are noted. If the patient experiences chest pains or arrhythmias, the test is discontinued
phlebography, venography	a radiograph of the veins to identify and locate thrombi in the venous system of the lower extremities. A radiopaque dye or contrast medium is injected into the venous system of the affected extremity, and a radiograph is taken. Incomplete filling of the vein indicates obstruction

SURGICAL PROCEDURES

TERM	DESCRIPTION	PRONUNCIATION
aneurysmectomy	removal of an aneurysm	ăn - ū - rĭz - MĔK - tō - mē

Continued on following page

SURGICAL PROCEDURES—*Continued*

TERM	DESCRIPTION	PRONUNCIATION
arterial anastomosis	end-to-end union of two different arteries or two separate segments of the same artery	ăr - tē - rē - ăl ăn - năs - tō - MŌ - sĭs
atriotomy	incision of the atrium	ā - trē - ŎT - ō - mē
cardiolysis	freeing pericardial adhesions to surrounding tissues, involving resection of ribs and sternum	kăr - dē - ŎL - ĭ - sĭs
cardioplasty	surgical repair of the heart to relieve spasm	kăr - dē - ō - PLĂS - tē
cardiorrhaphy	suture of the heart	kăr - dē - OR - ă - fē
cardiotomy	incision of the heart	kăr - dē - ŎT - ō - mē
ligation and stripping	tying off of a varicose vein followed by removal of the affected segment	lī - GĀ - shŭn
pericardiectomy	excision of a portion of the pericardium	pĕr - ĭ - kăr - dē - ĔK - tō - mē
phleborrhaphy, venorrhaphy	suturing of a vein	flĕb - OR - ă - fē vĕn - OR - ă - fē
phlebotomy, venesection, venipuncture	opening or piercing of a vein for removal of blood, or for the introduction of fluids or medications	flĕ - BŎT - ō - mē vĕn - ĕ - SĔK - shŭn
thrombectomy	removal of a thrombus	thrŏm - BĔK - tō - mē
valvotomy, mitral commissurotomy	surgical incision of a mitral valve to increase the size of the orifice; used in treating mitral stenosis	văl - VŎT - ō - mē MĪ - trăl kŏm - ĭ - shūr - ŎT - ō - mē
venotomy	surgical incision of a vein	vē - NŎT - ō - mē

LABORATORY PROCEDURES

TERM	DESCRIPTION
arterial biopsy	carried out to examine a specimen of an arterial vessel wall. Most frequently the temporal artery is selected, but other arteries may be biopsied as indicated. Arterial biopsy most often confirms inflammation of the vessel wall, or arteritis, a type of vasculitis. It is performed under local anesthesia in the operating room
cardiac enzyme studies	heart muscle tissue contains three important enzymes: creatine phosphokinase (CPK), also called creatine kinase (CK), glutamic

Continued on following page

162 LABORATORY PROCEDURES—Continued

TERM	DESCRIPTION
	oxaloacetic transaminase (GOT), also called aspartate transaminase (AST), and lactic dehydrogenase (LDH). When heart muscle is damaged or destroyed, these three enzymes are released into the blood. Each enzyme rises, peaks, and declines at predictable times following myocardial infarction. Blood serum studies that assess their levels, along with a clinical evaluation and an ECG, help in establishing a diagnosis and the extent of myocardial infarction
diagnostic pericardiocentesis	the pericardium is surgically punctured in order to remove a small sample of the pericardial fluid for laboratory examination. This test is performed while the patient is in a semisitting position and under constant ECG monitoring. The fluid removed is tested for protein, sugar, and LDH. Most often this procedure is used to determine the cause of pericarditis (bacterial, fungal, tubercular, or viral), or to confirm suspected carcinomatous infiltration of the pericardium

PHARMACOLOGY RELATED TO THE CARDIOVASCULAR SYSTEM

MEDICATION	ACTION
antihypertensives	reduce blood pressure
diuretics	reduce body fluid volume by stimulating the flow of urine. These drugs are considered the first-line, also called "step one," drugs in the management of hypertension
beta-adrenergic blocking agents (systemic), "beta blockers"	block the activity of epinephrine and norepinephrine, causing dilation of blood vessels and decreased heart rate and cardiac output, thereby reducing the workload on the heart
calcium channel blockers	a group of drugs that act by slowing the influx of calcium ions into muscle cells. This results in decreased arterial resistance and decreased myocardial oxygen demand. These drugs must be carefully monitored because they can cause hypotension. Because of this ability, these drugs are also used in the treatment of hypertension
inotropics (cardiotonics)	drugs that affect the force of muscular contraction of the heart. Positive inotropics increase contractility, while negative inotropics decrease contractility. These drugs are used to treat cardiac arrhythmias and cardiac failure
vasodilators	expand blood vessels. These medications are used in the treatment of angina and hypertension
antianginals	medications used to relieve angina pectoris by expanding the

Continued on following page

PHARMACOLOGY RELATED TO THE CARDIOVASCULAR SYSTEM—*Cont.*

MEDICATION	ACTION
	blood vessels of the heart. The most common drug in this category is nitroglycerin
peripheral vasodilators	these drugs expand the blood vessels in the extremities, thereby decreasing blood pressure. In addition, these drugs are used to treat poor peripheral circulation, thereby reducing pain due to atherosclerosis, and in the treatment of Raynaud's phenomenon

ABBREVIATIONS RELATED TO THE CARDIOVASCULAR SYSTEM

ABBREVIATION	MEANING
ACG	angiocardiography
AS	aortic stenosis
ASD	atrial septal defect
ASHD	arteriosclerotic heart disease
BBB	bundle-branch block
BP	blood pressure
CAD	coronary artery disease
CC	cardiac catheterization
CCU	coronary care unit
CHF	congestive heart failure
CPR	cardiopulmonary resuscitation
CV	cardiovascular
DVT	deep vein thrombosis
ECG, EKG	electrocardiogram
HDL	high-density lipoprotein
ICU	intensive care unit
LDL	low-density lipoprotein
MI	myocardial infarction
MS	mitral stenosis
MVP	mitral valve prolapse
OHS	open heart surgery
PAT	paroxysmal atrial tachycardia
PVC	premature ventricular contraction
S-A	sinoatrial (node)
VSD	ventricular septal defect

WORKSHEET 1

A. Using the word root/combining form ather/o (fatty plaque), build medical words to mean:

1. _____ a tumor of fatty plaque

2. _____ formation of fatty plaque

3. _____ condition of hardening associated with fatty plaque

B. Using the word root/combining form phleb/o (vein), build medical words to mean:

1. _____ inflammation of a vein

2. _____ hardening of a vein (wall)

3. _____ dilation of a vein

4. _____ stone in a vein

5. _____ veinlike

6. _____ rupture of a vein

7. _____ condition of clotting in a vein

C. Using the word root/combining form ven/o (vein), build medical words to mean:

1. _____ hardening of a vein

2. _____ spasm of a vein

3. _____ pertaining to a vein

4. _____ narrowing of a vein

D. Using the word root/combining form cardi/o (heart), build medical words to mean:

1. _____ enlargement of the heart

2. _____ inflammation of the inner heart

3. _____ inflammation of the epicardium

4. _____ pertaining to the heart and lung

5. _____ pertaining to the vessels of the heart

6. _____ inflammation of the heart muscle

7. _____ disease of the heart muscle

E. Using the word root/combining form arteri/o (artery), build medical words to mean:

1. _____ hardening of the artery

2. _____ spasm of an artery

3. _____ rupture of an artery

4. _____ pertaining to an artery

166   WORKSHEET 2

Fill in the correct word from the right hand column that matches the definitions in the statements below.

1. _____ lower heart chambers   Aorta

2. _____ pacemaker   Arteries

3. _____ smallest blood vessels   Atria

4. _____ top layer of heart tissue   Capillaries

5. _____ blood vessels with valves   Epicardium

6. _____ sac enclosing the heart   Pericardium

7. _____ upper heart chambers   Septum

8. _____ largest artery of the body   S-A node

9. _____ blood vessels with thick muscular   Veins
                             walls

10. _____ muscular wall dividing the right and   Ventricles
                              left sides of the heart

WORKSHEET 3

Build surgical terms for the following:

1. _____ incision of the heart

2. _____ surgical puncture of the heart

3. _____ fixation of vein (in varicocele)

4. _____ suturing of an artery

5. _____ (partial) excision of the pericardium

6. _____ incision of a vein

7. _____ surgical repair of an artery

8. _____ removal of an aneurysm

9. _____ removal of an embolus

10. _____ surgical puncture of a vein

168   WORKSHEET 4

Define the following diagnostic and symptomatic terms. Use the dictionary as a reference.

1. necrosis _____

2. ischemia _____

3. hypertension _____

4. fibrillation _____

5. phlebogram _____

6. arrhythmia _____

7. aortostenosis _____

8. electrocardiogram _____

9. aortography _____

10. vasoconstriction _____

11. hemangiomatosis _____

12. tachycardia _____

WORKSHEET 5

Special Procedures, Pharmacology, and Abbreviations

Choose the word(s) that best describes the following statements:

antianginals   impedance plethysmography
arterial biopsy   inotropics
beta blockers   MI
calcium channel blockers   MS
cardiac enzyme studies   phlebography
diagnostic pericardiocentesis   phonocardiography
echocardiography   stress/exercise testing
electrocardiography

1. _____ procedure that uses ultrasound to assess the structures of the heart

2. _____ procedure that graphically records the electrical impulses of the heart on a strip of paper

3. _____ surgical puncturing of the pericardium to remove fluid in order to test for protein, sugar, and LDH, or to determine the causative organism of pericarditis

4. _____ mitral stenosis

5. _____ vasodilator that expands the vessels of the heart to relieve chest pain

6. _____ drugs that affect the force of muscular contraction of the heart

7. _____ series of tests that establish a diagnosis and the extent of myocardial infarction by checking the release of cardiac enzymes into the blood

8. _____ radiographic study to identify and locate thrombi in the veins of the legs

9. _____ reduces the workload on the heart by blocking the activity of epinephrine and norepinephrine

10. _____ measures the efficiency of the heart when subjected to a predetermined exercise

11. _____ specialized microphone records and graphically displays the sounds of the heart to assess abnormal acoustic events

12. _____ myocardial infarction

170   WORKSHEET 6

Grammar Review—Cardiovascular System

Provide the plural form for each of the singular words listed below.

1. cardium   cardia

2. atrium   _____

3. aorta   _____

4. hemangioma   _____

5. myocardium   _____

Provide the adjective form for each of the nouns listed below.

6. atheroma   _____

7. artery   _____

8. aorta   _____

9. vein   _____

10. aneurysm   _____

WORKSHEET 7

Label the structures indicated on the diagram, and check your answers with Figure 8-3.

Aorta

Inferior vena cava

Right ventricle

Left pulmonary artery

Left atrium

Left pulmonary veins

Left ventricle

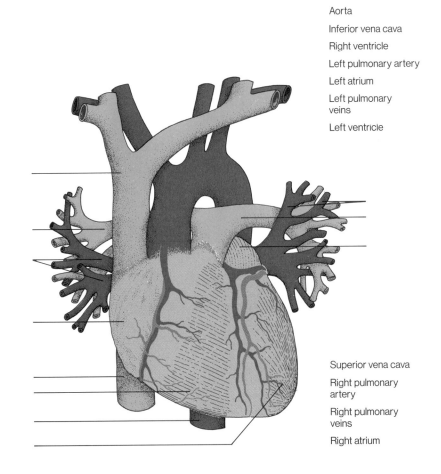

Superior vena cava

Right pulmonary artery

Right pulmonary veins

Right atrium

C H A P T E R   9

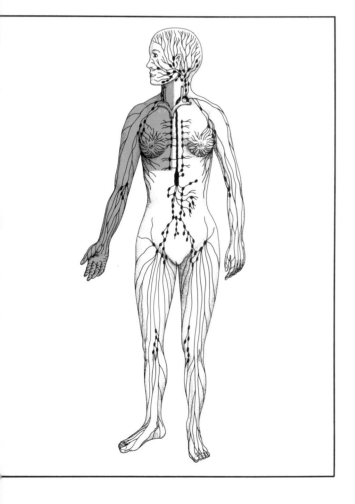

CHAPTER OUTLINE

Hematic and Lymphatic Systems

STUDENT OBJECTIVES

Upon completion of this chapter, you will be able to do the following:

Describe the appearance and function of each of the blood cells.

List the components of blood plasma, and briefly explain the function plasma serves.

Describe the functions of the lymphatic system, and explain the relationship that exists between plasma and lymph.

Briefly describe how protection is provided by each of the five types of white blood cells.

List the major blood groups, and explain compatibility/incompatibility.

Identify the word roots/combining forms and suffixes associated with the hematic and lymphatic systems.

Identify and discuss associated pathology related to the hematic and lymphatic systems.

Identify surgical and laboratory procedures and abbreviations related to the hematic and lymphatic systems.

Explain the pharmacology related to the treatment of disorders of the hematic and lymphatic systems.

Build and analyze diagnostic, symptomatic, and surgical terms related to the blood and lymph by completing the worksheets.

174 ANATOMY AND PHYSIOLOGY OF THE HEMATIC AND LYMPHATIC SYSTEMS

Blood and lymph are specialized tissues of the body (Fig. 9-1). Each is composed of cells that are suspended in a liquid medium. Both of these tissues play a vital role in defending the body against infection. Since blood and lymph have the ability to move throughout the entire body, they provide a transportation system for body cells. They transport nourishment, water, vitamins, electrolytes (sodium, potassium, and calcium), immune substances, heat, and oxygen to all parts of the body. Conveyance of waste products to appropriate body organs for removal, and distribution of hormones from the endocrine glands to numerous organs are some of the other vital functions performed by blood and lymph.

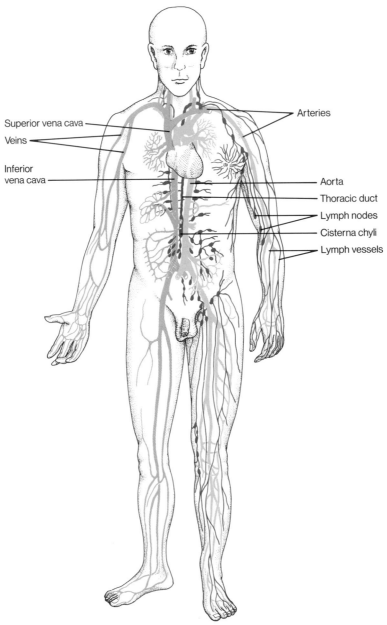

Figure 9-1. Diagram of veins, arteries, and lymph vessels.

Blood

Blood is composed of a liquid medium called plasma and a solid portion that consists of three major blood cells: red blood cells (erythrocytes), white blood cells (leukocytes), and platelets (thrombocytes). All blood cells develop from an undifferentiated cell, the hemocytoblast, also called stem cell (Fig. 9-2). The maturation of the different blood cells is called hematopoiesis. The immature forms are found in the bone marrow; the mature forms circulate in the peripheral blood. The composition of whole blood is represented by the following diagram:

Whole blood = Liquid portion + Solid portion

Plasma + Erythrocytes
Leukocytes
Thrombocytes (Platelets)

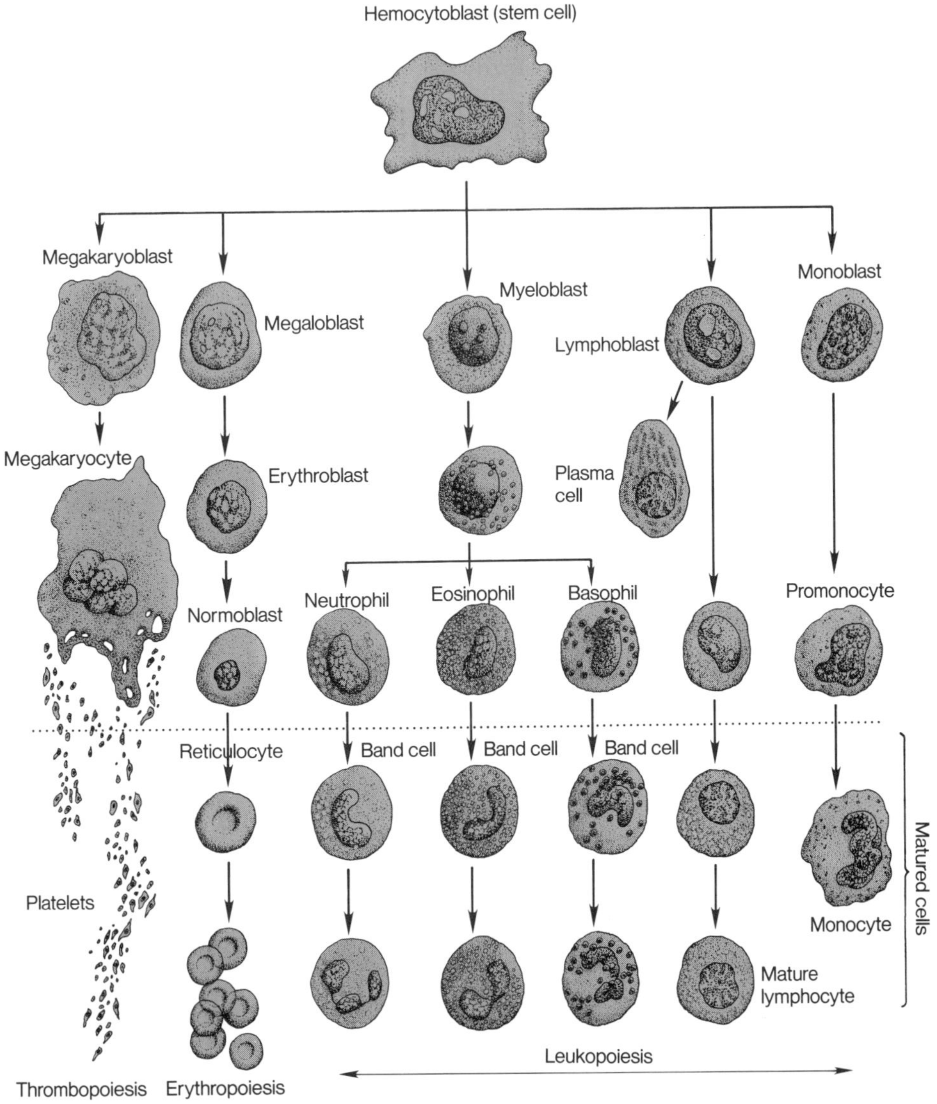

Figure 9-2. The maturation of blood cells—hematopoiesis.

Plasma accounts for about 55 percent and blood cells account for about 45 percent of the total blood volume.

ERYTHROCYTES

Erythrocytes are the most numerous of the circulating blood cells. They are formed in the red bone marrow (myeloid tissue) of the spongy bones of the skull, ribs, sternum, vertebrae, pelvis, and at the ends of the long bones of the arms and legs. Red blood cell development is called erythropoiesis.

During erythropoiesis, red cells develop a specialized compound called hemoglobin, which is an iron-containing pigment that gives the erythrocyte its red color. Hemoglobin carries oxygen (O_2) to body tissues, where it is exchanged for carbon dioxide (CO_2). (The fact that there are millions of hemoglobin molecules in each of the trillions of red blood cells can help you to appreciate the magnitude of the job that is accomplished by erythrocytes.) The size of the red cell and its nucleus decreases during erythropoiesis. Just prior to maturity, the nucleus is extruded from the cell, leaving behind a small vestige of nuclear material (DNA). This DNA resembles a fine, lacy net, giving this cell its name, reticulocyte. Eventually, the DNA disappears and the now mature erythrocyte enters the circulatory system.

The mature erythrocyte appears as a smooth, biconcave structure with the cytoplasm filled with hemoglobin. It is thin in the center where the nucleus was extruded, while the periphery of the cell is thicker.

Erythrocytes live about 120 days and then rupture, releasing hemoglobin and cell fragments. The hemoglobin breaks down into hemosiderin, a compound that contains iron, and several bile pigments. Most of the hemosiderin returns to the bone marrow and is re-used to manufacture new blood cells. The bile pigments are eventually excreted by the liver.

LEUKOCYTES

The chief function of the leukocytes is protection of the body against invasion by bacteria and other foreign substances. Their amoebic nature permits them to leave the blood stream in order to search for and destroy harmful substances. Leukocytes also play a role in tissue repair, but this activity is still not fully understood.

Leukocytes are classified into two categories: the granulocytes (those with granules in the cytoplasm) and the agranulocytes (those without granules). Each of these categories can be further subdivided, as shown in Table 9-1.

Granulocytes

Granulocytes are formed in the red bone marrow from stem cells, which give rise to myeloblasts. Myeloblasts differentiate into neutrophils, eosinophils, and basophils, as was illustrated in Figure 9-2. These names are derived from a polychromatic dye used to stain blood smears in the laboratory. The dye imparts specific colors to the granules of each of these cell types: eosinophils take up the acid dye eosin; basophils stain with a basic, or alkaline, dye; and neutrophils stain with both the acid and basic dyes and hence are "neutral" in their staining preference. In addition to the presence of granules, these cells are further characterized by a nucleus that is composed of several lobes in their mature form; hence these cells are also called polymorphonuclear cells.

Table 9-1.   LEUKOCYTE CLASSIFICATION

GRANULOCYTES	AGRANULOCYTES
neutrophils	monocytes
eosinophils	lymphocytes
basophils	

The neutrophil is the most numerous of the circulating white cells. It is very motile and highly phagocytic, permitting it to ingest and devour bacteria and other particulate matter. In some infections, it is not uncommon to find that one neutrophil has ingested as many as 20 bacteria.

The eosinophils and basophils, although capable of phagocytosis, rarely display this activity. Eosinophils protect the body by releasing many substances that are capable of detoxifying foreign protein and other material, especially of a chemical nature. They also are capable of destroying antigen/antibody complexes. Their number usually increases during allergic reactions.

Basophils release histamines and heparin in the area of damaged tissue. Histamines initiate the inflammation reaction, which increases blood flow. Therefore, additional neutrophils for phagocytosis are brought to the damaged area.

Agranulocytes

Agranulocytes include both monocytes and lymphocytes. These cells are characterized by the absence of granules in their cytoplasm. In addition, they both have a single large nucleus and are therefore called mononuclear cells. Agranulocytes develop from reticuloendothelial cells, the same cells that give rise to both erythrocytes and granulocytes (see Fig. 9-2). However, in early development, monocytes and lymphocytes migrate from the bone marrow and enter the lymphatic system, where they undergo change and maturation. Some of these changes still are not fully understood.

Monocytes provide protection for the body in much the same manner as neutrophils, that is, they engage in phagocytosis. Monocytes migrate into tissue to become macrophages. In this form, they are able to consume large numbers of bacteria or other invaders. They can phagocytize as many as 40 or 50 bacteria before they die.

Lymphocytes, on the other hand, provide protection through immunologic activity. An immune response is the body's ability to distinguish foreign material as harmful and invasive, and then neutralize, eliminate, or metabolize it, thereby rendering it harmless. The harmful invader is called the **antigen**; the defense provided by the body is called the **antibody**.

The immunologic response can be divided into two categories: humoral immunity and cellular immunity.

Humoral immunity is provided by a specialized type of lymphocytes called B-cells or B-lymphocytes. Humoral immunity involves the production of a substance called an antibody, which seeks out and renders harmless the invading substance called an antigen. As a general rule, the antigen-antibody reaction is specific, that is, the antibody reacts only with the antigen that induces its formation. For example, if the body has developed antipolio antibodies in response to the presence of polio antigens (a situation that occurs after the

Table 9–2.   PROTECTION PROVIDED BY LEUKOCYTES

GRANULOCYTES	AGRANULOCYTES
neutrophils (phagocytic)	monocytes (phagocytic)
eosinophils (detoxification)	lymphocytes (immunologic)
basophils (release of substances that increase circulation)	B-cells (humoral immunity) T-cells (cellular immunity)

administration of polio vaccine), these antipolio antibodies provide no protection against any other antigen except polio. In order to produce antibodies, certain B-cells are activated in the presence of an antigen to become plasma cells. Plasma cells synthesize and export antibodies. Some activated B-cells do not develop into plasma cells but remain as "memory cells." These cells stay in the lymphoid tissue. In the event of a future encounter by the same antigen, the memory cells immediately produce the plasma cells that are capable of manufacturing a specific antibody. It is believed that each plasma cell can manufacture specific antibodies at a rate of 2000 per second for about 4 or 5 days.

The other type of protection provided by lymphocytes is **cellular immunity**. This immunity is a function of T-lymphocytes, also called T-cells. T-cells mature in the thymus gland, hence the designation T-cells. When they encounter an antigen, T-cells become sensitized and change into "killer cells." They produce a lymphotoxin or cytotoxin that damages or ruptures the cell membranes of the antigen. T-cells also aid in the production of interferon, a protein released from cells that have been invaded by a virus or other antigen. Interferon induces noninfected cells to form an antiviral protein that inhibits viral multiplication within the cell. Table 9-2 summarizes the five types of leukocytes and their corresponding modes of protection.

THROMBOCYTES

The smallest formed elements within the blood are thrombocytes, or platelets. They are known as platelets because of their small platelike appearance. Their chief function is to initiate blood clotting when injury occurs.

Blood clotting is not a single reaction, but rather a chain of interlinked reactions. At least 13 separate steps are involved, but this complex reaction can be described as essentially three major reactions.

Thromboplastin is either released by traumatized tissue at the site of injury or formed when platelets rupture. The action of thromboplastin causes prothrombin, a blood protein, to convert to thrombin. Eventually, thrombin converts a soluble blood protein, fibrinogen, to fibrin, an insoluble protein. Fibrin forms a meshwork in which blood cells become entangled. This jellylike mass of protein and blood cells is a blood clot.

The following reaction, simplified below, shows the formation of a clot.

$$\text{Prothrombin} \xrightarrow{\text{Thromboplastin}} \text{Thrombin}$$

$$\text{Fibrinogen (soluble)} \xrightarrow{\text{Thrombin}} \text{Fibrin (insoluble)}$$

PLASMA

Plasma is the liquid portion of the blood in which the corpuscles are suspended. It is composed of about 92 percent water and contains the plasma proteins (albumins, globulins, and fibrinogen), gases, nutrients, salts, hormones, and excretory products. Plasma makes possible the chemical communication between all body cells by carrying these products to different parts of the body. When free of corpuscles, plasma is thin and colorless or has a faint yellow tinge.

Blood serum is a product of blood plasma. It differs from plasma in that serum does not contain fibrinogen. This can be represented as follows:

Plasma — Fibrinogen = Serum

When a blood sample is placed in a test tube and permitted to clot, the resulting clear fluid that remains after the removal of the clot from the test tube is serum. The formation of the clot has removed fibrinogen from the plasma.

BLOOD GROUPS

Human blood is divided into four groups based on the presence or absence of blood antigens on the surface of the red blood cells. These four groups are A, B, AB, and O. Type A blood has A antigen; type B blood, B antigen; type AB blood, both A and B antigens; and type O has neither A nor B antigens. In each of these four blood groups, the plasma does *not* contain the antibody against the antigen that is present on the red cells. Rather, the plasma contains the opposite antibodies. For example, A blood contains A antigen on the surface of the red cells; therefore its plasma contains B antibodies. B blood contains B antigen on the surface of the red blood cells; therefore its plasma contains A antibodies.

In clinical situations, the mode in which an antibody/antigen interacts provides a more specific way of identifying the antibody/antigen complex. The mode in which this antigen/antibody complex reacts when the clinician serologically identifies blood types is agglutination (clumping); therefore, the antigen may be called an **agglutinogen** and the antibody may be called an **agglutinin**. Hence, type B blood contains B agglutinogens (antigens) on the surface of the red blood cells and A agglutinins (antibodies) in the plasma. Table 9-3 summarizes the four major blood groups.

In addition to the blood groups listed above, there are numerous other antigens that may be present on the red blood cells. One such factor includes the Rh-hr system. This particular factor may be involved in hemolytic diseases of the newborn because of an incompatibility existing between the maternal blood and the fetal blood (refer to Chapter 12).

Although more than 90 blood factors have been identified by hematologists, most of these are not highly antigenic. Consequently, these factors generally do not cause concern in pregnancy or in a clinical situation in which blood is transfused into a patient.

Table 9–3. BLOOD GROUPS

AGGLUTINOGEN ON RBC (ANTIGEN)	AGGLUTININ IN PLASMA (ANTIBODY)
A	B
B	A
AB	none
O	A and B

180   Lymphatic System

The lymphatic system consists of lymph, a network of transporting structures called lymph vessels, lymph nodes, and the spleen, thymus, and tonsils. The primary function of the lymphatic system is to drain fluid from tissue spaces and return it to the blood. Other functions provided by the lymphatic system include transporting materials (nutrients, hormones, and oxygen) to body cells and carrying waste products from body tissues back to the blood stream. It also conveys lipids, or fats, away from the digestive organs. Finally, it aids in the control of infection by providing lymphocytes and monocytes, which are used to defend against infections caused by microorganisms.

Lymph originates from blood plasma. As whole blood circulates through the capillaries, some of the plasma seeps out of these thin-walled vessels. This fluid, now called interstitial, or tissue, fluid, resembles plasma, except it contains less protein.

Interstitial fluid nourishes and cleanses the body tissues through which it circulates. It also collects cellular debris, bacteria, and particulate matter. Eventually, interstitial fluid (plasma) enters into blind-ended vessels called lymph capillaries (Fig. 9-3). Once it enters a capillary

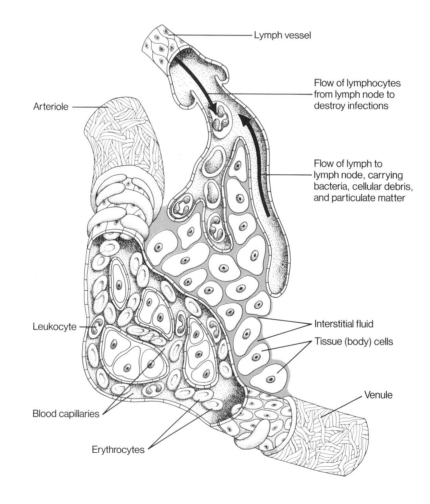

Figure 9–3. As plasma seeps from capillaries into surrounding tissue, it is referred to as interstitial fluid, or tissue fluid. When it finally enters into the blind-ended lymph vessels, it is called lymph.

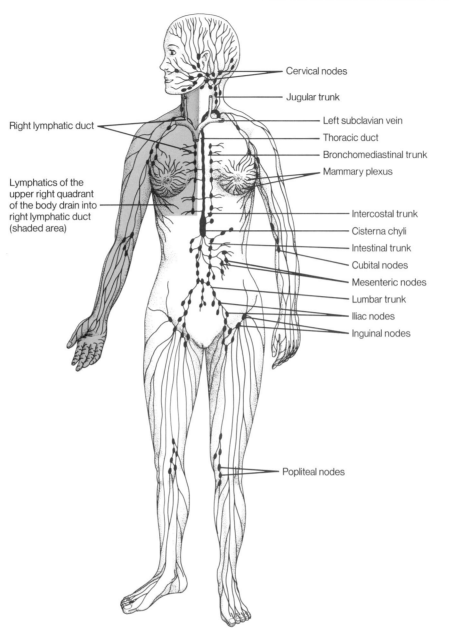

Figure 9-4. Lymphatic system.

it is called lymph. Lymph passes from the capillaries to larger vessels and finally to lymph nodes, which serve as depositories for cellular debris. As lymph passes through the nodes it is filtered and replenished with lymphocytes, globulins, and antibodies. Bacteria and debris are phagocytized by macrophages that line the nodes. At times, the number of bacteria entering a node is so great that the node enlarges and becomes tender.

Lymph vessels from the right chest and arm join the right lymphatic duct. This duct drains into the right subclavian vein, a major vessel in the cardiovascular system (Figs. 9-4 and 9-5). Lymph from all other parts of the body enters the thoracic duct, which drains into

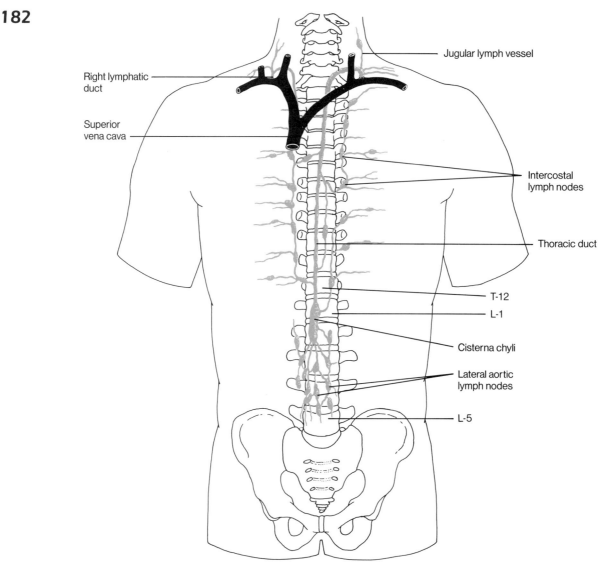

Figure 9–5. Deep lymph nodes.

the left subclavian vein. In this fashion, lymph is redeposited into the circulating blood in order to begin the cycle, once again, throughout the body.

Three organs are associated with the lymphatic system: the spleen, thymus gland, and tonsils. Like the lymph nodes, the spleen acts as a filter for lymph. Phagocytic cells within the lining of the spleen remove cellular debris, bacteria, parasites, and other infectious agents, thereby cleansing the lymph. The spleen also functions in the destruction of old red blood cells and serves as a repository for healthy blood cells, to be put into circulation when needed.

The thymus gland is located in the mediastinum, the upper part of the chest. It partially controls the immune system. The thymus changes lymphocytes to T-cells, which provide cellular immunity.

Three sets of tonsils, the palatine, pharyngeal, and lingual tonsils, contain T and B lymphocytes. They guard against infection at the entrance of the digestive and respiratory tracts.

WORD ROOTS/COMBINING FORMS RELATED TO THE HEMATIC AND LYMPHATIC SYSTEMS

WORD ROOT/ COMBINING FORM	MEANING	EXAMPLE	PRONUNCIATION
aden/o	gland	aden/o/pathy disease	ăd - ĕ - NŎP - ăh - thē
agranul/o	without granules	agranul/o/cyte cell	ă - GRĂN - ū - lō - sīt
bas/o	basic or alkaline	bas/o/phil attraction for	BĀ - sō - fĭl
blast/o	primitive, germ cell, embryonic	erythr/o/blast/osis red abnormal condition of	ĕ - rĭth - rō - blăs - TŌ - sĭs
chrom/o	color	hypo/chrom/ic decrease pertaining to	hī - pō - KRŌM - ĭk
eosin/o	red, rosy, dawn-colored	eosin/o/phil attraction for	ē - ō - SĬN - ō - fĭl
erythrocyt/o	red cell	erythrocyt/o/lysis destroy	ĕ - rĭth - rō - sī - TŎL - ĭ - sĭs
granul/o	granule	granul/o/cyte cell	GRĂN - ū - lō - sīt
hemat/o hem/o	blood	hemat/oma tumor hem/o/stasis standing still	hē - mă - TŌ - mă hē - mō - STĀ - sĭs
heter/o	different	heter/o/phil attraction for	HĔT - ĕr - ō - fĭl
hom/o	same	hom/o/log/ ous study pertain- of ing to	hō - MŎL - ō - gŭs
immun/o	safe, protected	immun/o/log/ ist study one of who special- izes	ĭm - ū - NŎL - ō - jĭst
is/o	equal	is/o/chromat/o/phil color attraction	ī - sō - krō - MĂT - ō - fĭl
kary/o	nucleus	mega/kary/o/cyte large cell	mĕg - ă - KĂR - ē - ō - sīt

Continued on following page

WORD ROOTS/COMBINING FORMS RELATED TO THE HEMATIC AND LYMPHATIC SYSTEMS—*Continued*

WORD ROOT/ COMBINING FORM	MEANING	EXAMPLE	PRONUNCIATION
leukocyt/o	white cell	leukocyt/osis abnormal increase	loo - kō - sǐ - TŌ - sǐs
lymph/o	lymph, lymph tissue	lymph/oma tumor	lǐm - FŌ - măh
mon/o	one	mon/o/cyte cell	MŎN - ō - sīt
morph/o	shape	morph/o/logy study	mŏr - FŎL - ō - jē
myel/o	bone marrow, spinal cord	myel/oid resemble	MĪ - ě - loid
neutr/o	neutral dye	neutr/o/phil attraction for	NŪ - trō - fǐl
phag/o	swallow, eat	phag/o/cyte cell	FĂG - ō - sīt
poikil/o	varied, irregular	poikil/o/cyte cell	POI - kǐl - ō - sīt
reticul/o	net, mesh (immature RBC)	reticul/o/cyte cell	rě - TǏK - ū - lō - sīt
sider/o	iron	hem/o/sider/osis blood abnormal increase	hē - mō - sǐd - ěr - Ō - sǐs
spher/o	globe, round	spher/o/cyt/ osis cell abnormal increase	sfē - rō - sǐ - TŌ - sǐs
splen/o	spleen	splen/o/megaly enlargement	splē - nō - MĚG - ăh - lē
thromb/o	clot	thromb/o/lysis destroy	thrŏm - BŎL - ǐ - sǐs
thrombocyt/o	platelet, thrombocyte	thrombocyt/o/penia decrease	thrŏm - bō - sǐ - tō - PĒ - nē - ăh
thym/o	thymus	thym/ectomy excision	thǐ - MĚK - tō - mē

SUFFIX	MEANING	EXAMPLE	PRONUNCIATION
-blast	embryonic, germ cell, primitive	myel/o/blast bone marrow	MĪ - ĕl - ō - blăst
-globin	protein	hem/o/globin blood	hē - mō - GLŌ - bĭn
-osis	abnormal condition, increase (used primarily with blood cells)	erythrocyt/osis red cell	ĕ - rĭth - rō - sī - TŌ - sĭs
-penia	decrease	leuk/o/penia white (cell)	loo - kō - PĒ - nē - ăh
-phil	to love, attraction for	hem/o/phil/ia blood noun ending	hē - mō - FĬL - ē - ăh
-phoresis	borne, carried	electr/o/phoresis electricity	ē - lĕk - trō - fō - RĒ - sĭs
-poiesis	formation, production	hem/o/poiesis blood	hē - mō - poi - Ē - sĭs
-stasis	standing still	hem/o/stasis blood	hē - mō - STĀ - sĭs

PATHOLOGY OF THE HEMATIC AND LYMPHATIC SYSTEMS

Anemias

Anemia results when there is a reduction in the number of circulating red blood cells (RBCs), a decrease in the amount of hemoglobin, or a decrease in the volume of packed erythrocytes **(hematocrit)**. Anemias may be identified according to the shape and form **(morphology)** of the erythrocytes in the affected individual. Normally, RBCs have a specific size **(normocytic)** and contain a specific quantity of hemoglobin **(normochromic)**. Many anemias cause these values to vary. The associated signs and symptoms of anemia include difficulty in breathing **(dyspnea)**, muscular weakness, and a rapid heart beat **(tachycardia)**. The patient shows paleness **(pallor)**, has low blood pressure **(hypotension)**, and often has a slight fever.

Pernicious anemia (PA) gives rise to RBCs that are larger than normal **(macrocytic)** and contain excessive amounts of hemoglobin **(hyperchromic)**, but the absolute number of RBCs is decreased **(erythropenia)**, These cells do not mature properly, are often nucleated, and function poorly in the circulatory system. In PA there is a deficiency of vitamin B_{12} (folic acid). Although the normal diet generally contains sufficient amounts of B_{12}, it cannot be absorbed by certain individuals because they lack a substance known as intrinsic factor.

This factor is required for intestinal absorption of vitamin B$_{12}$. Treatment consists of injections of B$_{12}$.

Hemorrhagic anemia results from any excessive bleeding (e.g., large wounds, stomach ulcers, or heavy menstrual flow). There is marked erythropenia, but the cells are normochromic normocytic.

Another type of normochromic normocytic anemia is hemolytic anemia. This anemia results when red blood cells rupture within the body. Causes include hemoglobin abnormalities **(hemoglobinopathies)**, abnormal red cell enzymes, or defective red cell membranes. In addition, toxins, parasites, or blood incompatibilities from transfusions or erythroblastosis fetalis may also cause hemolytic anemia.

An anemia that produces RBCs that are very small in size **(microcytic)** and lacking in hemoglobin **(hypochromic)** is iron deficiency anemia. Iron deficiency anemia occurs when the body lacks iron, a vital mineral component for the production of hemoglobin. This may be caused by inadequate iron intake, faulty absorption, defective storage in the liver, continuous loss of blood, or an excessive demand for iron by the body.

Aplastic anemia results when there is a destruction or inhibition of red bone marrow. Included in the causes of bone marrow failure are the presence of toxins, radiation, tumor cells, and the use of some medications. Aplastic anemia generally leads to a decrease in white blood cells **(leukopenia)** and platelets **(thrombocytopenia)**.

Two important inherited anemias are sickle-cell anemia and thalassemia. In both of these genetic disorders, the cause of anemia is due to hemoglobinopathy. In sickle-cell anemia, a decrease in oxygen causes the red cell to form a stiff rod, or sickle. This cell ruptures easily or, in many instances, blocks the capillaries, causing tissue ischemia. Sickle-cell anemia is found almost exclusively in the black race. In thalassemia (Cooley's anemia), the symptoms include hemolysis, with resulting jaundice, hypochromic, microcytic RBCs, and enlargement of the liver and spleen **(hepatosplenomegaly)**. Thalassemia is found most commonly in the people who either live near the Mediterranean Sea or have their origin from that area of the world.

Acquired Immune Deficiency Syndrome (AIDS)

Acquired immune deficiency syndrome is a transmissible infection caused by human T-cell leukemia virus type III (HTLV-III). It was first identified in 1981 in homosexual men. Since that time, it has been found throughout the world. In the United States, homosexuals, bisexuals, and intravenous drug users are in the highest risk group. It is believed that the disease is transmitted primarily through the exchange of body fluids, mostly semen and blood. This implicates sexual intercourse (anal) and blood transfusions as common routes of infection.

Since the disease ultimately destroys the cellular immune system, opportunistic infections (infections that result when normally non-pathogenic organisms are able to cause infection) become established in the patient. Kaposi's sarcoma, a neoplastic disorder, is also found in many patients afflicted with AIDS.

Associated with AIDS is a condition called AIDS-related complex (ARC). This syndrome is characterized by unexplained lymphadenopathy, fatigue, fever, night sweats, and weight loss. These symptoms parallel those experienced by AIDS patients. ARC is believed to be a milder form of AIDS or a prodrome to the development of Kaposi's sarcoma or opportunistic infections.

Research into the treatment of AIDS or the production of a vaccine is currently being undertaken by the federal government, but effective treatment is not anticipated until the 1990s.

Autoimmune Diseases

Failure of the body to accurately distinguish between what is "self" and what is "non-self" leads to a phenomenon called autoimmunity. In this abnormal immunological response, the body produces antibodies against itself to such an extent that it causes tissue injury. Certain diseases, such as hemolytic anemia, some forms of myasthenia gravis, rheumatoid arthritis, idiopathic thrombocytopenic purpura (ITP), and systemic lupus erythematosus, are believed to be a result of autoimmunity. Treatment consists of attempting to reach a balance between the suppressing of the autoimmune response in order to avoid tissue damage while at the same time maintaining the immune mechanism to protect against foreign invaders.

Edema

Edema is an abnormal accumulation of fluids in the intercellular spaces of the body. One of the major causes of edema is a condition in which there is a decrease in the blood protein level **(hypoproteinemia)**. This lowers the osmotic pressure within the blood. Consequently, abnormally large amounts of fluid and lymph pass out of the blood plasma and into the surrounding tissues. Other causes of edema include poor lymph drainage, increased capillary permeability, and congestive heart failure.

Edema limited to a specific area **(local edema)** may be relieved by the elevation of that body part and the application of cold packs. Generalized edema **(systemic edema)** may be treated with medications that remove tissue fluids through urination **(diuretics)**.

Closely associated with edema is a condition called ascites, in which fluid collects within the peritoneal cavity. The chief causes of ascites are interference in venous return during cardiac disease, obstruction of lymphatic flow, or disturbances in electrolyte balance.

Hemophilia

Classic hemophilia is a hereditary disorder in which there is an impairment of the blood-clotting mechanism. It results from the failure of thrombin formation from prothrombin. The disease is sex-linked and is most often found in men. Women are the carriers of the trait and generally do not have symptoms of the disease. In hemophilia, there is a lack of an essential blood clotting factor, Factor VIII **(AHF, or antihemophilic factor)**, within the blood plasma of the individual.

Hodgkin's Disease

Hodgkin's disease is a malignant lymphatic disease that primarily affects the lymph nodes. However, the spleen, gastrointestinal tract, liver, or bone marrow may also be involved.

Hodgkin's disease usually begins with a painless enlargement of lymph nodes, generally on one side of the neck. Other symptoms include itching **(pruritus)**, weight loss, progressive anemia, and fever. If the nodes in the neck become excessively large and start pressing on the trachea or esophagus, the patient may experience difficulty in breathing **(dyspnea)** or difficulty in swallowing **(dysphagia)** or both.

Radiation and chemotherapy are important methods of controlling the disease.

188   Infectious Mononucleosis

One of the acute infections caused by the Epstein-Barr virus (EBV) is infectious mononucleosis. This virus attacks only the B-cells but causes the proliferation of T-cells. The patient experiences a sore throat, fever, and enlarged cervical lymph nodes. Sometimes the patient develops a gum infection **(gingivitis)**, headache, tiredness, loss of appetite **(anorexia)**, and general malaise. Occasionally, the liver and spleen may enlarge **(hepatomegaly** and **splenomegaly)**. Many patients show some liver involvement. Other, less common, clinical findings include hemolytic anemia with jaundice, thrombocytopenia, and occasionally a ruptured spleen **(splenorrhexis)**. Recovery usually ensures a lasting immunity.

Polycythemia

Primary polycythemia occurs as a result of increased development **(hyperplasia)** of bone marrow. In this disorder, there is marked erythrocytosis and thrombocytosis but little or no change in plasma volume, causing the blood to become "thick" and "sticky" **(viscous)**. The blood's ability to flow through vessels decreases, causing hypertension. Erythrocytosis and thrombocytosis lead to the frequent formation of thrombi. Symptoms of this disease include dizziness **(vertigo)**, splenomegaly, and redness of the skin **(erythema)**. There is no permanent cure for polycythemia, but treatment includes the surgical opening of a vein for withdrawal of blood **(venesection, phlebotomy)**.

OTHER TERMS RELATED TO THE HEMATIC AND LYMPHATIC SYSTEMS

TERM	MEANING	PRONUNCIATION
agammaglobulinemia	a rare disease characterized by the absence of gamma globulin from blood plasma with resulting loss of the ability to produce antibodies	ā - găm - ăh - glŏb - ū - lĭ - NĒ - mē - ăh
anisocytosis	a condition in which a marked variation in cell sizes occurs (macrocytic and microcytic cells are present)	ăn - ī - sō - sī - TŌ - sĭs
anticoagulant	an agent that delays or inhibits blood clotting	ăn - tĭ - kō - ĂG - ū - lănt
antiserum, antisera (pl.)	blood serum that contains antibodies (e.g., antiserum A and antiserum B are used to determine ABO blood type)	ăn - tĭ - SĒ - rŭm
dyscrasia	any blood abnormality	dĭs - KRĀ - zē - ăh

Continued on following page

**OTHER TERMS RELATED TO THE HEMATIC AND
LYMPHATIC SYSTEMS**—*Continued*

TERM	MEANING	PRONUNCIATION
graft versus host reaction (GVHR)	pathological reaction between the host and grafted tissue; it occurs when the host immune system identifies the graft as "not self" and produces antibodies to the graft, resulting in tissue rejection	grăft
hematoma	a localized collection of blood, usually clotted, in an organ or within tissue space due to a break in a blood vessel	hē - mă - TŌ - măh
heterophile antibody	an antibody that reacts with other than its specific antigen	HĔT - ĕr - ō - fĭl/ăn - tĭ - BŎD - ē
hydrops, hydropsy, dropsy	edema	HĪ - drŏps hĭ - DRŎP - sē DRŎP - sē
immunoglobulin (Ig)	one of a family of five blood proteins capable of antibody activity. They are produced by plasma cells and include IgA, IgD, IgE, IgG, and IgM	ĭm - ū - nō - GLŎB - ū - lĭn
lymphosarcoma	a malignant neoplastic disorder of lymphatic tissue but not related to Hodgkin's disease	lĭm - fō - săr - KŌ - măh
purpura	hemorrhagic disease characterized by the seepage of blood under skin and mucous membranes; may be caused by thrombocytopenia	PŬR - pū - răh
serology	the study of blood serum, especially antigen-antibody reactions	sē - RŎL - ō - jē

SPECIAL PROCEDURES RELATED TO THE HEMATIC AND LYMPHATIC SYSTEMS

SURGICAL PROCEDURES

TERM	DESCRIPTION	PRONUNCIATION
autologous transfusion	a transfusion prepared from the recipient's own blood	ăw - TŎL - ō - gŭs trăns - FŪ - zhŭn
bone marrow aspiration	use of a surgical aspirating needle to obtain a specimen of bone marrow for examination	bōn/MĂR - ō ăs - pĭ - RĀ - shŭn
homologous transfusion	a transfusion prepared from another individual whose blood is compatible with that of the recipient	hō - MŎL - ō - gŭs trăns - FŪ - zhŭn
lymphadenectomy	excision of a lymph node	lĭm - făd - ĕ - NĔK - tō - mē
lymphoidectomy	excision of lymphoid tissue	lĭm - foi - DĔK - tō - mē
splenectomy	excision of a spleen	splē - NĔK - tō - mē
splenopexy	surgical fixation of a movable spleen	SPLĒ - nō - pĕk - sē

LABORATORY PROCEDURES

TERM	DESCRIPTION
bleeding time	a small stab wound is made in the earlobe or forearm, and the time required for it to stop bleeding is recorded. This test evaluates the vascular and platelet factors associated with hemostasis. Failure of either of these components leads to a prolonged bleeding time. An increase is noted in thrombocytopenia, ingestion of anti-inflammatory drugs, and infiltration of bone marrow by primary or metastatic tumors
complete blood count (CBC)	a routine hematologic test that assesses the cellular components of blood. A CBC consists of five distinct tests that are so closely interrelated that their absolute values can be meaningless unless the whole CBC is taken into consideration. The five tests that constitute a CBC are the red blood count, white blood count, hemoglobin, hematocrit, and the white blood cell differential
red blood count (RBC)	approximates the number of erythrocytes in a cubic millimeter of blood. A decrease in red cells often indicates anemia; an increase may indicate a polycythemia, especially one that results from disorders not associated with the blood-forming organs
white blood count (WBC)	approximates the number of leukocytes in a measured and diluted sample of blood. An increase often is noted when infection

Continued on following page

TERM	DESCRIPTION
	is present. In leukemia, the number of leukocytes is greatly increased. Chemotherapy and x-ray therapy often cause a decrease
hemoglobin (hb, hgb)	the iron-containing pigment that gives red blood cells their color. It functions in transporting oxygen within the body. A low hemoglobin is one of the classic symptoms of anemia
hematocrit (ht, hct, crit)	the volume of packed red blood cells expressed as a percentage of whole blood. A sample of blood in a capillary tube is placed in a centrifuge in order to separate the cellular components from the plasma. The hematocrit, along with the hemoglobin and red blood count, helps in differentiating the many types of anemias
differential	provides the percentage of the five major white blood cells present in the blood. A blood smear is stained with a polychromatic stain and 100 white cells are differentiated according to the five types of leukocytes. The test must be interpreted in relation to the white blood count. The differential values change considerably in pathology, and this test often is the first step in diagnosing a disease
erythrocyte sedimentation rate (ESR)	measures the speed at which red blood cells settle when placed in a narrow tube. The blood is first collected in a tube that contains an anticoagulant. This rate increases in inflammatory diseases, cancer, and pregnancy, and decreases in liver disease
Monospot	detects the presence of a nonspecific antibody called the heterophile antibody. It is present in the serum of patients with infectious mononucleosis. It occurs shortly after the appearance of the symptoms of the disease. When the heterophile antibody is present, it provides presumptive evidence of the disease
prothrombin time (pro-time, PT)	the time required for a clot to form in a test tube containing the patient's plasma after the addition of calcium. Prothrombin is a protein produced in the liver and is required for the clotting process. This test is commonly ordered in conjunction with the management of patients who are undergoing anticoagulant therapy. Delayed prothrombin time is also found in vitamin K deficiency, hemorrhagic disease of the newborn, liver disease, and biliary obstruction. When blood clotting is prolonged, the patient is at risk of hemorrhage

PHARMACOLOGY RELATED TO THE HEMATIC AND LYMPHATIC SYSTEMS

MEDICATION	ACTION
anticoagulants	inhibit or delay the clotting process and are used clinically to prevent clots from forming in blood vessels

Continued on following page

PHARMACOLOGY RELATED TO THE HEMATIC AND
LYMPHATIC SYSTEMS—*Continued*

MEDICATION	ACTION
fibrinolytics	trigger the body to produce plasmin, an enzyme that dissolves clots. Fibrinolytics are used to treat acute pulmonary embolism and, occasionally, deep vein thromboses
hemostatics	used to control excessive bleeding; blood coagulants. If the medication is on a pad that is applied directly to the bleeding area to form a blood clot, it is referred to as an absorbable hemostatic

ABBREVIATIONS RELATED TO THE HEMATIC AND LYMPHATIC SYSTEMS

ABBREVIATION	MEANING
AHF	antihemophilic factor VIII
AHG	antihemophilic globulin factor VIII
baso	basophil
CBC	complete blood count
diff	(white cell) differential
EBV	Epstein-Barr virus
eosin	eosinophil
ESR, SR	erythrocyte sedimentation rate; sedimentation rate
HCT, Hct	hematocrit
HGB, Hgb, Hb	hemoglobin
Ig	immunoglobulin
lymphs	lymphocytes
MCH	mean corpuscular hemoglobin
MCHC	mean corpuscular hemoglobin concentration
MCV	mean corpuscular volume
mono	monocyte
PCV	packed cell volume (hematocrit)
PMN, seg, poly	polymorphonuclear neutrophil
PT	prothrombin time
RBC	red blood cell; red blood count
WBC	white blood cell; white blood count

WORKSHEET 1

A. Using the suffix -phil (attraction), build medical words to mean:

1. _____ attraction to red (eosin dye)

2. _____ attraction to alkaline (basic dye)

3. _____ attraction to neutral (dye)

4. _____ attraction to blood

B. Using the suffix -osis (increase), build medical words to mean:

1. _____ increase in RBC

2. _____ increase in WBC

3. _____ increase in agranulocytes

4. _____ increase in granulocytes

5. _____ increase in thrombocytes

6. _____ increase in lymphocytes in the blood

7. _____ increase in reticulocytes

C. Using the suffix -o/penia (deficiency), build medical words to mean:

1. _____ decrease in red blood cells

2. _____ decrease in white blood cells

3. _____ decrease in platelets

4. _____ decrease in granulocytes

5. _____ decrease in lymphocytes

D. Using the word root/combining form lymphaden/o (lymph gland), build medical words to mean:

1. _____ inflammation of a lymph gland

2. _____ disease of a lymph gland

3. _____ tumor of a lymph gland

E. Using the suffix -o/poiesis (production or formation), build medical words to mean:

1. _____ production of blood

2. _____ production of red cells

3. _____ production of white cells

4. _____ production by bone marrow

5. _____ production of lymph

F. Using the word root/combining form immun/o (protection, safety, immunity), build medical words to mean:

1. _____ one who specializes in immunity

2. _____ the study of immunity

G. Using the word root/combining form splen/o (spleen), build medical words to mean:

1. _____ herniation of the spleen

2. _____ inflammation of the spleen

3. _____ pertaining to the spleen

4. _____ pertaining to the spleen and colon

WORKSHEET 2 **195**

Fill in the correct word from the right column that matches the definitions in the statements below.

1. _____ stringy substance in clots   Antigens

2. _____ soluble plasma protein   Fibrin

3. _____ liquid portion of blood   Fibrinogen

4. _____ liquid portion of blood without fibrino- Macrocyte
gen

5. _____ stimulate the production of antibodies   Microcyte

6. _____ provide cell-mediated immunity   Phagocyte

7. _____ abnormally small red blood cell   Plasma

8. _____ unusually shaped RBC   Poikilocyte

9. _____ very large RBC   Serum

10. _____ neutrophil   T-cells

196   WORKSHEET 3

Build a surgical term for the following:

1. _____ excision of a lymph node

2. _____ incision (for draining) of a lymph node

3. _____ excision of the spleen

4. _____ destruction of splenic tissue

5. _____ incision of the spleen

6. _____ removal of the thymus

7. _____ destruction of the thymus

WORKSHEET 4

Define the following diagnostic or symptomatic words. Consult the dictionary for assistance.

1. splenohepatomegaly _____

2. splenonephric _____

3. splenoptosis _____

4. splenectopia _____

5. splenicterus _____

6. splenoma _____

7. splenalgia _____

8. myelopoiesis _____

9. myeloma _____

10. myelogenic _____

11. thymitis _____

12. aplastic anemia _____

13. hemolytic anemia _____

WORSHEET 5

Special Procedures, Pharmacology, and Abbreviations

Choose the word(s) that best describes the following statements:

anticoagulant
baso
bleeding time
complete blood count
EBV
erythrocyte sedimentation rate
fibrinolytic
hematocrit

hemoglobin determination
hemostatic
Ig
mono
Monospot
PMN, seg, poly
prothrombin time

1. _____ blood coagulant

2. _____ test that assesses the amount of iron-containing pigment in RBCs

3. _____ measures the speed at which RBCs settle when placed in a narrow tube

4. _____ the volume of packed RBCs expressed as a percentage of whole blood

5. _____ immunoglobulin

6. _____ polymorphonuclear neutrophil

7. _____ time required for a clot to form in a test tube; often used in conjunction with management of anticoagulant therapy

8. _____ a nonspecific test for the presence of the heterophile anti-body, present in patients with infectious mononucleosis

9. _____ time required for a small puncture wound to stop bleeding

10. _____ a series of blood tests that includes WBC, RBC, diff, Hgb, and Hct

11. _____ triggers the body to produce plasmin, an enzyme that dissolves clots

12. _____ an agent that delays or inhibits clotting

WORKSHEET 6

Grammar Review—Hematic and Lymphatic Systems

Using the nouns listed below, build adjectives for each.

NOUN	ADJECTIVE
1. thymus	thymic
2. spleen	_____
3. anemia	_____
4. hemophilia	_____
5. lymphedema	_____
6. nucleus	_____

Using the word part listed below, build medical words to mean persons or people who

7. hemat/o ____hematologist____ specialize in the study of blood

8. immun/o _____ specialize in the study of immunity

9. ser/o _____ specialize in the study of blood serum

10. path/o _____ specialize in the study of diseases

CHAPTER 10

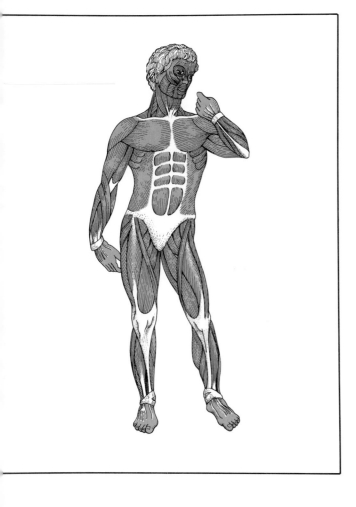

CHAPTER OUTLINE

Musculoskeletal System

STUDENT OBJECTIVES

Upon completion of this chapter, you will be able to do the following:

Describe the functions of the skeletal system.

Locate and identify the major bones of the body.

Identify the two main divisions of the skeletal system.

List the four main types of bones.

Explain the function of the vertebral column, and list the five main groups of bones in the vertebral column.

Describe the function of the thorax, and list five main parts that compose its skeletal framework.

List the three main classifications of joints, and describe the function of joints.

Explain the purpose of bone markings.

Describe three types of bone projections and depressions.

List the three main functions of muscles.

Identify word roots/combining forms and suffixes of the musculoskeletal system.

Identify and discuss associated pathology related to the musculoskeletal system.

Identify radiographic, endoscopic, surgical, and laboratory procedures and abbreviations related to the musculoskeletal system.

Explain the pharmacology related to the treatment of musculoskeletal disorders.

Build and analyze diagnostic, symptomatic, and surgical terms related to the musculoskeletal system by completing the worksheets.

202 ANATOMY AND PHYSIOLOGY OF THE MUSCULOSKELETAL SYSTEM

The musculoskeletal system consists of bones, joints, and muscles. Bones are the principal organs of support and protection for the body. Joints are the places at which two bones meet (articulate). Because bones are incapable of movement without the help of muscles, contraction must be provided by muscular tissue. In the human skeleton, muscles are usually attached to two articulating bones, and during contraction, one bone is drawn toward another. Muscles, therefore, produce movement by exerting a force on the bones to which they are attached. Stated more simply, skeletal muscles produce movement by pulling on bones.

This chapter is devoted to the study of bones, joints, and muscles.

Skeletal System

FUNCTIONS

Besides **support** and **protection** of the vital organs from injury, the skeletal system provides a number of other important functions. **Movement** is possible because bones act as points of attachment for muscles, joints, tendons, and ligaments. Bone marrow, which is found within the larger bones, is responsible for blood cell formation, or **hematopoiesis**. Bone marrow continuously produces millions of red and white blood cells to replace worn out cells. The bones serve as a **storehouse for minerals**, particularly phosphorus and calcium. When the body experiences a deficiency in a mineral salt, such as calcium during pregnancy, it is withdrawn from the bones.

STRUCTURE AND TYPES OF BONES

Bones consist of mineral deposits embedded with living cells that must continually receive food and oxygen. Bone cells also require a system to carry away accumulated waste products. In order to provide these vital functions, there is an extensive vascular system within bones. Fundamentally, all bones are composed of the same basic substances, but bones vary in both size and shape. Thus bones can be distinguished from each other by classifying them in four main categories: long bones, short bones, flat bones, and irregular bones.

Long bones are found in the extremities of the body; for example, arms and legs. Typical long bones consist of the following parts, as shown in Figure 10-1:

1. (1) **Diaphysis**, which is the shaft, or long main portion, of the bone, consists mainly of **compact bone**.
2. (2) **Epiphyses**, which are the two ends, or extremities, of the bone, have a somewhat bulbous shape to provide space for muscle and ligament attachments near the joints. **Proximal** and **distal epiphyses** are the two terms used for the ends of a long bone.
3. (3) **Articular cartilage** is a thin layer of resilient hyaline cartilage. The elasticity of the hyaline cartilage provides the joints with a cushion against jars and blows.
4. (4) **Periosteum**, which is a dense white fibrous membrane that covers the remaining surface of the bone, contains numerous blood and lymph vessels and nerves. In growing bones, the inner layer contains the bone-forming cells, or osteoblasts. Since the blood vessels and osteoblasts are located here, the periosteum provides a means for bone repair and general bone nutrition. It also serves as a point of attachment for muscles, ligaments, and tendons.

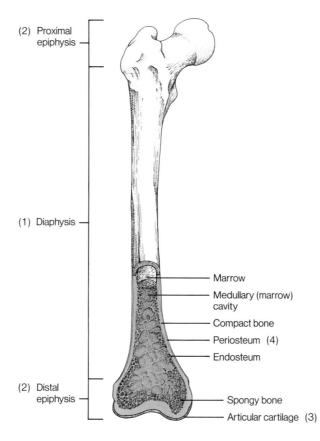

(2) Proximal epiphysis

(1) Diaphysis

(2) Distal epiphysis

Marrow
Medullary (marrow) cavity
Compact bone
Periosteum (4)
Endosteum

Spongy bone
Articular cartilage (3)

Figure 10-1. Longitudinal section of a typical long bone.

Flat bones are exactly what their name suggests. They provide broad surfaces for muscular attachment and extensive protection for internal organs. Examples are bones of the skull, shoulder blades, and sternum.

Short bones are irregularly shaped and consist of a core of cancellous, or spongy, bone enclosed in a thin layer of compact tissue. Examples are bones of the ankles, wrists, and toes.

Irregular bones are all of the other bones that cannot be grouped under the previous headings because of their peculiar shapes. Examples are the bones of the ear and the vertebrae.

DIVISIONS OF THE SKELETAL SYSTEM: AXIAL AND APPENDICULAR SKELETON

The skeleton can be divided into two main parts: the axial skeleton and the appendicular skeleton (Fig. 10-2).

The **axial skeleton** comprises the bones of the skull, the thorax, and the vertebral column. These bones contribute to the formation of body cavities and provide protection for internal organs.

The **appendicular skeleton** consists of the bones of the shoulder, the upper extremities, the hips, and the lower extremities. They attach to the axial skeleton as appendages.

Since the human skeleton consists of 206 bones, only the major bones have been identified in Figure 10-2.

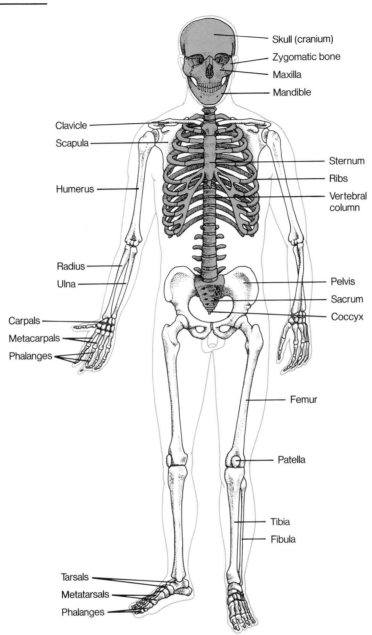

Figure 10–2. The skeleton can be divided into the axial (shaded) and appendicular portions.

Vertebral Column

The vertebral column of the adult is composed of 26 bones called vertebrae. The vertebral column supports the body and provides a protective bony canal for the passage of the spinal cord. (For a better understanding of the backbone structures, refer to Figure 10-3 as you continue to read the text.) Vertebrae are separated by flat, round structures, or (1) **intervertebral disks**, which are composed of a fibrocartilagenous substance with a gelatinous mass in the center (nucleus pulposus). When the disk material protrudes into the neural canal, pressure on the adjacent nerve root is manifested by pain. This condition is referred to as

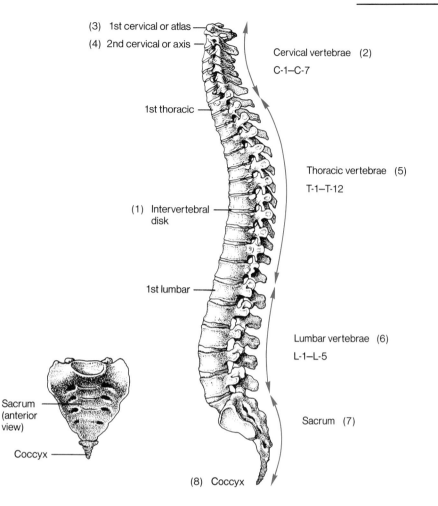

(3) 1st cervical or atlas
(4) 2nd cervical or axis

Cervical vertebrae (2)
C-1–C-7

1st thoracic

Thoracic vertebrae (5)
T-1–T-12

(1) Intervertebral disk

1st lumbar

Lumbar vertebrae (6)
L-1–L-5

Sacrum (anterior view)

Sacrum (7)

Coccyx

(8) Coccyx

Figure 10-3. *Spinal column (vertebral column), indicating individual vertebrae at various levels.*

herniation of an intervertebral disk, herniated nucleus pulposus (HNP), ruptured disk, or slipped disk.

Basically, the vertebral column is divided into five groups of bones, and each group derives its name from its location within the spinal column. The seven (2) **cervical vertebrae** form the skeletal framework of the neck. The first cervical vertebra is called the (3) **atlas** and supports the skull. The second cervical vertebra, the (4) **axis**, makes possible rotation of the skull on the neck. Under these are the twelve (5) **thoracic** or **dorsal vertebrae**, which support the chest and serve as a point of articulation for the ribs. The next five vertebrae, the (6) **lumbar vertebrae**, are situated in the lower back area and carry most of the weight of the torso. Below this area, the five sacral vertebrae are fused into a single bone in the adult and are referred to as the (7) **sacrum**. The tail of the vertebral column consists of four or five fragmented vertebrae fused together, referred to as the (8) **coccyx**.

Thorax

Two of the more important internal organs of the chest are the heart and lungs. Together with other soft tissue, they are enclosed and protected by the thorax, or rib cage. As you read the following paragraph, refer to Figure 10-4.

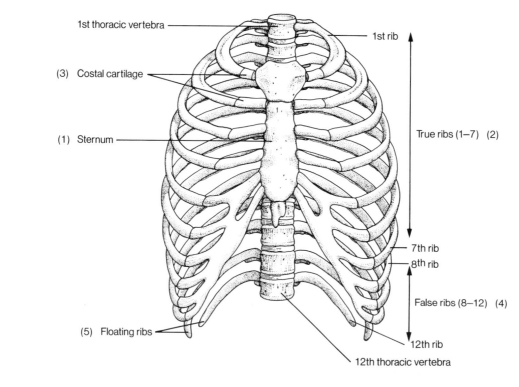

1st thoracic vertebra

1st rib

(3) Costal cartilage

True ribs (1–7) (2)

(1) Sternum

7th rib
8th rib

False ribs (8–12) (4)

(5) Floating ribs

12th rib

12th thoracic vertebra

Figure 10–4. The thorax.

The ribs, the (1) **sternum**, or chest plate, and the thoracic vertebrae form the skeletal framework of the rib cage. The normal set of ribs in both sexes consists of 12 pairs, or a total of 24 ribs. Twelve ribs are situated on each side of the thoracic cavity. The (2) **true ribs** are the first seven pairs of ribs. These are attached directly to the sternum by a strip of (3) **costal cartilage** (hyaline cartilage). The costal cartilages of the next five pairs of ribs are not fastened directly to the sternum. These are known as (4) **false ribs**. The last two pairs of false ribs are not joined, even indirectly, to the sternum but attach posteriorly to the thoracic vertebrae and are known as (5) **floating ribs**.

Pelvic Girdle (Pelvis)

The pelvis is a basin-shaped structure that supports the sigmoid colon, the rectum, the urinary bladder, and other soft organs of the abdominopelvic cavity. It also provides a point of attachment for the legs, as shown in Figure 10-5.

Male and female pelves differ considerably in size and shape. Some of the differences are attributable to the function of the female pelvis during the stages of childbearing. The female pelvis is more shallow than the male pelvis but wider in every direction. Not only does the female pelvis support the enlarged abdomen as the fetus matures, but it also must provide a large enough opening to allow the infant to pass through during the process of birth.

Both the female and male pelves are divided into the (1) **ilium**, (2) **ischium**, and (3) **pubis**. These are fused together in the adult to form a single bone called the innominate bone. Nevertheless, the individual names are retained in order to identify the respective

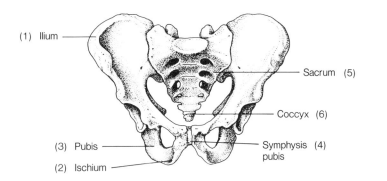

(1) Ilium

Sacrum (5)

Coccyx (6)

(3) Pubis

Symphysis (4) pubis

(2) Ischium

Figure 10–5. *The male pelvis.*

areas of the hipbone. The bladder is located behind the (4) **symphysis pubis**; the rectum is in the curve of the (5) **sacrum** and (6) **coccyx**. In the female, the uterus, fallopian tubes, ovaries, and vagina are located between the bladder and the rectum.

BONE MARKINGS

Surfaces of bones have both projections and depressions to provide attachments for muscles, to join one bone to another, or to furnish cavities and pathways for nerve and blood supplies.

The portion of the bone that projects is called a process. Various types of projections, or processes, are evident in bones. They may be rounded, sharp, and narrow or have a larger ridge, called a **crest**. The anatomical terms for the most common types of processes are discussed below.

A **condyle** is a rounded process at the end of a bone that forms an articulation. An example is the condyles of the humerus. A **tubercle** is a small, rounded elevation from the surface of a bone, while its larger counterpart is known as a **tuberosity**. These elevations provide points of attachment for muscles and ligaments. The **trochanter** is a very large projection and serves the same purpose as the smaller projections. An example of a trochanter is the greater trochanter of the femur.

Depressions are cavities or openings in a bone. There are several distinct types. **Sinus** is a term applied to a bone cavity, and an example is the frontal sinus. A **foramen** is an opening, or orifice, for passage of blood vessels and nerves. **Fissure** (also called sulcus) indicates a narrow slit, often between two bones. A **fossa** is a depression in a bone surface. The line of bone union in an immovable articulation, as in between the skull bones, is known as a **suture**. **Fontanelle** is a soft spot—one of the membrane-covered spaces remaining at the junction of the sutures in the incompletely ossified skull of the fetus or infant.

JOINTS OR ARTICULATIONS

In order to allow body movements, all bones must have articulating surfaces. These surfaces form joints, or articulations, with various degrees of mobility. Some are freely movable (diarthroses); others are only slightly movable (amphiarthroses); and the remaining are totally immovable (synarthroses). All three types are necessary for smooth, coordinated body movements.

Every joint is covered with connective tissue and cartilage. The ligaments and connective tissue in these areas permit bones to be connected to each other. Muscles attached to freely movable joints permit a great deal of body movement. The synovial membrane that

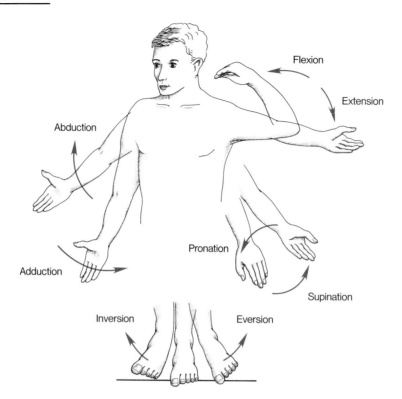

Figure 10-6. *Movements of the body at the joints.*

lines the joint cavity secretes synovial fluid, which acts as a lubricant of the joints. The bones in a synovial joint are separated by a joint capsule. The joint capsule is strengthened by ligaments (fibrous bands, or sheets, of connective tissues) that often anchor bones to each other. All of the above factors, working together in a complementary manner, make various body movements possible (Fig. 10-6).

Muscles

Muscular tissue refers to all of the contractile tissue of the body. It includes the cardiac muscle of the heart, the smooth muscles that compose the viscera, and the skeletal muscles that attach to bones. The first two categories of muscles are referred to as involuntary, because there is no discretionary control over them. In contrast, the skeletal muscles are voluntary, since their contractions are fully controllable. Some examples of other types of voluntary muscles are those that move the tongue or eyeballs and those that control facial expressions.

All muscles, through contraction, provide the body with motion or body posture. The less apparent motions provided by muscles are the passage and elimination of food through the digestive system, propulsion of blood through the arteries, and contraction of the bladder to eliminate urine.

Motions such as running and lifting originate with the skeletal muscles, which act upon the system of levers formed by the bones and joints. This engineering relationship needs further explaining. One end of a muscle, usually the proximal end (also called the origin), must attach to a rather immovable bone surface, while its remaining part spans across a joint. The other end of the muscle, the distal end (or insertion) is attached to a movable bone. As the muscle contracts, the insertion pulls toward the origin and draws the second bone toward the immovable, or first, bone. This produces motion. Often, motion is produced when several muscles spanning over the same joint are contracted. Each of these muscles provides for slight variations in a particular movement.

Whether acting singly or in groups, the muscle or muscles that produce the movement are referred to as **prime movers**, or **agonists**. Once a motion has occurred, such as bending an arm at the elbow, the arm does not return to its original position even after the contraction has stopped. Instead, an opposing muscle, called the **antagonist**, must contract to bring the arm back to its original position. The need for both agonist and antagonist muscles implies that muscles possess only contracting, or pulling, capabilities, not those of pushing. This means that a prime mover is not able to reverse its activity and push a bone away from the origin. Opposite motions are accomplished by muscles that act antagonistically to the prime movers.

When other muscles contribute indirectly to a specific movement, they are called **synergists**. They aid the prime movers in their activity, but only indirectly.

Finally, a **fixator** is a muscle that stabilizes, or fixes, one end of a muscle, so that all of the force exerted by it occurs only at one end.

CONNECTIVE TISSUE COVERINGS

Skeletal muscles are enclosed in a sheath of connective tissue (Fig. 10-7). This connective tissue is part of the deep **fascia** of the body, which is continuous with adjacent muscles,

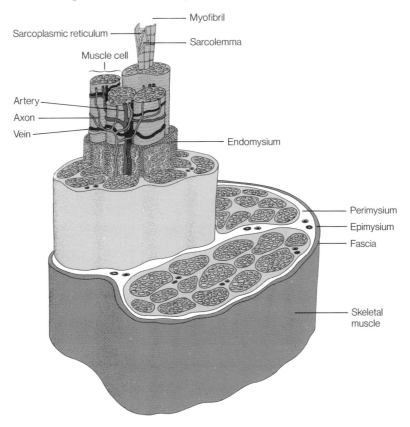

Figure 10-7. *Skeletal muscles are enclosed in a sheath of connective tissue.*

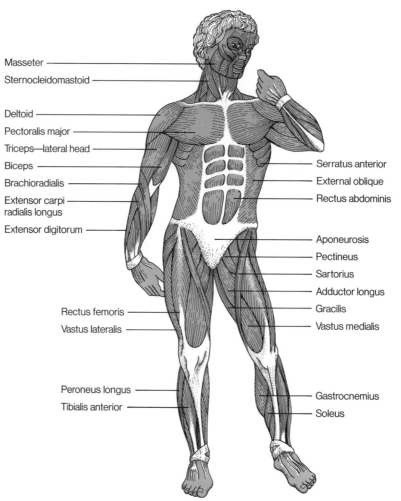

Masseter

Sternocleidomastoid

Deltoid

Pectoralis major

Triceps—lateral head

Biceps

Brachioradialis

Extensor carpi
radialis longus

Extensor digitorum

Serratus anterior

External oblique

Rectus abdominis

Aponeurosis

Pectineus

Sartorius

Adductor longus

Gracilis

Vastus medialis

Rectus femoris

Vastus lateralis

Peroneus longus

Tibialis anterior

Gastrocnemius

Soleus

Figure 10-8. Anterior view of muscles.

periosteum, and subcutaneous connective tissue. The outer sheath of the muscle is the **epimysium**. Within a given muscle, a **perimysium** surrounds small bundles of muscles. The **endomysium** covers each single muscle fiber. These layers of connective tissue contain the nerves and supply blood to the muscles.

ATTACHMENTS

Muscles attach to bones either by fleshy or fibrous attachments. In **fleshy attachments**, muscle fibers arise directly from bone. These fibers distribute force over wide areas, but a fleshy attachment is weaker than a fibrous attachment. In **fibrous attachments**, the connective tissue of the epimysium, perimysium, and endomysium converges at the end of the muscle to become continuous and indistinguishable from the periosteum. In some instances, this connective tissue penetrates the very bone itself. When these connective tissue fibers form a cord or strap, it is referred to as a **tendon**. This provides for a great deal of force to be localized in a small area of bone. Ligaments are composed of connective tissue and attach one bone to another. When the fibrous attachment spans over a large area of a partic-

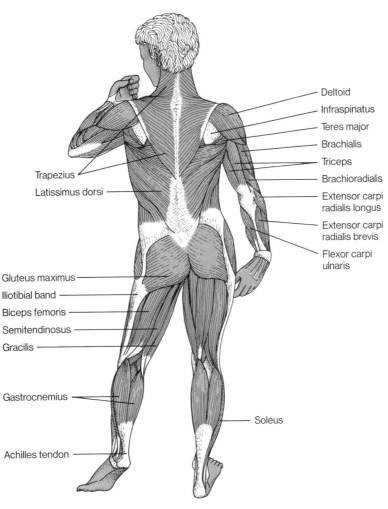

Figure 10-9. *Posterior view of muscles.*

Deltoid
Infraspinatus
Teres major
Brachialis
Triceps
Brachioradialis
Extensor carpi radialis longus
Extensor carpi radialis brevis
Flexor carpi ulnaris

Trapezius
Latissimus dorsi

Gluteus maximus
Iliotibial band
Biceps femoris
Semitendinosus
Gracilis

Gastrocnemius

Soleus

Achilles tendon

ular bone, the attachment is called an **aponeurosis**. Such attachments are found in the lumbar region of the back.

You should become familiar with some of the names of the major muscles of the body by studying Figures 10-8 and 10-9.

WORD ROOTS/COMBINING FORMS RELATED TO THE MUSCULOSKELETAL SYSTEM

WORD ROOT/ COMBINING FORM (BONES)	MEANING	EXAMPLE	PRONUNCIATION
Upper Extremities			
cephal/o	head	cephal/ad toward	SĔF - ăh - lăd

Continued on following page

WORD ROOTS/COMBINING FORMS RELATED TO THE MUSCULOSKELETAL SYSTEM—*Continued*

WORD ROOT/ COMBINING FORM (BONES)	MEANING	EXAMPLE	PRONUNCIATION
Upper Extremities			
crani/o	skull bones, cranium	crani/o/malacia softening	krā - nē - ō - măh - LĀ - shē - ăh
cervic/o	neck	cervic/o/facial face	sĕr - vĭ - kō - FĀ - shē - ăl
lamin/o	lamina (part of vertebral arch)	lamin/ectomy excision	lăm - ĭ - NĔK - tō - mē

vertebr/o (used to make words that describe the structure)	vertebrae (backbone)	cost/o/vertebr/al
		 ribs adjec-
		        tive
		        ending
			kŏs - tō - VĔR - tĕ - brăl

spondyl/o (used to make words about the condition of the structure)	vertebrae (backbone)	spondyl/itis inflammation	spŏn - dĭl - Ī - tĭs
rachi/o } rach/o }	vertebrae (spinal column)	rach/itis inflammation	rā - KĪ - tĭs
thorac/o	chest	thoraco/dynia pain	thō - răk - ō - DĬN - ē - ă
cost/o	ribs	cost/ectomy excision	kŏs - TĔK - tō - mē
stern/o	sternum, breastbone	sub/stern/al under adjective ending	sŭb - STĔR - năl

arthr/o	joint	arthr/o/desis
		     binding,
		     stabilization
			ăr - thrō - DĒ - sĭs

humer/o	humerus	humer/o/uln/ ar
		      ul- pertain-
		      na ing to
			hū - mĕr - ō - ŬL - năr

Continued on following page

WORD ROOTS/COMBINING FORMS RELATED TO THE MUSCULOSKELETAL SYSTEM—*Continued*

WORD ROOT/ COMBINING FORM (BONES)	MEANING	EXAMPLE	PRONUNCIATION
Upper Extremities			
brachi/o	arm	brachi/o/cephal/ic head pertaining to	brăk - ē - ō - sĕ - FĂL - ĭk
carp/o	wrist, carpus	carp/al pertaining to	KĂR - păl
metacarp/o	metacarpus (bones of the hand)	metacarp/ectomy excision	mĕt - ă - kăr - PĔK - tō - mē
phalang/o	phalanges (bones of fingers and toes)	phalang/eal relating to	fā - LĂN - jē - ăl
dactyl/o	digit (a finger or toe)	syn/dactyl/ism joined condition together	sĭn - DĂK - tĭl - ĭzm
Lower Extremities			
pelv/i	pelvis	pelv/i/metry to measure	pĕl - VĬM - ĕt - rē
lumb/o	loins	lumbo/dynia pain	lŭm - bō - DĬN - ē - ăh
ili/o	ilium (lateral flaring portion of hip bone)	ili/ac pertaining to	ĬL - ē - ăk
ischi/o	ischium (lower portion of hip bone)	ischi/al adjective ending	ĬS - kē - ăl
pub/o	pubis anterior (inferior portion of hip bone)	pub/ic pertaining to	PŪ - bĭk

femor/o	femur (thigh bone)	femor/o/tibi/ al
		         tib- pertaining
		         ia to
			fĕm - ō - rō - TĬB - ē - ăl

Continued on following page

WORD ROOTS/COMBINING FORMS RELATED TO THE
MUSCULOSKELETAL SYSTEM—*Continued*

WORD ROOT/ COMBINING FORM (BONES)	MEANING	EXAMPLE	PRONUNCIATION
Lower Extremities			
patell/o	patella, kneecap	<u>patell</u>/a/pexy fixation	păh - TĔL - ăh - pĕk - sē
fibul/o	fibula (smaller and outer bone of lower leg)	<u>fibul</u>/a noun ending	FĬB - ū - lă
tibi/o	tibia (larger and inner bone of lower leg)	<u>tibi</u>/o/femor/al fe- pertain- mur ing to	tĭb - ē - ō - FĔM - ŏr - ăl
calcane/o	calcaneum, heel bone	<u>calcane</u>/o/dynia pain	kăl - kā - nē - ō - DĬN - ē - ăh
ped/i ⎫	foot	<u>ped</u>/i/cure care	PĔD - ĭ - kūr
pod/o ⎭		<u>pod</u>/iatry treatment	pō - DĪ - ă - trē

WORD ROOTS/COMBINING FORMS RELATED TO THE
MUSCULOSKELETAL SYSTEM

WORD ROOT/ COMBINING FORM	MEANING	EXAMPLE	PRONUNCIATION
Miscellaneous			
acromi/o	acromion (projection of scapula)	<u>acromi</u>/o/clavic/ular col- relat- lar ing to bone	ă - krō - mē - ŏ - klă - VĬK - ū - lăr
ankyl/o	stiff joint, fusion or growing together of parts	<u>ankyl</u>/osis abnormal condition (of)	ăng - kĭ - LŌ - sĭs

Continued on following page

WORD ROOTS/COMBINING FORMS RELATED TO THE MUSCULOSKELETAL SYSTEM—*Continued*

WORD ROOT/ COMBINING FORM	MEANING	EXAMPLE	PRONUNCIATION
Miscellaneous			
chondr/o	cartilage	chondr/itis inflammation	kŏn - DRĪ - tĭs
condyl/o	condyle (rounded protuberance at the end of a bone forming an articulation)	condyl/ectomy excision	kŏn - dĭl - ĔK - tō - mē
lamin/o	lamina (part of vertebral arch)	lamin/ectomy excision	lăm - ĭ - NĔK - tō - mē
leiomy/o	smooth (visceral) muscle	leiomy/oma tumor	lī - ō - mī - Ō - mă
myel/o	bone marrow, spinal cord	myel/o/cele hernia	MĪ - ĕl - lō - sēl
my/o	muscle	myo/scler/ osis hard- abnormal en- condition ing (of)	mī - ō - sklĕ - RŌ - sĭs
orth/o	straight	orth/o/ped/ ic child pertain- ing to	ŏr - thō - PĒ - dĭk
oste/o	bone	oste/oma tumor	ŏs - tē - Ō - mă
rhabd/o	rod	rhabd/oid resemble	RĂB - doyd
rhabdomy/o	striated (skeletal) muscle	rhabdomy/oma tumor	răb - dō - mī - Ō - mă
ten/o		ten/o/tomy incision	tĕn - ŎT - ō - mē
tend/o	tendon	tend/o/tome instrument to cut	TĔN - dō - tōm
tendin/o		tendin/itis inflammation	tĕn - dĭn - Ī - tĭs

SUFFIXES RELATED TO THE MUSCULOSKELETAL SYSTEM

SUFFIX	MEANING	EXAMPLE	PRONUNCIATION
-blast	germ cell, primitive, embryonic	oste/o/blast bone	ŎS - tē - ō - blăst
-clast	to break	oste/o/clast bone	ŎS - tē - ō - klăst
-desis	binding, stabilization, fusion	arthr/o/desis joint	ăr - thrō - DĒ - sis
-malacia	softening	oste/o/malacia bone	ŏs - tē - ō - măh - LĀ - shē - ăh
-physis	to grow	epi/physis upon	ĕ - PĬF - ĭ - sĭs
-plasty	formation, surgical repair, plastic repair	arthr/o/plasty joint	ĂR - thrō - plăs - tē
-porosis	pores or cavities	oste/o/porosis bone	ŏs - tē - ō - pŏ - RŌ - sĭs
-scopy	visual examination	arthr/o/scopy joint	ăr - THRŎS - kō - pē

PATHOLOGY OF THE MUSCULOSKELETAL SYSTEM

Bones

Inflammation of the bone, especially of the bone marrow (**osteomyelitis**), is due to a pyogenic infection. This infection is more difficult to cure than a soft-tissue infection and can eventually result in bone destruction (**necrosis**) and stiffening, or freezing, of the joints (**ankylosis**). Osteomyelitis may be acute or chronic.

Bone tumors (**osteomas**), which are composed of bony tissue, can be either benign (**exostoses**) or malignant. Some of the bone tumors are common and some are exceedingly rare. Some present no problem, while others rapidly become life-threatening. Generally, benign tumors are slow growing and are usually treated by surgical excision. Malignant tumors that arise from bone (**sarcoma**) are rare. They usually develop rapidly and metastasize through lymph channels. Sarcomas are named for the specific tissue that they affect, for example, sarcomas in fibrous connective tissue (**fibrosarcoma**), sarcomas in lymphoid tissue (**lymphosarcoma**), or sarcomas in cartilage (**chondrosarcoma**). A sarcoma that often attacks the shafts rather than the ends of the long bones is called **Ewing's sarcoma**. This highly malignant tumor is found primarily in young males. Included in the treatment of malignant bone tumors are chemotherapy for management of metastasis and radiation when the tumor is radiosensitive.

Osteitis deformans, which is a slowly progressive bone disorder, is a rare osteitis of unknown origin that leads to bowing of long bones and deformation of flat bones. It is usually found in persons over the age of 35. The long bones of the legs, the lower spine, the pelvis, and the skull are most commonly affected. This disorder is also known as **Paget's disease**.

Joints

Because of their location and constant use, joints are prone to stress, injuries, and inflammation. The main diseases affecting the joints are rheumatoid arthritis, osteoarthritis, and gout.

Rheumatoid arthritis, which is a systemic disease characterized by inflammatory changes in joints and their related structures, results in crippling deformities. This form of arthritis is believed to be caused by an autoimmune reaction of joint tissue. It begins most often in women between 23 and 35, but can affect people of any age group. Exacerbations of this disease are frequently associated with periods of increased physical or emotional stress. In addition to the joint changes, there is atrophy of muscles, bones, and skin adjacent to the affected joint. There is no specific cure, but nonsteroidal anti-inflammatory drugs (NSAIDs), physical therapy, and orthopedic measures are used in treatment.

Gout is a metabolic disease marked by acute arthritis and inflammation of the joints. It usually begins in the knee or foot, but the joints affected may be at any location. The joint chiefly affected is the big toe, and the disorder is known as podagra (excessive foot pain). An attack of gout is marked by swelling, inflammation, and extreme pain.

Another chronic disease involving the joints is characterized by destruction of articular cartilage, overgrowth of bone, and spur formation **(osteoarthritis)**. Even though osteoarthritis is less crippling than rheumatoid arthritis, it may result in fusion of two bone surfaces, thereby completely immobilizing the joint. Also, there may be formation of small, hard nodules at the distal interphalangeal joints of the fingers **(Heberden's nodes)**.

Fractures

A fracture is a breakage of a bone, due to trauma or a disease such as cancer, that results in decalcification of the bone. Pain, swelling, and deformity are common symptoms of a fracture. Although a fracture primarily affects the bone, it may also produce injury to the muscles surrounding the injured bone and to the blood vessels and nerves in the vicinity of the fracture. Fractures are classified according to the type of break sustained and according to the cause of the fracture (Fig. 10-10).

A (1) **closed** or **simple fracture** is one in which the bone is broken, but there is no external wound (see Fig. 10-10). An (2) **open** or **compound fracture** involves a broken bone and an external wound that leads down to the site of the fracture. Many times, fragments of bone protrude through the skin. A (3) **complicated fracture** occurs when the broken bone has injured some internal organ, such as a broken rib piercing a lung. (4) **Comminuted fractures** are evident when a bone has broken or splintered into pieces. An (5) **impacted fracture** takes place when the bone is broken and one end is wedged into the interior of the other. An (6) **incomplete fracture** occurs when the line of fracture does not include the whole bone. Fractures in children, especially children with rickets, are known as (7) **greenstick fractures**. The bone is partially bent and partially broken. **Pathological** (spontaneous) **fractures** are usually caused by a disease process such as neoplasm or osteoporosis.

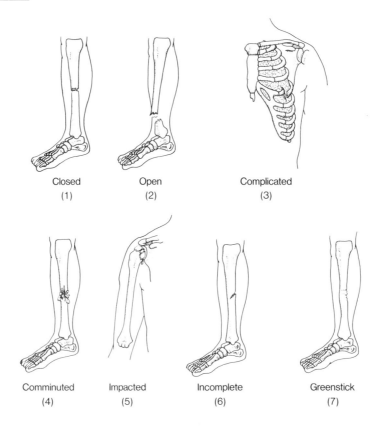

Closed (1)   Open (2)   Complicated (3)

Comminuted (4)   Impacted (5)   Incomplete (6)   Greenstick (7)

Figure 10–10. Types of fractures.

Unlike other repairs of the body, bones sometimes require months to heal. Several factors influence the rate at which fractures heal. The closer together the ends of the broken bone are, the faster the bone will heal. That is the main reason for setting fractured bones in a cast. Some bones have a natural tendency to heal more rapidly than others. For instance, the long bones of the arms have an inclination to mend twice as fast as the ones in the legs. Lastly, age plays an important role in the healing rate. The older the person is, the more time is required for the bones to heal.

Osteoporosis

Osteoporosis (porous bone) is a general term for bone disorders that commonly occur in older persons, especially women past 60. It is characterized by a rate of bone resorption (loss of substance) that exceeds bone formation. This, in turn, results in a decrease in the bone density. Among the many causes of osteoporosis are disturbances of protein metabolism or protein deficiency, disuse of bones or prolonged periods of immobilization, estrogen deficiencies associated with menopause, a diet deficient in vitamins or calcium, and long-term administration of high doses of corticosteroids.

Patients with osteoporosis frequently complain of bone pain, most commonly in the back, which may be caused by repeated microscopic fractures. Thin areas of porous bone are also evident. Deformity associated with osteoporosis is usually the result of pathological fractures.

Spinal Disorders

Because of various conditions, the normal curvature of the spine may become abnormally bent or may slope away. These cases are referred to as **curvatures** of the spine. When a lateral curvature (usually consisting of two curves) of the spine takes place, the disorder is identified as **scoliosis** (bent). Scoliosis may be congenital, or it may develop in the early teens. Poor posture over a long period of time is a contributing factor. Surgery, braces, casts, and corrective exercise may alleviate this condition. Untreated scoliosis may result in pulmonary insufficiency (curvature may decrease lung capacity), back pain, sciatica, disk disease, or degenerative arthritis.

The exaggeration or angulation of the thoracic curve of the vertebral column gives rise to **kyphosis** (hunchback or humpback). This condition may be caused by rheumatoid arthritis, rickets, poor posture, or chronic respiratory diseases. Treatment for kyphosis caused by poor posture may consist of bed rest, therapeutic exercise, and a brace to straighten the kyphotic curve until growth is completed. Treatment for both adolescent and adult kyphosis includes appropriate measures for the underlying cause and, possibly, spinal arthrodesis for relief of symptoms. Surgery may be necessary when kyphosis causes neurological damage or intractable and disabling pain, but it is rarely necessary.

Lordosis (swayback) is a forward curvature of the lumbar spine. It may be caused by increased weight of the abdominal contents. This could be due to obesity or excessive weight gain during pregnancy.

Spina bifida is a genetic disorder that results in various malformations of the spine due to imperfect joining of the vertebrae. These defects usually occur in the lumbosacral area but are occasionally found in the sacral, thoracic, and cervical areas. The most common and least severe spinal cord defect is **spina bifida occulta**. With this defect, there is no protrusion of the spinal cord or meninges (intraspinal contents). In more severe forms of spina bifida, incomplete closure of one or more vertebrae causes protrusion of the spinal contents to form a saclike structure that contains meninges and cerebrospinal fluid. This condition is called **spina bifida with meningocele**. However, when the sac contains meninges, cerebrospinal fluid, and a portion of the spinal cord or nerve roots, the defect is known as **spina bifida with myelomeningocele**. **Spina bifida occulta** usually does not cause neurological dysfunction but is occasionally associated with foot weakness or bowel and bladder disturbances. These same dysfunctions may be apparent in **spina bifida with meningocele** and **spina bifida with myelomeningocele**. Treatment varies with the severity of the defect. Surgery may be required to remove the meningocele or myelomeningocele. Continual assessment of growth and development is necessary.

Spondylitis, which is an inflammation of the vertebrae, is almost always a serious chronic disorder. It may be associated with tuberculosis of the bones, in which case it is called Pott's disease. The vertebrae become eroded and collapse, causing kyphosis. Spondylitis may also be associated with other infectious diseases, such as brucellosis, or undulant fever. The intervertebral disks and the vertebrae are affected and sometimes destroyed, and permanent stiffening, or ankylosis, of the back results.

Muscular Disorders

Myasthenia gravis (MG) is a disease of the neuromuscular junction characterized by fluctuating weakness of certain skeletal muscle groups (of the eyes, face, and to a lesser degree, the limbs). It is caused by failure of the neurons to release **acetylcholine** (which helps transmit nerve impulses across the myoneural junction). Acetylcholine is quickly destroyed

220

by an enzyme, cholinesterase, which is released from the muscle fibers. Either excessive or deficient action of acetylcholine at the motor end-plates may result in neuromuscular block. As the disease progresses, more neuromuscular junctions become affected. The muscle becomes increasingly weaker and may eventually cease to function altogether. Women are affected slightly more than men. Initial symptoms include a weakness of the eye muscles and difficulty in swallowing. Later, the individual has difficulty chewing and talking. Eventually, the muscles of the limbs may become involved. Anticholinesterase drugs have been the primary treatment for the disease.

Muscular dystrophy is a group of genetically determined degenerative myopathies that are progressively crippling because muscles are gradually weakened and eventually atrophy. This childhood-type disease—unfortunately the most common type—is known as the Duchenne type or progressive muscular dystrophy. It is also called pseudohypertrophic muscular dystrophy because at the beginning, the muscles, especially those in the calves, appear healthy and bulging when actually they are already weakened and their size is due to an excess of fat.

OTHER TERMS RELATED TO THE MUSCULOSKELETAL SYSTEM

TERM	MEANING	PRONUNCIATION
carpal tunnel syndrome	soreness, tenderness, and weakness of the muscles of the thumb caused by pressure on the median nerve at the point at which it goes through the carpal tunnel of the wrist	
claudication	lameness, limping	klăw - dǐ - KĀ - shŭn
crepitation	a dry, crackling sound or sensation, such as that produced by the grating of the ends of a fractured bone	krĕp - ĭ - TĀ - shŭn
exacerbation	increase in severity of a disease or any of its symptoms	ĕks - ăs - ĕr - BĀ - shŭn
genu valgus	knock-knee; a condition where knees are very close to each other and the ankles are apart	JĒ - nū/VĂL - gŭs
genu varus	bowleg; a condition of curving out of the legs	JĒ - nū/VĀ - rŭs
hemarthrosis	effusion of blood into a joint cavity	hĕm - ăr - THRŌ - sǐs
hyperkinesia	increased muscular movement and physical activity	hǐ - pĕr - kǐ - NĒ - zē - ăh
multiple myeloma	a primary malignant tumor of plasma cells usually arising in bone marrow, usually progressive, and generally fatal	MŬL - tǐ - p'l/mǐ - ĕ - LŌ - măh
paraplegia	paralysis of lower spine; paralysis of lower portion of the trunk and of both legs	păr - ă - PLĒ - jē - ăh

Continued on following page

OTHER TERMS RELATED TO THE MUSCULOSKELETAL SYSTEM—*Cont.*   **221**

TERM	MEANING	PRONUNCIATION
phantom limb	an illusion, following amputation of a limb, that the limb still exists. The sensation that pain exists in the removed part is known as phantom-limb pain.	
quadriplegia	paralysis of upper spine; paralysis of all four extremities and, usually, the trunk	kwŏd - rĭ - PLĒ - jē - ăh
rickets, rachitis	a form of osteomalacia in children, caused by deficiency of vitamin D	RĬK - ĕts rā - KĪ - tĭs
sequestrum	fragment of necrosed bone that has become separated from surrounding tissue	sē - KWĔS - trŭm
sprain	wrenching or twisting of a joint, with partial rupture of its ligaments. There may also be damage to the associated blood vessels, muscles, tendons, and nerves. A sprain is more serious than a **strain**, which is simply the overstretching of a muscle, without swelling. Severe sprains are so painful that the joint cannot be used. There is much swelling, with reddish to blue discoloration owing to hemorrhage from ruptured blood vessels	
subluxation	a partial or incomplete dislocation	sŭb - lŭk - SĀ - shŭn
talipes	any number of deformities of the foot, especially those occurring congenitally; clubfoot	TĂL - ĭ - pēz
torticollis, wryneck	stiff neck caused by spasmodic contraction of neck muscles drawing the head to one side with the chin pointing to the other side	tŏr - tĭ - KŎL - ĭs RĪ - nĕk

SPECIAL PROCEDURES RELATED TO THE MUSCULOSKELETAL SYSTEM

RADIOGRAPHIC AND CLINICAL PROCEDURES

TERM	DESCRIPTION
arthrocentesis	performed to obtain synovial fluid, especially from the knee or

Continued on following page

RADIOGRAPHIC AND CLINICAL PROCEDURES—*Continued*

TERM	DESCRIPTION
	shoulder, for the purpose of examination
arthrography	injection of a radiopaque substance or air into a joint cavity, especially the knee or shoulder, in order to outline the contour of the joint. The joint is passively ranged while a series of radiographs are taken
bone scan	used to evaluate skeletal involvement related to connective tissue disease. Camera scans the entire body front and back, and a recording is made on paper
electromyography (EMG)	used to determine the presence of muscle inflammation or degeneration when skeletal muscle is directly affected by connective tissue disease
joint scan	the most sensitive study for the detection of early disease. This procedure allows determination of joint damage throughout the body
lumbosacral spinal radiograph (L.S. Spine)	a radiological study of the five lumbar vertebrae and the fused sacral vertebrae. This radiographic series includes anteroposterior, lateral, and oblique views of the lower spine. The most common indication for this test is lower back pain. The test is used to identify or differentiate traumatic fractures, spondylosis (stress fractures of the vertebrae), spondylolisthesis (slipped vertebrae), and metastatic tumor
myelography	a radiograph of the spinal subarachnoid space taken after an opaque medium or air is injected into the spinal subarachnoid space through a spinal puncture. It outlines the spinal subarachnoid space and shows any distortion of the spinal cord or spinal dural sac caused by tumors, cysts, herniated intervertebral disks, or other lesions
radiography	the most common diagnostic study used to assess musculoskeletal problems and to follow the progress and effectiveness of treatment. Bone films determine bone density, texture, erosion, and changes in bone relationships. Radiographs of the bone cortex detect widening, narrowing, and signs of irregularity. Joint radiographs reveal the presence of fluid excess, irregularity, bone overgrowth, narrowing, and changes in the joint structure
thermography	measures the degree of heat radiating from the skin surface. It is used to investigate the pathophysiology of inflamed joints and to assess the patient's response to anti-inflammatory drug therapy

ENDOSCOPIC PROCEDURE

TERM	DESCRIPTION
arthroscopy	allows direct visualization of a joint, especially the knee. Although it is used primarily to detect trauma or lesions, it may be used to obtain a biopsy of synovial tissue for microscopic examination. A synovial biopsy may also be obtained by needle or surgical incision

SURGICAL PROCEDURES

TERM	DESCRIPTION	PRONUNCIATION
amputation	partial or complete removal of a limb	ăm - pū - TĀ - shŭn
arthrocentesis	surgical puncture of a joint space by using a needle. This procedure is usually done in order to remove accumulated fluid from a joint	ăr - thrŏ - sĕn - TĒ - sĭs
arthrotomy	surgical opening of a joint	ăr - THRŎT - ō - mē
arthroclasia	artificial breaking of an ankylosed joint to provide movement	ăr - thrō - KLĀ - zē - ăh
arthrodesis	surgical immobilization of a joint	ăr - thrō - DĒ - sĭs
bone grafting	transplantation of bone	bōn/GRĀFT - ĭng
bursectomy	excision of bursa (a padlike sac or cavity found in connecting tissue, usually in the vicinity of joints)	bĕr - SĔK - tŏ - mē
capsulotomy	incision of a capsule, as that of a joint	kăp - sū - LŎT - ō - mē
closed reduction	repair of fracture by manipulation and application of cast, or application of splint or traction apparatus in selected cases when the fractured ends are not in alignment	rē - DŬK - shŭn
coccygectomy	excision of the coccyx	kŏk - sē - JĔK - tō - mē
laminectomy	surgical excision of the posterior arch of a vertebra. This procedure is most often performed to relieve the symptoms of a ruptured intervertebral disk (slipped disk)	lăm - ĭ - NĔK - tō - mē
myorrhaphy	suture of a muscle	mī - ŌR - ăh - fē
myotasis	stretching of a muscle	mī - ŎT - ă - sĭs
open reduction	surgical repair of a fracture; manipulation and insertion of plate, screws,	Ō - pĕn/rē - DŬK - shŭn

Continued on following page

SURGICAL PROCEDURES—*Continued*

TERM	DESCRIPTION	PRONUNCIATION
	or nail with occasional prosthesis for severe fractures of the upper or lower end of the humerus or femur	
osteoplasty	plastic surgery of the bones	ŎS - tē - ō - plăs - tē
prosthesis	replacement of a missing part by an artificial substitute, such as an artificial extremity	PRŎS - thē - sĭs
rachicentesis, rachiocentesis	puncture into the spinal column	rā - kē - sĕn - TĒ - sĭs rā - kē - ō - sĕn - TĒ - sĭs
sequestrectomy	excision of a sequestrum (segment of necrosed bone)	sē - kwĕs - TRĔK - tō - mē
synovectomy	excision of synovial membrane	sĭn - ō - VĔK - tō - mē
tenodesis	surgical fixation of a tendon	tĕn - ŎD - ě - sĭs

LABORATORY PROCEDURES

TERM	DESCRIPTION
rheumatoid factor (latex fixation)	the serum of a patient with rheumatoid arthritis contains this antibody in elevated levels. The test, however, is not specific since rheumatoid factor is present in aging, scleroderma, acute pulmonary tuberculosis, systemic lupus erythematosus, and other disorders
skin biopsy	performed to confirm inflammatory connective tissue diseases, such as lupus erythematosus or progressive systemic sclerosis (scleroderma). A specimen may be lightly scraped from the patient's skin without discomfort. Deeper skin biopsies may need to be performed when scraping is not sufficient

PHARMACOLOGY RELATED TO THE MUSCULOSKELETAL SYSTEM

MEDICATION	ACTION
nonsteroidal anti-inflammatory drugs (NSAIDs) (antirheumatics)	reduce pain, fever, and swelling of musculoskeletal inflammatory diseases (e.g., rheumatoid arthritis, osteoarthritis). The main antirheumatic is aspirin. It is given in much larger amounts for arthritis than for fever and other types of pain
antihyperuricemics	used to treat gout by suppressing formation or increasing elimination of uric acid
corticosteroids	major anti-inflammatory drugs used for bone and joint disorders

Continued on following page

PHARMACOLOGY RELATED TO THE MUSCULOSKELETAL SYSTEM—*Cont.*   **225**

MEDICATION	ACTION
gold therapy (chrysotherapy)	oral or injectable gold salts may be useful when rheumatoid activity is uncontrolled by conventional therapy
muscle relaxants	relieve pain and stiffness of skeletal muscles; used extensively for various orthopedic disorders, injuries, and back pain. These drugs are really various types of sedatives and tranquilizers that affect the central nervous system (CNS) rather than directly relaxing the muscles
uricosuric agents	drugs that increase the urinary excretion of uric acid (often used in the treatment of gout)

ABBREVIATIONS RELATED TO THE MUSCULOSKELETAL SYSTEM

ABBREVIATION	MEANING
Amputations	
A.C.	acromioclavicular (joint)
AE	above the elbow
AK	above the knee
BE	below the elbow
BK	below the knee
HD	hip disarticulation
HP	hemipelvectomy
KD	knee disarticulation
SD	shoulder disarticulation
THA	total hip arthroplasty
THR	total hip replacement
TKA	total knee arthroplasty
TKR	total knee replacement
General	
AP	anteroposterior
LAT, lat.	lateral
CDH	congenital dislocation of the hip
C-1	first cervical vertebra

Continued on following page

ABBREVIATIONS RELATED TO THE MUSCULOSKELETAL SYSTEM—*Cont.*

ABBREVIATION	MEANING
General	
C-2	second cervical vertebra
C-3	third cervical vertebra
EMG	electromyography
HNP	herniated nucleus pulposus (herniated disk)
IM	intramuscular
IS	intracostal space
L-1	first lumbar vertebra
L-2	second lumbar vertebra
L-3	third lumbar vertebra
NSAID	nonsteroidal anti-inflammatory drug
Ortho, ORTH	orthopedics, orthopaedics
OA	osteoarthritis
RA	rheumatoid arthritis
SLE	systemic lupus erythematosis
T-1	first thoracic vertebra
T-2	second thoracic vertebra
T-3	third thoracic vertebra

WORKSHEET 1

A. Using the word root/combining form cephal/o (head), build medical words to mean:

1. ____cephalic____ pertaining to the head

2. _____ concerning the (fetal) head and (maternal) pelvis

3. _____ inflammation of the brain

4. _____ disease of the head or brain

B. Using the word root/combining form crani/o (skull bones), build medical words to mean:

1. _____ softening of the skull bones

2. _____ protrusion or herniation (of the brain) from the skull

3. _____ plastic repair of the skull

4. _____ incision through the cranium

C. Using the word root/combining form cervic/o (neck), build medical words to mean:

1. _____ pertaining to the neck

2. _____ pertaining to the neck and arm

3. _____ pertaining to the neck and face

D. Using the word root/combining form myel/o (bone marrow, spinal cord), build medical terms to mean:

1. _____ hemorrhage into the spinal cord

2. _____ sarcoma of bone marrow (cells)

3. _____ softening of the spinal cord

4. _____ tumor containing myeloblasts

E. Using the word root/combining form cost/o (ribs) or stern/o (breastbone), build medical terms to mean:

1. _____ pertaining to a rib and its cartilage

2. _____ pain in a rib (or in the intercostal spaces)

3. _____ relating to above the sternum

4. _____ resembling the breastbone

F. Using the word root/combining form arthr/o (joint) or chondr/o (cartilage), build medical words to mean:

1. _____ a germ cell that forms cartilage

2. _____ the science or study of cartilage

3. _____ cartilage in an angioma

4. _____ cartilaginous sarcoma

5. _____ inflammation of a joint

6. _____ instrument to cut into a joint

7. _____ joint disease

8. _____ pertaining to a rib and its cartilage (junction)

G. Using the word root/combining form pelv/i (pelvic bone) or lumb/o (lumbar, loins), build medical terms to mean:

1. _____ instrument for measuring the pelvis

2. _____ pain in the loin or lower back

3. _____ pertaining to the loins and ribs

H. Using the word root/combining form pub/o (pubic bone, os pubis) or condyl/o (condyle), build medical words that mean:

1. _____ pertaining to the os pubis and femur

2. _____ resembling a condyle

3. _____ excision of a condyle

I. Using the word root/combining form my/o (muscle), build medical words that mean:

1. _____ tumor containing muscle tissue

2. _____ hardening of a muscle

3. _____ plastic repair of muscle tissue

4. _____ rupture of a muscle

5. _____ a bony (growth or) tumor in muscle tissue

WORKSHEET 2

Fill in the correct word from the right hand column that matches the definition in the statements below.

1. _____ incomplete or partial dislocation   Claudication

2. _____ softening of the bones due to lack of vitamin D   Myasthenia gravis

3. _____ a contracted state of the cervical muscles   Muscular dystrophy

4. _____ limping   Rickets

5. _____ degeneration of the muscles   Sequestrum

6. _____ a congenital deformity of the foot, which is twisted out of shape or position   Subluxation

7. _____ part of a dead or necrosed bone that has become separated from surrounding tissue   Talipes

8. _____ chronic neuromuscular disorder characterized by weakness manifested in ocular muscles, resulting in bilateral ptosis of the eyelids   Wryneck

230

WORKSHEET 3

Build a surgical term for the following:

1. _____ excision of one or more of the phalanges (bones of a finger or toe)

2. _____ surgical incision of the thorax (chest wall)

3. _____ surgical puncture of the chest wall (to remove fluids)

4. _____ excision of a vertebra or part of one

5. _____ surgical binding of a joint; artificial ankylosis

6. _____ artificial breaking of an ankylosed joint to provide movement

7. _____ plastic repair of the bones

8. _____ surgical fracture of a bone

9. _____ plastic repair of muscle tissue

10. _____ partial or complete removal of a limb

WORKSHEET 4

Define the following diagnostic terms. Use the dictionary as a reference.

1. greenstick fracture _____

2. simple fracture _____

3. compound fracture _____

4. rickets _____

5. gout _____

6. kyphosis _____

7. scoliosis _____

8. lordosis _____

9. Paget's disease _____

10. Ewing's sarcoma _____

232   WORKSHEET 5

Label the diagram below, and check your answers with Figure 10-2.

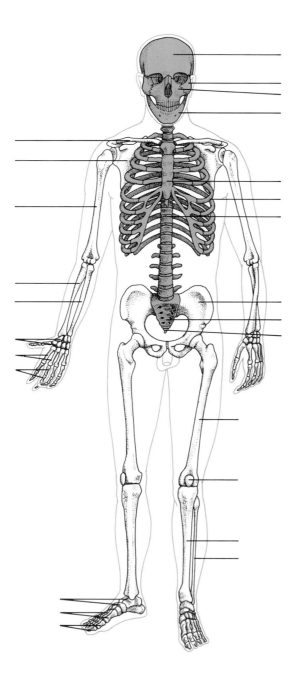

Skull (cranium)

Zygomatic bone

Maxilla

Mandible

Sternum

Ribs

Vertebral
column

Pelvis

Sacrum

Coccyx

Femur

Patella

Tibia

Fibula

Clavicle

Scapula

Humerus

Radius

Ulna

Carpals

Metacarpals

Phalanges

Tarsals

Metatarsals

Phalanges

WORKSHEET 6

Label the diagram below, and check your answers with Figure 10-1.

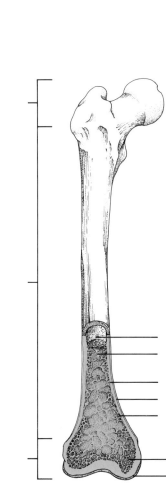

Proximal
epiphysis

Diaphysis

Distal
epiphysis

Marrow

Medullary (marrow)
cavity

Compact bone

Periosteum

Endosteum

Spongy bone

Articular cartilage

234   WORKSHEET 7

Label the diagram below, and check your answers with Figure 10-8.

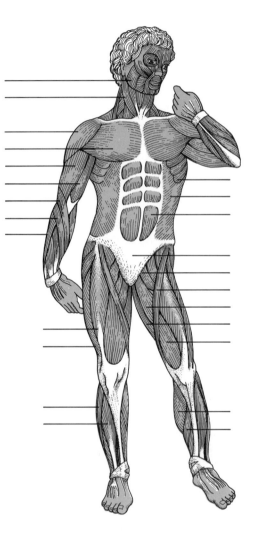

Masseter

Sternocleidomastoid

Deltoid

Pectoralis major

Triceps—lateral head

Biceps

Brachioradialis

Extensor carpi
radialis longus

Extensor digitorum

Rectus femoris

Vastus lateralis

Peroneus longus

Tibialis anterior

Serratus anterior

External oblique

Rectus abdominis

Aponeurosis

Pectineus

Sartorius

Adductor longus

Gracilis

Vastus medialis

Gastrocnemius

Soleus

WORKSHEET 8

Label the diagram below, and check your answers with Figure 10-9.

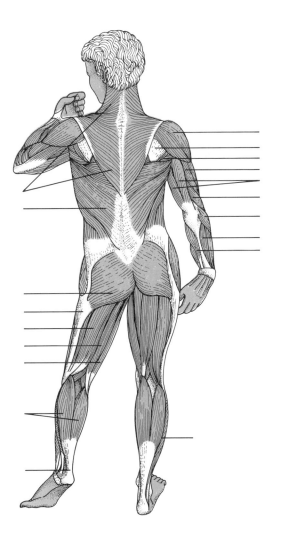

Deltoid

Infraspinatus

Teres major

Brachialis

Triceps

Brachioradialis

Extensor carpi
radialis longus

Extensor carpi
radialis brevis

Flexor carpi
ulnaris

Soleus

Trapezius

Latissimus dorsi

Gluteus maximus

Iliotibial band

Biceps femoris

Semitendinosus

Gracilis

Gastrocnemius

Achilles tendon

WORKSHEET 9

Special Procedures, Pharmacology, and Abbreviations

Choose the word(s) that best describes the following statements:

amputation	EMG
antihyperuricemics	HPN
arthrocentesis	L-3
arthroclasia	myelography
arthrodesis	myotasis
arthrography	prosthesis
bone scan	rachicentesis
chrysotherapy	skin biopsy
corticosteroids	thermography

1. _____ a radiograph of the spinal subarachnoid space taken after an opaque medium or air is injected into the spinal subarachnoid space. It shows distortions of the spinal cord caused by tumors, cysts, herniated intervertebral disks, or other lesions

2. _____ puncture into the spinal column

3. _____ a specimen is lightly scraped from patient's skin to confirm inflammatory connective tisue diseases

4. _____ stretching of a muscle

5. _____ oral or injectable gold salts are administered as a treatment for rheumatoid arthritis

6. _____ a major anti-inflammatory drug used for bone and joint disorders

7. _____ used to treat gout by suppressing formation or increasing elimination of uric acid

8. _____ third lumbar vertebra

9. _____ electromyography

10. _____ the joint is passively ranged while a series of radiographs are taken. This is preceded by injection of a radiopaque substance or air into the joint cavity

11. _____ replacement of a missing part by an artificial substitute such as an artificial extremity

12. _____ surgical immobilization of a joint

13. _____ partial or complete removal of a limb

14. _____ herniated nucleus pulposus

15. _____ measures the heat radiating from the skin surface, and is used to investigate the pathophysiology of inflamed joints

CHAPTER 11

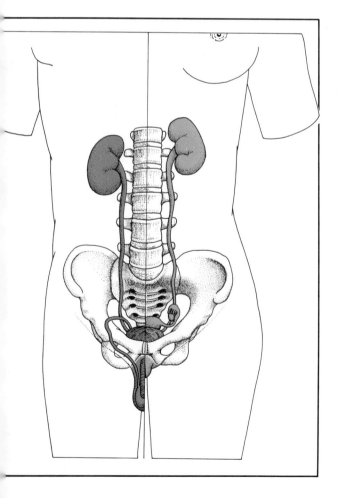

Urogenital System

STUDENT OBJECTIVES

Upon completion of this chapter, you will be able to do the following:

List the macroscopic structures of the urinary system, and describe how each of these function.

Describe the structure and function of the nephron.

Explain the physiological activities involved in the formation of urine.

Identify the structures associated with the reproductive process in the male.

Identify the word roots/combining forms and suffixes associated with the urogenital system.

Identify and discuss the pathology related to the urogenital system.

Identify radiographic, endoscopic, laboratory, and surgical procedures and abbreviations related to the urogenital system.

Discuss the pharmacology related to the treatment of disorders associated with the urogenital system.

Build and analyze diagnostic, symptomatic, and surgical terms related to the urogenital system by completing the worksheets.

240 ANATOMY AND PHYSIOLOGY OF THE UROGENITAL SYSTEM

The male and female urinary systems consist of four major structures: a pair of kidneys, two ureters, a bladder, and a urethra. This chapter presents information on these structures. In addition, it includes a discussion of the male reproductive system, since some of the male reproductive organs use urinary structures (Fig. 11-1).

Urinary System

The urinary system acts as the regulator of extracellular products of the body by determining the harmful products in the blood plasma and selectively filtering them from the blood. Included in the products that must be removed from the body are nitrogenous wastes and excess fluid electrolytes (sodium, potassium, and calcium). One of the nitrogenous prod-

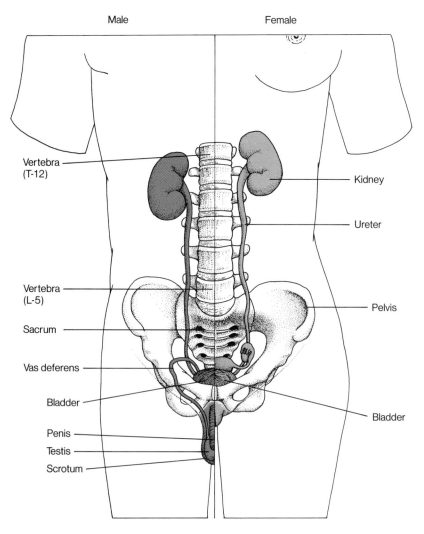

Figure 11-1. Macroscopic structures of the urogenital system.

ucts is urea. This substance is produced when body tissues metabolize protein. High concentrations of urea in the blood cause a toxic condition known as uremia. The blood collects urea and other waste materials from body tissues and conveys these materials to the kidneys. In the kidneys, microscopic structures called nephrons filter these substances from the blood as they form a complex fluid called urine. Urine is eventually expelled from the body.

MACROSCOPIC STRUCTURES OF THE URINARY SYSTEM

Figure 11-2 illustrates the macroscopic structures of the urinary system. Study and identify each structure as you read the following material.

Two (1) **kidneys**, each about the size of a fist, are located in the retroperitoneal area of the abdominal cavity. A concave medial border gives the kidney its beanlike shape. Near the medial border is a slitlike aperture, the (2) **hilus** or **hilum**. It serves as an opening for a (3) **renal vein** and a (4) **renal artery** to enter the kidney. The renal artery carries blood that is laden with waste products to the microscopic filtering tubules located within the kidney for purification. After the blood is cleansed, it leaves the kidney by way of the renal vein. The waste material, now in the form of urine, is carried to a hollow chamber, the (5) **renal**

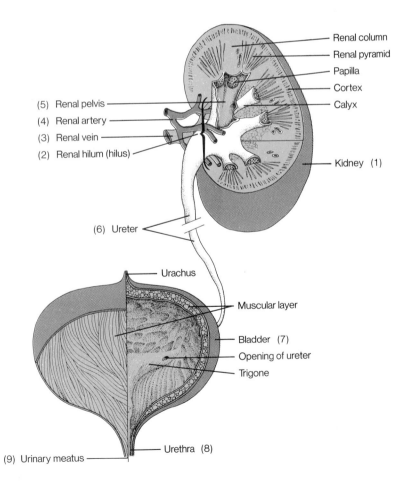

Figure 11–2. Macroscopic urinary structures.

pelvis, located at the hilus. This chamber is an enlarged funnel-shaped extension of the ureter at the entrance to the kidney. Each (6) **ureter** is a slender tube about 10 to 12 inches long that conveys urine, in peristaltic waves, to the bladder. The (7) **bladder**, which is an expandable hollow organ, acts as a temporary reservoir for urine. During micturition (voiding), urine is expelled from the bladder through the (8) **urethra**, a membranous tube that terminates at the (9) **urinary meatus**. The urethra is approximately 1¹/₂ inches in women and about 7 inches in men.

MICROSCOPIC STRUCTURES OF THE URINARY SYSTEM

Microscopic examination of kidney tissue reveals the presence of approximately 1 million tiny functional structures called **nephrons**. These little filtering units are responsible for maintaining homeostasis (a stable optimal internal environment) by continually adjusting the conditions that are necessary for survival. When the level of various products in the blood becomes elevated beyond a normal range, or reaches the renal threshold, nephrons selectively remove those products from the blood to re-establish a level that can sustain life. The substances that are removed by nephrons are the end products of metabolism—urea, uric acid, and creatinine. Nephrons also extract any excess electrolytes. Some pathological

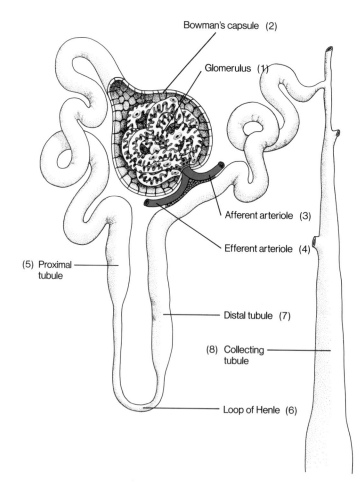

Figure 11–3. A nephron.

states may cause certain undesirable substances to appear in the blood. These may also be removed by the nephrons. For example, when the blood sugar level becomes elevated, as in diabetes mellitus, the excess sugar is filtered from the blood and is removed from the body in the urine.

Figure 11-3 is an illustration of a nephron. Locate each structure as you read the following material.

Each nephron includes a **renal corpuscle** and a **renal tubule**. The renal corpuscle is composed of a tuft of capillaries, the (1) **glomerulus**, and a modified, funnel-shaped end of the renal tubule, (2) **Bowman's capsule**. This capsule encases the glomerulus. An (3) **afferent arteriole** conveys blood to the glomerulus, and a smaller (4) **efferent arteriole** carries blood away from the glomerulus. As the efferent arteriole passes behind the renal corpuscle, it forms the **peritubular capillaries**.

Each renal tubule consists of four sections: the (5) **proximal tubule**, followed by the narrow (6) **loop of Henle**, then a larger portion, the (7) **distal tubule**, and finally, the (8) **collecting tubule**.

The nephron removes waste products from the blood by three physiological activities: filtration, reabsorption, and secretion. All of these activities are performed by different sections of the nephron.

The first phase of urine production, filtration, takes place in the renal corpuscle. Here, water, electrolytes, sugar, amino acids, and other compounds pass from the blood in the glomerulus into Bowman's capsule. The fluid that is formed is called filtrate. The next phase of urine production starts with the passing of filtrate through the four sections of the tubule. As the filtrate travels the long and twisted pathway, most of the water and some of the electrolytes and amino acids are absorbed by the peritubular capillaries, thus re-entering the circulating blood. The final stage of urine production occurs when specialized cells of the collecting tubules secrete ammonia, uric acid, and other substances directly into the lumen of the tubule. The formation of urine is now completed. It is passed from the collecting tubules to the renal pelvis, or the basin of the kidney.

Male Reproductive System

The male reproductive system serves two important functions. First, it produces sperm, the male sex cell, which contains one half of the genetic material necessary to produce a living being. Second, it provides the structures necessary to transport and maintain viable sperm. As you read this section, identify the structures in Figure 11-4.

The primary male reproductive organ consists of a pair of (1) **testes** (singular, **testis**), which are located in an external sac, the (2) **scrotum**. Within the testes are numerous small tubes that twist and coil to form the **seminiferous tubules**. These structures produce sperm, which is the male sex cell. The testes also secrete testosterone, an androgenic hormone that develops and maintains secondary sex characteristics and influences adult male sexual behavior. Lying over the superior surface of each testis is a single, tightly coiled tube, the (3) **epididymis**. This structure stores sperm after it leaves the seminiferous tubules. The epididymis is the first duct through which sperm passes after its production in the testes. Tracing the duct upward, the epididymis forms the (4) **vas deferens (seminal duct** or **ductus deferens)**, which is a narrow tube that passes through the inguinal canal into the abdominal cavity. The vas extends over the top and down the posterior surface of the bladder, where it joins a duct leading from an accessory sex gland, the (5) **seminal vesicle**. The union of the vas and the duct from the seminal vesicle forms the (6) **ejaculatory duct**.

The seminal vesicle secretes approximately 60 percent of the fluid that is ultimately ejaculated during sexual climax. This fluid contains nutrients that support sperm viability.

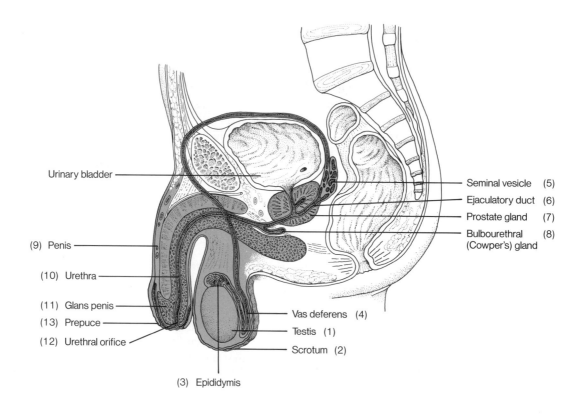

Urinary bladder

Seminal vesicle (5)
Ejaculatory duct (6)
Prostate gland (7)
Bulbourethral (8)
(Cowper's) gland

(9) Penis

(10) Urethra

(11) Glans penis
(13) Prepuce
(12) Urethral orifice

Vas deferens (4)
Testis (1)
Scrotum (2)

(3) Epididymis

Figure 11–4. *The male reproductive system.*

The ejaculatory duct passes at an angle through the (7) **prostate gland**, which is a triple-lobed organ fused to the base of the bladder where it joins the urethra. The prostate secretes a thin, alkaline substance that accounts for about 30 percent of the seminal fluid. Its alkalinity helps protect the sperm from the acidic environments of both the male urethra and the female vagina. Two pea-shaped glands, (8) **Cowper's glands**, or **bulbourethral glands**, are located below the prostate. They are connected by a small duct to the urethra. Cowper's glands also provide an alkaline fluid that is necessary for the viability of the sperm. The (9) **penis** is the male organ of copulation. It is a cylindrical organ composed of erectile tissue, and it encloses the (10) **urethra**. The urethra expels both semen and urine from the body. During ejaculation, the sphincter at the base of the bladder is closed. This not only stops the urine from being expelled with the semen, but also prevents the sperm from entering the bladder.

The enlarged tip of the penis is the (11) **glans penis**. It contains the (12) **urethral orifice (meatus)**. A movable hood of skin, called (13) **prepuce** or **foreskin**, covers the glans penis.

WORD ROOTS/COMBINING FORMS RELATED TO THE
UROGENITAL SYSTEM

WORD ROOT/ COMBINING FORM	MEANING	EXAMPLE	PRONUNCIATION
Urinary			

cyst/o		cyst/o/scopy
		    visual
		    examination
			sĭs - TŎS - kō - pē

vesic/o	bladder	vesic/o/tomy incision	věs - ĭ - KŎT - ō - mē

glomerul/o	glomerulus	glomerul/o/nephr/itis
		    kid- inflam-
		    ney mation
			glō - měr - ū - lō - ně - FRĪ - tĭs

nephr/o		nephr/o/pexy suspension	NĚF - rō - pěk - sē
ren/o	kidney	ren/al pertaining to	RĒ - năl
pyel/o	renal pelvis	pyel/itis inflammation	pī - ě - LĪ - tĭs
ureter/o	ureter	ureter/ectasis dilation	ū - rē - těr - ĔK - tăh - sĭs
urethr/o	urethra	urethr/itis inflammation	ū - rē - THRĪ - tĭs

ur/o	urine	ur/o/log/ ist
		    study one who
		    of specializes
			ū - RŎL - ō - jĭst

Male Reproductive			
andr/o	male	andr/o/gen to produce	ĂN - drō - jěn
balan/o	glans penis	balan/itis inflammation	băl - ă - NĪ - tĭs
epididym/o	epididymis	epididym/itis inflammation	ěp - ĭ - dĭd - ĭ - MĪ - tĭs
orchid/o		orchid/ectomy excision	ŏr - kĭ - DĔK - tō - mē
orchi/o		orchi/ectomy excision	ŏr - kē - ĔK - tō - mē
orch/o	testes	orch/itis inflammation	ŏr - KĪ - tĭs
test/o		test/itis inflammation	těs - TĪ - tĭs

Continued on following page

WORD ROOTS/COMBINING FORMS RELATED TO THE UROGENITAL SYSTEM—*Continued*

WORD ROOT/ COMBINING FORM	MEANING	EXAMPLE	PRONUNCIATION
Urinary			
prostat/o	prostate	prostat/ectomy excision	prŏs - tăh - TĔK - tō - mē
spermat/o	sperm	spermat/ic pertaining to	spĕr - MĂ - tĭk
vas/o	vas deferens, vessel	vas/ectomy excision	văh - SĔK - tō - mē
vesicul/o	seminal vesicle	vesicul/itis inflammation	vĕ - sĭk - ū - LĪ - tis
Miscellaneous			
albumin/o	albumin, white protein	albumin/oid resemble	ăl - BŪ - mĭ - noid
bacteri/o	bacteria	bacteri/al pertaining to	băk - TĒ - rē - ăl
crypt/o	hidden	crypt/orchid/ism testes abnormal condition	krĭpt - ŎR - kĭd - ĭzm
glyc/o		glyc/o/gen to produce	GLĪ - kŏ - jĕn
gluc/o	sugar	gluco/gen/ ic for- pertain- mation ing to	gloo - kō - JĔN - ĭk
glucos/o		glucos/uria urine	gloo - kō - SŪ - rē - ăh
noct/o	night	noct/uria urine	nŏk - TŪ - rē - ăh
olig/o	scanty	olig/uria urine	ŏl - ĭg - Ū - rē - ăh
py/o	pus	py/uria urine	pĭ - Ū - rē - ăh

SUFFIX	MEANING	EXAMPLE	PRONUNCIATION
-chrome	color	ur/o/chrome urine	Ū - rō - krōm
-genesis	origin, beginning process	spermat/o/genesis sperm	spĕr - măt - ō - GĔN - ĕ - sĭs
-lith	calculus, stone	nephr/o/lith kidney	NĔF - rō - lĭth
-lithiasis	presence, condition, or formation of calculi	nephr/o/lithiasis kidney	nĕf - rō - lĭth - Ī - ă - sĭs
-uria	urine	dys/uria pain-ful	dĭs - Ū - rĕ - ăh

PATHOLOGY OF THE UROGENITAL SYSTEM

Pyelonephritis

Pyelonephritis is one of the most common forms of kidney disease. In this disorder, bacteria invade the renal pelvis and the tissue of the kidney. In many instances, pyelonephritis is often a consequence of a lower-urinary-tract infection that has ascended to the kidney via the ureters. When the infection is severe, lesions form in the renal pelvis.

Characteristic of this disease is urine that contains large quantities of bacteria **(bacteri-uria)** and white blood cells **(pyuria)**. When lesions are present, blood is found in the urine **(hematuria)**. The onset of the disease is usually sudden, and the symptoms include chills, fever, nausea, and vomiting. Treatment includes the use of antibiotics.

Glomerulonephritis

Glomerulonephritis occurs when the walls of the glomeruli become inflamed. The most common cause of glomerular inflammation is a reaction to the toxins given off by pathogenic streptococci that have recently infected another part of the body, especially the throat. Glomerulonephritis is also associated with the autoimmune diseases, such as systemic lupus erythematosus, polyarthritis nodosa, and scleroderma.

When the glomerular membrane is inflamed, it becomes highly permeable and permits blood cells and protein to enter the filtrate. This results in the presence of protein in the urine **(proteinuria)** and hematuria. In some cases, protein solidifies in the tubules of the nephrons and forms solid masses that take the shape of the tubules in which they develop. These masses are called casts. They often pass out of the kidney by way of the urine and may be visible during the microscopic examination of the urine. The majority of patients with acute glomerulonephritis associated with a streptococcal infection recover with no residual kidney damage.

Nephrolithiasis

Nephrolithiasis, or kidney stones **(renal calculi)**, form when certain urine salts, which are normally dissolved in urine, become solidified. As these stones increase in size, they may obstruct the urinary structures. When they lodge in the ureters, urine is hindered from flowing into the bladder, often causing spasms of the ureters **(colic)**. The urine now accumulates both in the renal pelvis and the tubules, causing them to dilate. This distention of the renal pelvis and kidney is known as **hydronephrosis**. For calculi that cannot be dislodged or dissolved, surgical removal **(lithotomy)** may be necessary.

Bladder Neck Obstructions

Bladder neck obstruction occurs when there is a blockage of the bladder outlet. This obstruction may be the result of an enlarged prostate gland **(prostatic hypertrophy)** or it may be caused by the presence of an obstructive mass, such as a calculus, blood clot, or tumor. The resulting distention of the bladder may lead to hydronephrosis accompanied by bladder infection **(cystitis)**. The patient experiences a need to void but is only able to void small quantities at a time. This is referred to as **retention with overflow**. Correction of bladder neck obstruction includes surgery to either relieve or remove the obstruction.

Benign Prostatic Hypertrophy

Benign prostatic hypertrophy is often associated with the aging process. The prostate enlarges and decreases the lumen of the urethra. Inability to empty the bladder completely may cause cystitis, which may lead to nephritis. Surgical removal of the prostate may be necessary. The different operative procedures include the removal of the prostate through the perineum **(perineal prostatectomy)**, excision through the urethra **(transurethral resection—TUR)**, or excision through an abdominal opening above the pubis and directly over the bladder **(suprapubic prostatectomy)**.

Phimosis

Phimosis is a narrowing **(stenosis)** of the opening of the foreskin **(prepuce)** that prevents the retraction of the foreskin over the glans penis. This may interfere with urination or cause infection. Treatment for this condition is the removal of the foreskin **(circumcision)**.

Cryptorchidism

Failure of the testes to descend into the scrotal sac prior to birth is called cryptorchidism. In about 80 percent of infants born with cryptorchidism, the testes will descend spontaneously by the end of the first year. If the testes do not descend by that time, correction of the disorder involves surgical suspension of the testes in the scrotum **(orchidopexy or orchiopexy)**. This is usually done between 1 and 5 years of age. Herniorrhaphy may accompany this operation since an inguinal hernia is often present in cryptorchidism.

Acute Tubular Necrosis

The two major causes of acute tubular necrosis (ATN) include ischemia and nephrotoxic injury. In ATN, the tubular portion of the nephron is injured either through a decreased blood supply or the presence of toxic substances (generally following ingestion of certain toxic chemical agents). Ischemia may be the result of circulatory collapse, severe hypotension, hemorrhage, dehydration, or other disorders that affect blood supply. In the hospital, the use of antibiotics or contrast media may be the source of nephrotoxic injury.

Symptoms include oliguria and increased calcium in the blood (**hypercalcemia**). Other possible complications of ATN are congestive heart failure, pulmonary edema, and uremic pericarditis.

When tubular damage is not too severe, the disorder is potentially reversible.

OTHER TERMS RELATED TO THE UROGENITAL SYSTEM

TERM	MEANING	PRONUNCIATION
Urinary		
anuria	complete absence of urine production	ăh - NŪ - rē - ăh
azotemia	metabolic wastes (urea, creatinine, and uric acid) in the blood	ăz - ō - TĒ - mē - ăh
enuresis	incontinence or involuntary discharge of urine: at night, nocturnal; during the day, diurnal	ĕn - ū - RĒ - sĭs
frequency	voiding at frequent intervals either in small or large amounts	FRĒ - kwĕn - sē
hemodialysis	removal of chemical substances from the blood by passing it through tubes made of semipermeable membranes. The tubes are continually bathed by solutions that selectively remove harmful products	hē - mō - dī - ĂL - ĭ - sĭs
hesitancy	an involuntary delay in or the inability to start the urinary stream	HĔZ - ĭ - tĕn - sē
lithotriptor	device that destroys urinary stones by employing laser technology	LĬTH - ō - trĭp - tŏr
oliguria	production of less than 200 ml of urine per 24 hours	ŏl - ĭg - Ū - rē - ăh
peritoneal dialysis	removal of toxic substances from the body by perfusing the peritoneal cavity with specific warm sterile chemical solutions	pĕr - ĭ - tō - NĒ - ăl dī - ĂL - ĭ - sĭs
uremia	toxic condition associated with renal	ū - RĒ - mē - ăh

Continued on following page

OTHER TERMS RELATED TO THE UROGENITAL SYSTEM—Continued

TERM	MEANING	PRONUNCIATION
Urinary		
	insufficiency in which nitrogenous products are found within the blood	
urgency	the need to void immediately. Urgency commonly accompanies frequency in persons with urinary tract infections	ŬR - jĕn - sē
Genital		
aspermia	lack of or failure to ejaculate semen	ăh - SPĔR - mē - ăh
epispadias	a malformation in which the urethra opens on the dorsum of the penis	ĕp - ĭ - SPĀ - dē - ăs
hydrocele	the accumulation of serous fluid in a saclike cavity, especially the testes and associated structures	HĪ - drō - sēl
hypospadias	a developmental anomaly in the male where the urethra opens on the underside of the penis, or in extreme cases, on the perineum	hī - pō - SPĀ - dē - ăs
impotence	condition characterized by the inability to achieve an erection	ĬM - pō - tĕns
semen	the thick, white secretion of the reproductive organs of the male. This fluid is composed of spermatozoa and the mixed product of various glands, including the prostate and bulbourethral glands	SĒ - mĕn
varicocele	swelling and distention of veins of the spermatic cord	VĂR - ĭ - kō - sēl

SPECIAL PROCEDURES RELATED TO THE UROGENITAL SYSTEM

RADIOGRAPHIC PROCEDURES

TERM	DESCRIPTION
intravenous pyelography (IVP), excretory urography	radiopaque contrast medium is injected intravenously. As it is filtered from the blood by the urinary structures, the kidneys, renal pelvis, ureters, and bladder are visualized on radiographs or by

Continued on following page

TERM	DESCRIPTION
	fluoroscopy. IVPs are used for diagnosing pathological and congenital abnormalities in the urinary structures. Tumors or cysts often distort the bean-shaped appearance of the kidney. Blockage in the renal artery will cause the kidney to remain unvisualized on the radiograph. These and other abnormalities, including those of the ureters and bladder, can be determined by intravenous pyelography
cystography	radiopaque contrast medium is introduced into the bladder through a catheter, providing visualization of the bladder. Shadows in the bladder frequently indicate the presence of tumors, while indentations of the bladder may indicate pelvic tumors and hematomas following pelvic bone fractures. Vesicoureteral reflux (abnormal backflow of urine from the bladder to the ureters) is determined by a distention of the ureters. A seepage of the contrast medium into the peritoneal cavity is seen in traumatic rupture of the bladder
retrograde pyelography (RP)	is more involved than cystography. It includes passing a catheter from the urethra to the urinary bladder, then to the right or left ureter, and injecting a contrast medium. This study provides detailed visualization of the urinary collecting system. It is chiefly used to diagnose obstruction
nephrotomography	a study in which several planes of the kidney are visualized. The purpose of this test is to differentiate solid renal and adrenal tumors from benign renal cysts. This test is performed in conjunction with intravenous pyelography

ENDOSCOPIC PROCEDURES

TERM	DESCRIPTION
cystoscopy	permits an examination for inflammation, calculi, tumors, and deformities of the bladder, ureters, and prostate
nephroscopy	examination of the kidney using a specialized three-channel endoscope. The three channels provide for telescope, fiberoptic light input, and irrigation. The nephroscope is passed through a small incision made in the renal pelvis. Kidney pathology and congenital deformities may be observed
resectoscopy	permits transurethral resection of the prostate
urethroscopy	permits the visualization of the urethra. It is often used for lithotripsy or for transurethral resection of the prostate

SURGICAL PROCEDURES

TERM	DESCRIPTION	PRONUNCIATION
Urinary		
cystectomy	excision of bladder	sĭs - TĔK - tō - mē
cystolithotomy	incision of the bladder for stone removal	sĭs - tō - lĭ - THŎT - ō - mē
cystostomy	surgical incision of the bladder to establish a temporary opening	sĭs - TŎS - tō - mē
cystoplasty	surgical repair of a cystocele	SĬS - tō - plăs - tē
lithotripsy	crushing of a calculus in the bladder or urethra	LĬTH - ō - trĭp - sē
nephrectomy	removal of a kidney	nĕ - FRĔK - tō - mē
nephrolysis	surgical separation of an inflamed kidney from perinephric adhesions	nĕ - FRŎL - ĭ - sĭs
nephrorrhaphy	suturing of a kidney	nĕf - RŎR - ăh - fē
nephrostomy	formation of an artificial fistula into the renal pelvis	nĕ - FRŎS - tō - mē
nephroureterectomy	surgical removal of the kidney and part or all of the ureter	nĕf - rō - ū - rē - tĕr - ĔK - tō - mē
pyelolithotomy	removal of a calculus from the renal pelvis by an incision	pĭ - ĕ - lō - lĭ - THŎT - ō - mē
pyeloplasty	surgical repair of the renal pelvis	PĪ - ĕ - lō - plăs - tē
renal biopsy	removal of a small piece of kidney tissue for microscopic evaluation	RĒ - năl/BĪ - ŏp - sē
renal transplant	incorporating a kidney from a compatible donor into a recipient	RĒ - năl/TRĂNS - plănt
ureteropyelostomy	anastomosis of ureter and renal pelvis	ū - rē - tĕr - ō - pĭ - ĕ - LŎS - tō - mē
ureterovesicostomy	reimplantation of a ureter into the bladder	ū - rē - tĕr - ō - vĕs - ĭ - KŎS - tō - mē
ureterectomy	removal of a ureter	ū - rē - tĕr - ĔK - tō - mē

Continued on following page

SURGICAL PROCEDURES—*Continued*

TERM	DESCRIPTION	PRONUNCIATION
Urinary		
urethrectomy	excision of part or all of the urethra	ū - rĕ - THRĔK - tō - mē
urethropexy	surgical fixation of the urethra	ū - RĒ - thrō - pĕk - sĕ
urethroplasty	surgical correction of the urethra	ū - RĒ - thrō - plăs - tē
Genital		
circumcision	surgical removal of the end of the prepuce of the glans penis	sĕr - kŭm - SĬZH - ŭn
epididymectomy	excision of the epididymis	ĕp - ĭ - dĭd - ĭ - MĔK - tō - mē
orchiectomy, orchidectomy, orchectomy	removal of the testes	ŏr - kē - ĔK - tō - mē ŏr - kĭ - DĔK - tō - mē ŏr - KĔK - tō - mē
orchidoplasty, orchiopexy	surgical transfer of an undescended testicle to the scrotum	ŎR - kĭ - dō - plăs - tē ŏr - kē - ō - PĔK - sē
orchotomy	incision of a testis	ŏr - KŎT - ō - mē
prostatectomy	removal of the prostate gland	prŏs - tă - TĔK - tō - mē
prostatomy	incision into the prostate	prŏs - TĂT - ō - mē
vasectomy	removal of all or a segment of the vas deferens; bilateral vasectomy results in sterility	vah - SĔK - tō - mē

LABORATORY PROCEDURES

TERM	DESCRIPTION
blood urea nitrogen (BUN)	a widely used test that assesses the excretory function of the kidney. Urea, which is an end product of protein catabolism, is formed in the liver and excreted into the blood. In normal kidney function, urea is constantly being filtered from the blood, resulting in a blood urea level that is relatively low. Nearly all primary kidney diseases will cause the blood urea level to elevate since the kidney is unable to remove this substance from the blood. The primary kidney diseases include glo-

Continued on following page

LABORATORY PROCEDURES—*Continued*

TERM	DESCRIPTION
	merulonephritis, pyelonephritis, acute tubular necrosis, and urinary obstruction due to calculi or tumors
urinalysis	one of the most widely used laboratory tests. It provides general information regarding the health of the body as a whole as well as specific information on the condition of the urinary structures
semen analysis	one of the most important aspects of the infertility work-up. Infertility of the male is the cause or contributing factor in 30 percent to 40 percent of the infertility cases. After 3 to 5 days of sexual abstinence, sperm is collected and analyzed for volume, sperm count, motility, and morphology. This test is also used to document adequate sterilization after a vasectomy. If any sperm are seen 6 weeks after vasectomy, the adequacy of the surgery must be questioned

PHARMACOLOGY RELATED TO THE UROGENITAL SYSTEM

MEDICATION	ACTION
diuretic	increases the production of urine either by increasing glomerular filtration or decreasing tubular reabsorption
estrogenic hormones (female hormones)	used to treat prostatic cancer in males who refuse to undergo castration or who have a recurrence of cancer after castration. These hormones suppress gonadotropic and testicular androgenic hormones. In females, these drugs are used for birth control and for reduction of discomfort at menopause
gonadotropin	hormonal preparation used to raise sperm count in cases of infertility
spermicidal preparations	substances that destroy sperm. They are used by the female within the vagina for contraceptive purposes
uricosuric agents	drugs that increase the urinary excretion of uric acid (often used in the treatment of gout)

ABBREVIATIONS RELATED TO THE UROGENITAL SYSTEM

ABBREVIATION	MEANING
A/G	albumin/globulin ratio
AGN	acute glomerulonephritis
ATN	acute tubular necrosis
BPH	benign prostatic hypertrophy
BUN	blood urea nitrogen

Continued on following page

ABBREVIATIONS RELATED TO THE UROGENITAL SYSTEM—*Continued*

ABBREVIATION	MEANING
cysto	cystoscopic examination
GU	genitourinary
IVP	intravenous pyelogram
KUB	kidney, ureter, bladder
pH	hydrogen ion concentration
PKU	phenylketonuria
RP	retrograde pyelogram
TUR; TURP	transurethral resection (for prostatectomy)
UA	urinalysis
UTI	urinary tract infection

WORKSHEET 1

A. Using the word root/combining form nephr/o (kidney), build medical words to mean:

1. _____ pertaining to the kidney

2. _____ inflammation of a kidney

3. _____ pertaining to the kidney and the heart

4. _____ dropping or prolapse of a kidney

5. _____ pertaining to originating or arising in the kidney

6. _____ calculus or stone in the kidney

7. _____ tumor of the kidney

8. _____ condition of pus in the kidney

9. _____ hardening of the kidney

10. _____ water in the kidney (due to reflux)

B. Using the word root/combining form pyel/o (renal pelvis), build medical words to mean:

1. _____ dilation of the renal pelvis

2. _____ inflammation of the renal pelvis

3. _____ inflammation of the renal pelvis and bladder

4. _____ disease of the renal pelvis

C. Using the word root/combining form ureter/o (ureter), build medical words to mean:

1. _____ dilation of the ureter

2. _____ calculus in the ureter

3. _____ enlargement of the ureter

4. _____ condition of pus in the ureter

D. Using the word root/combining form cyst/o (bladder), build medical words to mean:

1. _____ inflammation of the bladder

2. _____ herniation of the bladder (into vagina)

3. _____ an endoscope to visually inspect the bladder

4. _____ pertaining to the bladder

E. Using the word root/combining form vesic/o (bladder), build medical words to mean:

1. _____ concretion of the bladder

2. _____ hernia of the bladder

3. _____ pertaining to the bladder and prostate

F. Using the word root/combining form urethr/o (urethra), build medical words to mean:

1. _____ narrowing of the urethra

2. _____ an instrument for cutting a urethral stricture

3. _____ pertaining to the urethra and prostate

G. Using the word root/combining form ur/o (urine), build medical words to mean:

1. _____ pertaining to the urinary and reproductive (organs)

2. _____ radiograph of the urinary organs

3. _____ a concretion or calculus in the urine

4. _____ one who specializes in problems associated with the urinary system

5. _____ any disease associated with the urinary system

6. _____ inflammation of the urinary bladder

H. Using the suffix -uria (urine), build medical words to mean:

1. _____ excessive urination

2. _____ blood in the urine

3. _____ pus in the urine

4. _____ sugar (glucose) in the urine

5. _____ scanty urine formation

6. _____ absence of urine production

7. _____ (frequent) nightly urination

I. Using the word root/combining forms orchid/o, orchi/o (testes), build medical words to mean:

1. _____ inflammation of the testes

2. _____ disease of the testes

3. _____ testicular pain

4. _____ pertaining to the testes

5. _____ inflammation of the testes and epididymis

J. Using the word root/combining form epididym/o (epididymis), build medical words to mean:

1. _____ inflammation of the epididymis

2. _____ inflammation of the epididymis and the testicles

K. Using the word root/combining form vesicul/o (seminal vesicle), build medical words to mean:

1. _____ radiograph of the seminal vesicle

2. _____ disease of the seminal vesicle

3. _____ inflammation of the seminal vesicle

L. Using the word root/combining form prostat/o (prostate), build medical words to mean:

1. _____ pain in the prostate

2. _____ inflammation of the prostate

3. _____ flow from the prostate

4. _____ pertaining to the prostate gland

5. _____ instrument for measuring the prostate

6. _____ pain in the prostate and bladder

M. Using the word root/combining form balan/o (glans penis), build medical words to mean:

1. _____ pertaining to the glans penis

2. _____ discharge from the glans penis

WORKSHEET 2

Fill in the correct word from the right column that matches the definitions in the statements below.

1. _____ureter_____ structure that leads from the renal pelvis to the bladder Bladder

2. _____ structure that expels urine from the body Bowman's capsule

3. _____ hollow chamber of the kidney Glans penis

4. _____ enlarged portion of tubule responsible for selective filtration Glomerulus

5. _____ portion of nephron in which casts are formed Prepuce

6. _____ cluster of capillaries in nephron Prostate

7. _____ enlarged tip of penis Renal pelvis

8. _____ foreskin covering tip of penis Seminiferous tubule

9. _____ sperm-producing structure of testes Tubule

10. _____ temporary reservoir for urine Ureter

11. _____ triple-lobed gland at base of bladder Urethra

12. _____ structure that carries sperm from testes into pelvic region Vas deferens

WORKSHEET 3

Build surgical terms for the following:

1. __vasoepididymostomy__ creation of a new opening between vas and epididymis

2. _____ removal of (a portion of) the vas deferens

3. _____ suturing of the urethra

4. _____ surgical repair of ureter and renal pelvis

5. _____ removal of the kidney and its ureter

6. _____ excision of a stone from the bladder

7. _____ surgical repair of the bladder

8. _____ suturing of the bladder

9. _____ surgical connection between the kidney and the bladder

10. _____ removal of the prostate

11. _____ incision for removal of a stone in the prostate

12. _____ surgical repair of glans penis

WORKSHEET 4

Define the following diagnostic and symptomatic terms.

1. urinalysis _____ chemical, microscopic, and physical tests performed on urine _____

2. bacteriuria _____

3. cystoscopy _____

4. hydrocele _____

5. aspermia _____

6. spermaturia _____

7. phimosis _____

8. cryptorchidism _____

9. spermatocele _____

10. anorchism _____

262 WORKSHEET 5

Special Procedures, Pharmacology, and Abbreviations

Choose the word(s) that best describes the following statements:

ATN	pH
blood urea nitrogen	PKU
cystography	resectoscopy
diuretic	retrograde pyelography
estrogenic hormones	semen analysis
gonadotropin	spermicidal preparation
intravenous pyelography	urethroscopy
nephroscopy	uricosuric agent
nephrotomography	urinalysis
	UTI

1. _____ utilization of a radiopaque dye administered intravenously to visualize the urinary structures, especially the structures of the kidney

2. _____ one of the most widely used laboratory tests that provides information on the urinary structures as well as the body as a whole

3. _____ a test that determines kidney function by assessing its ability to remove the end product of protein catabolism (urea)

4. _____ drug that increases the excretion of uric acid by the kidney (used in the treatment of gout)

5. _____ hormonal preparation used to raise sperm count in cases of infertility

6. _____ hydrogen ion concentration

7. _____ acute tubular necrosis

8. _____ increases the production of urine

9. _____ substance that destroys sperm (used for birth control)

10. _____ analysis of volume, sperm count, motility, and morphology, usually performed as part of an infertility work-up

11. _____ a procedure that uses an endoscope to permit a transurethral resection of the prostate

12. _____ a study in which several planes of the kidney are visualized

13. _____ a visualization of the urinary collecting system that includes the passing of a catheter through the lower urinary tract to the ureters for the injection of a contrast medium

14. _____ a procedure that permits visualization of the urethra, often used for lithotripsy or TURP

15. _____ a radiographic procedure that involves the introduction of a contrast medium into the bladder to visualize this structure

16. _____ urinary tract infection

264 **WORKSHEET 6**

Grammar Review—Urogenital System

Provide the adjective form for each of the following. Use the dictionary, if necessary.

1. meatus   _meatal_

2. testicle   _____

3. tube   _____

4. medulla   _____

5. scrotum   _____

Provide the plural form for each of the following:

6. calyx   _____

7. papilla   _____

8. medulla   _____

9. pelvis   _____

10. scrotum   _____

WORKSHEET 7

Label the following diagram, and check your answers with Figure 11-2.

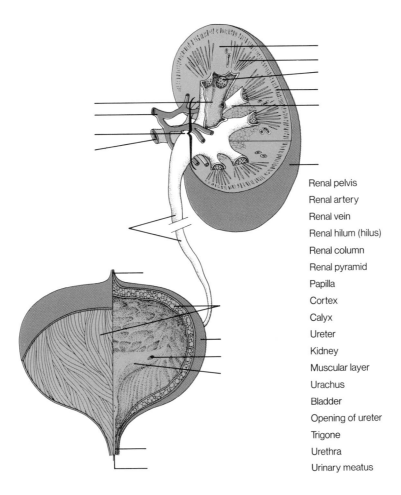

Renal pelvis

Renal artery

Renal vein

Renal hilum (hilus)

Renal column

Renal pyramid

Papilla

Cortex

Calyx

Ureter

Kidney

Muscular layer

Urachus

Bladder

Opening of ureter

Trigone

Urethra

Urinary meatus

CHAPTER 12

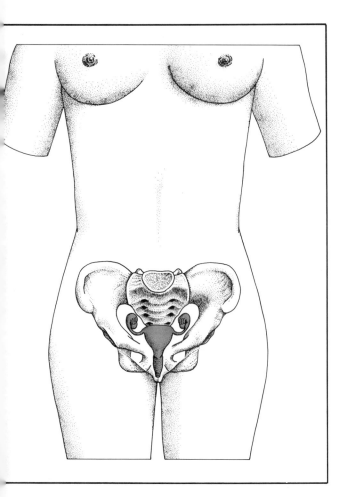

CHAPTER OUTLINE

Female Reproductive System

STUDENT OBJECTIVES

Upon completion of this chapter, you will be able to do the following:

List the organs of the female reproductive system.

Describe the position and function of each organ.

Explain the series of events associated with the maturation of the ovum.

Describe the condition and stages of pregnancy.

Identify the word roots/combining forms and suffixes associated with the female reproductive system.

Identify and discuss associated pathology related to the female reproductive system.

Identify radiographic, endoscopic, surgical, and laboratory procedures and abbreviations related to the female reproductive system.

Explain the pharmacology related to the treatment of female reproductive disorders.

Build and analyze diagnostic, symptomatic, and surgical terms related to the female reproductive system by completing the worksheets.

268 ANATOMY AND PHYSIOLOGY OF THE FEMALE REPRODUCTIVE SYSTEM

The female reproductive system (Fig. 12-1) consists of internal and external organs of reproduction, as illustrated in Figure 12-2. The internal, or essential, organs of reproduction are the (1) **ovaries**, (2) **fallopian tubes**, (3) **uterus**, and (4) **vagina**. The external genitalia include the (5) **labia majora**, (6) **labia minora**, (7) **clitoris**, **vestibule of the vagina**, and the **greater vestibular glands**, or (8) **Bartholin's glands**. The combined structures of the external genitalia are known as the vulva.

Both the cervix and vagina are lubricated by the mucus secretions of the Bartholin's glands. These glands provide lubrication during sexual intercourse by secreting a mucoid acid substance. Refer to Figure 12-3 as you read the following material.

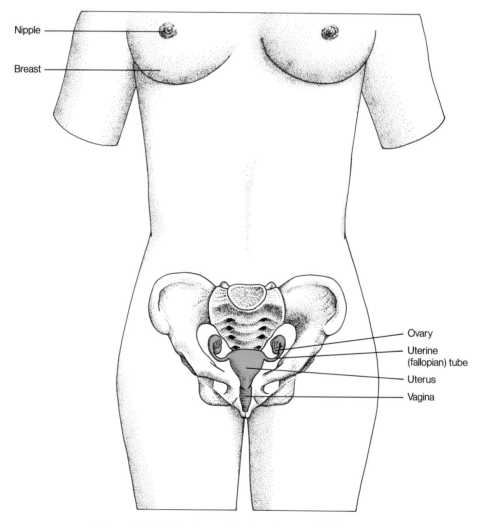

Figure 12–1. Overview of the female reproductive system.

Internal Organs of Reproduction

OVARIES

The (1) **ovaries** are almond-shaped glands located in the pelvic cavity, one on each side of the uterus. They produce both the ovum, or egg, which is the female reproductive cell, and various hormones.

Two of the hormones secreted by the ovaries are estrogen and progesterone. These hormones are responsible for the menstrual cycle and menopause. In addition, both hormones prepare the uterus for implantation of the fertilized egg, help maintain pregnancy, and promote growth of the placenta. Estrogen and progesterone also play an important role in the development of secondary sex characteristics. This is discussed in Chapter 5, Integumentary System, under Breasts.

FALLOPIAN TUBES OR OVIDUCTS

Two (2) **fallopian tubes**, or **oviducts**, extend laterally from superior angles of the uterus. They transport the ovum by a wavelike current (peristalsis) from the ovary to the uterus. In addition to conveying the ovum, an oviduct provides a passageway through which sperm travel from the uterus toward the ovary. Union of the ovum and sperm results in fertilization. Thus, a 9-month period of development (gestation, pregnancy within the uterus) begins with the fertilization of the egg.

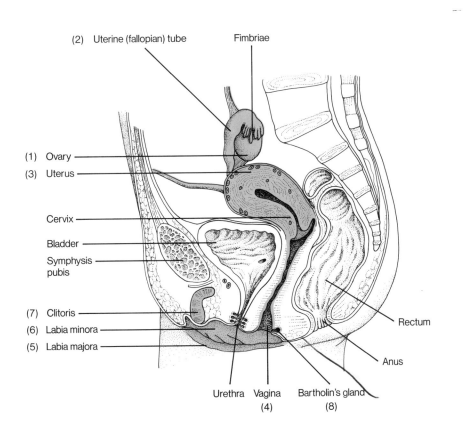

Figure 12–2. Anatomic view of the female reproductive system.

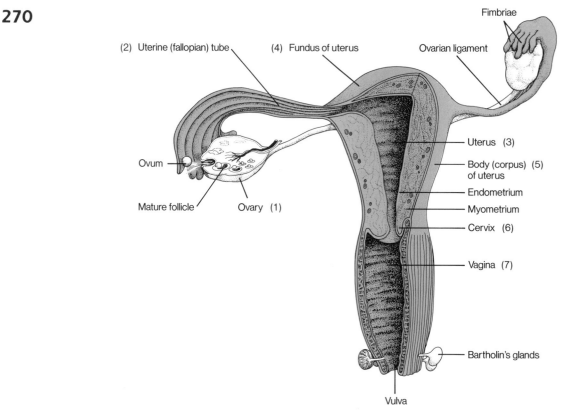

(2) Uterine (fallopian) tube

(4) Fundus of uterus

Fimbriae

Ovarian ligament

Ovum

Mature follicle

Ovary (1)

Uterus (3)

Body (corpus) (5) of uterus

Endometrium

Myometrium

Cervix (6)

Vagina (7)

Bartholin's glands

Vulva

Figure 12–3. *Female reproductive organs.*

UTERUS AND VAGINA

The (3) **uterus** is an organ that contains and nourishes the embryo from the time the fertilized egg is implanted until the fetus is born. It is a muscular, hollow, pear-shaped structure and is located in the pelvic area between the bladder and rectum. The uterus is normally in a position of anteflexion (bent forward), and it consists of three parts: the (4) **fundus**, which is the upper-rounded part; the (5) **corpus**, or body, which is the central part; and the (6) **cervix**. The cervix is sometimes referred to as the neck of the uterus, and it extends into the top portion of the vagina.

The (7) **vagina** is a muscular tube about 7½ cm long, and its lining consists of a mucous membrane fold that gives the organ an elastic quality. The vagina extends from the cervix to the exterior of the body. Besides serving as the organ of sexual intercourse and the receptor of semen, the vagina discharges the menstrual flow. The vagina also acts as a passageway for the delivery of the fetus.

Menstrual Cycle

The menstrual cycle consists of approximately 28 days and can be grouped into four phases, which are used in describing the events of the cycle. The initial menstrual period (menarche) occurs between the ages of 9 and 18, the average being 12 to 13 years of age.

PHASE 1

Menstrual phase
    (First 5 days)

A discharge that is a mixture of endometrium, blood, mucus, and vaginal cells passes from the uterine cavity to the cervix, through the vagina, and ultimately to the exterior.

PHASE 2

Pre-ovulatory phase
    (Days 6–13)

Ovarian follicles produce more estrogen, which stimulates the repair of the endometrium. During this phase, one of the secondary follicles matures into a graafian follicle, which is ready for ovulation.

PHASE 3

Ovulation
    (Day 14)

About the 14th day, the graafian follicle ruptures (ovulation), and the egg cell leaves the ovary and enters the peritoneal cavity. The egg cell is then drawn into the uterine tubes.

PHASE 4

Postovulatory phase
    (Days 15–28)

This represents the time between ovulation and the onset of the next menses.

Following ovulation, the graafian follicle collapses and forms a clot which is absorbed by the remaining follicular cells. These follicular cells enlarge, change character, and form the corpus luteum, or yellow body. The corpus luteum then secretes increasing quantities of estrogens and progesterone.

If fertilization and implantation do not occur, the decreased secretions of progesterone and estrogens (by the corpus luteum) then initiates another menstrual cycle.

Menopause

Menopause is the cessation of menses for the remainder of a woman's lifetime. It is usually diagnosed if amenorrhea (absence of menses) has persisted for 1 year and there are no other problems. The period of time in which symptoms of approaching menopause occur is known as the climacteric period. Some common manifestations during the climacteric are as follows:

Premenopausal

nervousness
irregular menses
vasomotor symptoms (due to an effect on
    the diameter of blood vessels)
instability (hot flashes)

Menopausal	frequent vasomotor symptoms
	cessation of menses
	atrophy of genitourinary tissue (wasting; a decrease in size of an organ or tissue)
Postmenopausal	occasional vasomotor symptoms
	atrophic vaginitis
	atrophy of genitourinary tissue with decreased support
	osteoporosis

Pregnancy

Pregnancy is the condition in which a zygote (fertilized ovum) develops in the uterus. The normal gestation period is approximately 9 calendar months. The product of conception up to the third month of pregnancy is referred to as the embryo. From the third month to the time of birth, the unborn offspring is referred to as the fetus.

During pregnancy, the uterus changes its shape, size, and consistency. The peritoneal covering becomes enlarged, and there is an enormous increase in the muscle mass. The vaginal canal becomes elongated by the rise of the uterus in the pelvis. The mucosa thickens and secretions increase, and there is a rise in the vascularity and elasticity of both the cervix and vagina.

Pregnancy also causes enlargement of the breasts, sometimes to the point of painfulness. On the whole, many changes are evident in all of the body systems in order to accommodate the development and birth of the fetus.

Labor and Birth

Labor is the physiological process by which the fetus is expelled from the uterus. Labor occurs in three stages, as follows: The first is the **stage of dilation**, which begins with uterine contractions and terminates when there is complete dilation (10 cm) of the cervix. The second is the **stage of expulsion**. This is the time from complete cervical dilation to the birth of the baby. The last is the **placental stage**, or afterbirth. It begins shortly after childbirth, when the uterine contractions discharge the placenta from the uterus. Barring complications, the actual birth usually occurs in a relatively short period of time.

WORD ROOTS/COMBINING FORMS RELATED TO THE FEMALE REPRODUCTIVE SYSTEM

WORD ROOT/ COMBINING FORM	MEANING	EXAMPLE	PRONUNCIATION
cervic/o	cervix, neck	cervic/itis inflammation	sĕr - vĭ - SĪ - tĭs
colp/o }	vagina	colp/o/rrhaphy suture	kŏl - PŎR - ă - fē
vagin/o }		vagin/itis inflammation	văj - ĭn - Ī - tĭs

Continued on following page

**WORD ROOTS/COMBINING FORMS RELATED TO THE
FEMALE REPRODUCTIVE SYSTEM**—*Continued*

WORD ROOT/ COMBINING FORM	MEANING	EXAMPLE	PRONUNCIATION
episi/o vulv/o	vulva	episi/o/tomy incision vulv/ectomy excision	ĕ - pĭz - ē - ŎT - ō - mē vŭl - VĔK - tō - mē
galact/o lact/o	milk	galact/o/rrhea flow lact/o/gen/ to produce ic relating to	gă - lăk - tō - RĒ - ăh lăk - tō - JĔN - ĭk
gynec/o	woman, female	gynec/o/log/ study of ist one who specializes	gī - nĕ - KŎL - ō - jĭst
hyster/o uter/o metr/o	uterus, womb	hyster/ectomy excision intra/uter/ine within adjective ending	hĭs - tĕr - ĔK - tō - mē ĭn - tră - Ū - tĕr - ĭn
labi/o	lip	labi/al pertaining to	LĀ - bē - ăl
mamm/o mast/o	breast	mamm/ary relating to gynec/o/mast/ia female noun ending	MĂM - ă - rē jī - nĕ - kō - MĂS - tē - ăh
men/o	menses, menstruation	men/o/rrhagia burst forth	mĕn - ō - RĀ - jē - ăh
nat/a	birth	nat/al pertaining to	NĀ - tăl
oo/o	egg, ovum	oo/cyte cell	Ō - ō - sīt
oophor/o ovari/o	ovary	oophor/itis inflammation	ō - ŏf - ō - RĪ - tĭs
perine/o	perineum	perine/al pertaining to	pĕr - ĭ - NĒ - ăl
salping/o	fallopian tubes, oviducts, uterine tubes	salping/o/oophor/ectomy ovary excision	săl - pĭng - gō - ō - ŏf - ō - RĔK - tō - mē

SUFFIXES RELATED TO THE FEMALE REPRODUCTIVE SYSTEM

SUFFIX	MEANING	EXAMPLE	PRONUNCIATION
-arche	beginning	men/arche menstru- ation	měn - ĂR - kē
-cyesis	pregnancy	pseud/o/cyesis false	sū - dō - sĭ - Ē - sĭs
-gravida	pregnancy	multi/gravida many	mŭl - tĭ - GRĂV - ĭ - dă
-para	to bear	nulli/para none	nŭh - LĬP - ăh - răh
-salpinx	fallopian tubes, oviducts, uterine tubes	hemo/salpinx blood	hē - mō - SĂL - pĭnks
-tocia	childbirth, labor	dys/tocia difficult, painful	dĭs - TŌ - sē - ăh

PATHOLOGY RELATED TO THE FEMALE REPRODUCTIVE SYSTEM

Disturbances of Menstruation

Menstrual disturbances are generally caused by hormonal dysfunctions or pathological conditions of the uterus. They produce a variety of symptoms.

Menstrual pain and tension (**dysmenorrhea**) may be the result of uterine contractions, a pathological growth, or general chronic disorders such as anemia, fatigue, diabetes, or tuberculosis. The female hormone estrogen is used to treat dysmenorrhea and also to regulate menstrual abnormalities.

Irregular uterine bleeding between menstrual periods (**metrorrhagia**) or after menopause is usually symptomatic of some disease, often benign or malignant uterine tumors. Consequently, early diagnosis and treatment is warranted. Metrorrhagia is probably the most significant form of menstrual dysfunction.

Profuse or prolonged bleeding during regular menstruation (**menorrhagia**) may, during early life, be caused by endocrine disturbances. However, in later life, it is usually due to inflammatory diseases, tumors, or emotional disturbances, which also affect bleeding.

Premenstrual Syndrome (PMS)

The effects of PMS range from minimal discomfort to severe, disruptive symptoms. PMS appears 7 to 14 days before menses and usually subsides with onset of menses. It occurs in 30 to 50 percent of women, usually between ages 25 and 40. The incidence seems to rise with age and parity (the fact of having borne offspring).

Currently, the direct cause of PMS is unknown. It is widely suspected that the precipitating factor is the loss of intravascular fluid into body tissues, which triggers an increase in antidiuretic hormone (ADH) and aldosterone. The final effect is retention of transient water, which in turn produces symptoms such as edema, weight gain, and breast tenderness. Edema induces central nervous system changes, which result in headaches and mood shifts.

Other possible contributing factors to PMS include estrogen-progesterone imbalance, progesterone allergy, and hypoglycemia, as well as psychogenic factors.

Treatment is primarily symptomatic. Tranquilizers and sedatives may be included to relieve behavioral symptoms. Diuretics and decreased salt intake are also recommended in order to reduce bloating and edema.

Toxic Shock Syndrome (TSS)

This condition is caused by a toxin of the bacteria *Staphylococcus aureus*. It is usually associated with women under age 30 who are using tampons during menstruation. However, it has also occasionally occurred in nonmenstruating women. The onset of TSS occurs with a sudden fever, vomiting, diarrhea, myalgia, hypotension, and signs that suggest the onset of shock. An erythematous macular rash often develops. In some patients, this rash makes its first appearance on the body. In other patients, this rash appears on the hands (palms and fingers) and feet (soles and toes); it may then desquamate in 7 to 10 days. Urine output is decreased, and blood urea nitrogen (BUN) becomes elevated. Hyperemia of mucous membranes may also result.

Endometriosis

Endometriosis is the presence of endometrial tissue outside the lining of the uterine cavity. Such ectopic tissue is generally confined to the pelvic area, most commonly around the ovaries, uterovesical peritoneum, uterosacral ligaments, and the cul-de-sac, but it can appear anywhere in the body. Active endometriosis is uncommon before the age of 20. Generally, this disorder becomes progressively severe during the menstrual years; after menopause, it tends to subside.

Infections

Pelvic inflammatory disease (PID) is an acute, subacute, recurrent, or chronic condition of the oviducts and ovaries with adjacent tissue involvement. It includes inflammation of the cervix **(cervicitis)**, uterus **(endometritis)**, fallopian tubes **(salpingitis)**, and ovaries **(oophoritis)**, which can extend to the connective tissue lying between the broad ligaments **(parametritis)**. Early diagnosis prevents damage to the reproductive system. If left untreated, PID may cause infertility and may lead to potentially fatal septicemia, pulmonary emboli, and shock.

Inflammation of the vagina **(vaginitis)** is most often caused by a parasite known as *Trichomonas* or a fungal infection caused by *Candida albicans*. Large amounts of white vaginal discharge **(leukorrhea)** result from *Trichomonas* infections. Even though this condition is difficult to control, vaginal suppositories, medications, and douches are helpful.

Candidiasis is a fungal infection caused by *Candida albicans*. The patient exhibits a curdy or cheeselike discharge and experiences extreme itching **(pruritus)**. Since the organism thrives in an environment rich in carbohydrates, it is commonly seen in patients with poorly controlled diabetes. Also, patients who have been on steroid therapy or antibiotics often develop a *Candida* infection. Steroids and antibiotics alter the normal flora of the vagina, thereby providing an environment conducive to this organism. Medications that suppress the growth of fungi **(mycostatics)** are used to treat this disease.

Sexually Transmitted Diseases (STD)

Any disease that is transmitted through sexual activity is referred to as a sexually transmitted disease (venereal disease). Gonorrhea, syphilis, and genital herpes are considered the three major venereal diseases.

In gonorrhea (GC), bacteria attack the mucous membranes of both the urinary and genital organs. Some women do not experience pain **(asymptomatic)** until the disease has spread to the ovaries **(oophoritis)** and uterine tubes **(salpingitis)**. The female may then develop PID. Nevertheless, the most common symptom of gonorrhea in females is a greenish-yellowish cervical discharge. In males, gonorrhea generally causes painful urination and a mucopurulent urethral discharge, symptoms of acute anterior urethritis. If untreated with antibiotics, the disease may infect the bladder **(cystitis)**, inflame the joints **(arthritis)**, and result in meningitis. In addition, sterility may result from the formation of scars that close the reproductive tubes of both sexes. Both sex partners must be treated since the infection can recur.

Syphilis is also caused by a microorganism that enters the body through a break in the skin or mucous membrane. The initial stage of the disease is referred to as primary syphilis. Within 90 days of contact, a chancre, which is a firm, hard, ulcerlike lesion, develops. In women, the chancre usually appears on the labia or within the vagina. The chancre is not painful and may go entirely unnoticed and may heal without treatment. The secondary stage occurs about 4 months after the disappearance of the chancre. During the second stage, the patient may have a rash, sore throat, or other mild symptoms suggestive of a viral infection. Again, the signs and symptoms disappear without treatment. The disease may be spread during either the first or second stage. By this time, the microorganisms may have gained entrance into vital organs such as the heart, liver, brain, and spinal cord. Signs of the third stage, in which permanent damage is done to vital organs, may not appear for many years. In pregnancy, the microorganisms can attack the fetus, causing it to die or to be seriously deformed. Penicillin and other antibiotics are used in the treatment of syphilis.

Herpes simplex II, also known as genital herpes, is an infectious disease caused by the herpes simplex virus. It is transmitted primarily through direct sexual contact. Red blister-like sores develop on the genitalia. The sores are associated with a burning sensation and usually heal in about 2 weeks. The fluid in the blisters is also infectious. Individuals with herpes infection may have only one episode or may have repeated attacks. There seems to be a greater incidence of cancer of the cervix and miscarriages when this disease is present. There is also the danger of seriously infecting children during childbirth. In males, lesions appear on the glans, foreskin, or penile shaft. Nongenital lesions may cause complications such as herpetic keratitis, which may lead to blindness. Although there is treatment that reduces the discomfort, there is no cure at the present time.

Microorganisms of the *Chlamydia* bacteria are transmitted primarily through sexual intercourse. This venereal disease is the fastest growing sexually transmitted disease in the United States. *Chlamydia* is rarely transmitted through nonsexual person-to-person contact or contact with contaminated objects. After a 1- to 3-week incubation period, a painless lesion appears on the genitalia, urethral meatus, or the labia in females, and on the glans penis in males. The lesion ranges from a slight erosion to a small macule or papule. It often goes undetected because of its location. This lesion heals spontaneously in a few days.

About 2 weeks later, the lymph nodes begin to swell and other complications begin to develop because of secondary bacterial infection. Systemic symptoms in both males and females include myalgia, headache, fever, chills, malaise, backache, and weight loss.

Tumors of the Uterus

About 30 percent to 40 percent of all women develop myomatous or fibroid tumors of the uterus, which are benign and arise from the muscle tissue of the uterus. These benign tumors develop slowly between the ages of 25 and 40, and often become large in size after this period. There are instances in which such a tumor causes no symptoms. However, the most common symptom is menorrhagia. Other symptoms are due to pressure on the surrounding organs—pain, backache, constipation, and urinary symptoms. In addition, such tumors often cause metrorrhagia and even sterility.

Treatment of uterine fibroid tumors depends to a large extent on their size and location. If the patient plans to have children, treatment is as conservative as possible. As a rule, large tumors that produce pressure symptoms should be removed. Usually, the uterus is removed **(hysterectomy)**, while the ovaries are preserved. A myomectomy may be performed to remove the tumor if it is small. However, when the tumor is producing excessive bleeding, both the uterus and the tumor are removed **(hysteromyomectomy)**.

Cancer of the Cervix

This is the third most common malignancy of the reproductive system. Although it rarely occurs before the age of 20, it is most common between the ages of 30 to 50. Statistics indicate that infection due to sexual activity has some relationship to the incidence of cancer of the cervix. It is more prevalent in those who have had many sex partners and several pregnancies. Studies made on the incidence of cervical cancer among prostitutes also tend toward this conclusion.

A cytological exam (Pap smear) can detect cervical cancer before clinical evidence appears. Abnormal cervical cytology routinely calls for colposcopy, which can detect the presence and extent of pre-clinical lesions requiring biopsy and histologic examination. Treatment for cervical cancer consists of surgery, radiation and/or chemotherapy. If left untreated, the condition will eventually lead to death.

OTHER TERMS RELATED TO THE FEMALE REPRODUCTIVE SYSTEM

TERM	MEANING	PRONUNCIATION
adnexa	accessory parts of a structure. The adnexa uteri (ovaries and uterine tubes) are the accessory parts of the uterus	ăd - NĔK - să
atresia	congenital absence or closure of a normal body opening	ăh - TRĒ - zē - ăh
choriocarcinoma	a malignant neoplasm of the uterus or at the site of an ectopic pregnancy. Although its actual cause is unknown, this rare tumor may occur following pregnancy or abortion	kō - rē - ō - kăr - sĭ - NŌ - măh

Continued on following page

OTHER TERMS RELATED TO THE FEMALE REPRODUCTIVE SYSTEM—*Cont.*

TERM	MEANING	PRONUNCIATION
corpus luteum	scar tissue of the ovary that results from the rupturing of a follicle during ovulation. This small, yellow body serves to produce progesterone following ovulation	KŎR - pŭs/LOO - tē - ŭm
dyspareunia	occurrence of pain during sexual intercourse	dĭs - pă - RŪ - nē - ăh
endocervicitis	a fairly common problem that results when organisms gain access to the cervical glands after delivery, abortion, or intrauterine manipulation. This inflammation, in the majority of patients, is caused by ordinary pyogenic organisms, but gonorrheal infection of the glands can occur. When left untreated, this infection may extend into the uterus, fallopian tubes, and pelvic cavity	ĕn - dō - sĕr - vĭ - SĪ - tĭs
fibroids, fibromyoma uteri	benign uterine tumors that are composed of muscle and fibrous tissue; leiomyomas. Myomectomy or hysterectomy may be indicated if the fibroids grow too large, causing symptoms such as metrorrhagia, pelvic pain, or menorrhagia	FĪ - broids fĭ - brō - mĭ - Ō - măh
parametrium	loose connective tissue around the uterus	păr - ă - MĒ - trē - ŭm
puberty	the period during which the secondary sex characteristics begin to develop and the capability of sexual reproduction is attained	PŪ - bĕr - tē
vaginismus	painful spasm of the vagina from contraction of the muscles surrounding the vagina	văj - ĭn - ĬZ - mŭs

OTHER TERMS RELATED TO OBSTETRICS

TERM	MEANING	PRONUNCIATION
abruptio placenta	premature separation of a normally situated placenta	ăb - RŬP - shē - ō plăh - SĔN - tăh

Continued on following page

OTHER TERMS RELATED TO OBSTETRICS—*Continued*

TERM	MEANING	PRONUNCIATION
abortion	a deliberate termination of pregnancy before the fetus is capable of surviving outside the uterus	ăh - BŎR - shŭn
amnion	the innermost membrane enclosing the developing fetus and the fluid in which the fetus is bathed	ĂM - nē - ŏn
Down's syndrome, trisomy 21	preferred terms for mongolism. A congenital condition characterized by physical malformations and some degree of mental retardation. Trisomy of chromosome 21 usually occurs in 1 of 700 live births	dŏwnz/SĬN - drōm
eclampsia toxemia	major disorder of pregnancy that may be manifested by high blood pressure, edema, convulsions, renal dysfunction, proteinuria, and in severe cases, coma	ĕ - KLĂMP - sē - ăh tŏks - Ē - mē - ăh
ectopic pregnancy	a pregnancy in which the fertilized ovum does not reach the uterine cavity, but becomes implanted on any tissue other than the lining of the uterine cavity. Areas in which the fertilized egg may implant are the uterine tube, ovary, abdomen, or even the cervix of the uterus. In a tubal pregnancy, as the fertilized ovum increases in size, the tube becomes more and more distended. About 4 to 6 weeks after conception, rupture occurs, and the ovum is discharged into the abdominal cavity	ĕk - TŎP - ĭk/PRĔG - năn - sē
gravida	a pregnant woman	GRĂV - ĭ - dă
hydrocephalu	increased accumulation of cerebrospinal fluid within the ventricles of the brain	hĭ - drō - SĔF - ăh - lŭs
IUD (intrauterine device)	a small coil is placed inside the uterus to prevent implantation of the fertilized egg in the uterine lining. This method is approximately 95 percent effective	
kernicterus	an extremely serious condition involving mental retardation, jaundice, and brain damage	kĕr - NĬK - tĕr - ŭs
menarche	establishment or beginning of the menstrual function	mĕn - ĂR - kē

Continued on following page

Female Reproductive System

280

OTHER TERMS RELATED TO OBSTETRICS—Continued

TERM	MEANING	PRONUNCIATION
miscarriage, spontaneous abortion	a natural, spontaneous termination of pregnancy before the fetus is able to survive outside the uterus	
multigravida	a woman who has been pregnant two or more times	mŭl - tĭ - GRĂV - ĭ - dăh
multipara	a woman who has borne more than one viable fetus, whether or not the offspring were alive at birth. May be written para II or III etc. according to the number of pregnancies	mŭl - TĬP - ăh - răh
obstetrician	a physician who specializes in the branch of medicine dealing with pregnancy, labor, and the puerperium	ŏb - stĕ - TRĬSH - ăn
parturition	the act or process of giving birth to a child	păr - tū - RĬSH - ŭn
pelvimetry	measurement of the pelvic dimensions or proportions; helps determine whether or not the fetus can be delivered by the normal route	pĕl - VĬM - ĕ - trē
placenta previa	a condition in which the placenta is attached near the cervix and is thus subject to rupture; may necessitate a cesarean section	plă - SĔN - tăh/PRĒ - vē - ăh
primigravida	a woman during her first pregnancy	prĭ - mĭ - GRĂV - ĭ - dăh
primipara	a woman who has produced one viable infant (500 grams or 20 weeks gestation)	prĭ - MĬP - ăh - răh
puerperium	the period of 42 days following childbirth and expulsion of the placenta and membranes. The reproductive organs usually return to normal during this time	pū - ĕr - PĒ - rē - ŭm
pruritus vulvae	disorders marked by severe itching of external female genitalia	proo - RĪ - tŭs/VŬL - vā
puberty	the period during which the secondary sex characteristics begin to develop and the capability of sexual reproduction is attained	PŪ - bĕr - tē
pyosalpinx	pus in the fallopian tube	pĭ - ō - SĂL - pĭnks

Continued on following page

TERM	DESCRIPTION

SPECIAL PROCEDURES RELATED TO THE FEMALE REPRODUCTIVE SYSTEM

RADIOGRAPHIC PROCEDURES

TERM	DESCRIPTION
hysterosalpingography, uterotubography, uterosalpingography	employs an injection of a contrast medium through the cervix for radiographic visualization of the uterus and oviducts. Primarily, this examination serves to determine the presence of pathology in the uterine cavity, to evaluate tubal patency, and to study fertility problems
ultrasonography	a noninvasive ultrasound technique used to evaluate the female genital tract and fetus in the obstetric patient. This procedure also helps detect pelvic inflammations, tubo-ovarian abscesses, ectopic pregnancies, ovarian masses, and other abnormalities of the female reproductive system

ENDOSCOPIC PROCEDURES

TERM	DESCRIPTION
culdoscopy	is performed in the operating room and permits direct visualization of the uterus, uterine tubes, broad ligaments, rectal wall, sigmoid colon, and small intestine. An incision is made in the posterior vaginal cul-de-sac to admit a **culdoscope**, which is a tubular, lighted endoscope. Culdoscopy is indicated in suspected ectopic pregnancy, in unexplained pelvic pain, and in the presence of undetermined pelvic masses
colposcopy, colpomicroscopy	utilization of optical instruments designed to permit three-dimensional views of stained or unstained cervical epithelium in situ (in position, localized). These instruments provide visual access to suspicious tissue areas, but in many instances, biopsy of the tissue is required for accurate diagnosis
laparoscopy, pelvic peritoneoscopy	examination of the abdominal cavity with a laparoscope through a small incision in the abdominal wall. The procedure is also used for examining the ovaries and fallopian tubes and as a gynecological sterilization technique for fulgurating (destruction of tissue by means of long, high-frequency electric sparks) the oviducts

Continued on following page

282   SURGICAL PROCEDURES RELATED TO THE FEMALE
REPRODUCTIVE SYSTEM

TERM	DESCRIPTION	PRONUNCIATION
cryosurgery, cryocautery	the process of freezing tissue for the purpose of destroying cells. This procedure is used for chronic cervical infections and erosions since the offending organisms may be entrenched in the cervical cells and glands. Cryocautery destroys these infected areas, and in the healing process, normal cells are replenished. It may also be used when a patient shows atypical or possible malignancy as seen on a Pap smear	krī - ō - SĔR - jĕr - ē krī - ō - KĂW - tĕr - ē
colpectomy, vaginectomy	excision of the vagina	kŏl - PĔK - tō - mē văj - ĭn - ĔK - tō - mē
colpocleisis	closure of the vaginal canal	kŏl - pō - KLĪ - sĭs
colpoperineoplasty, colpoperineorrhaphy	plastic surgery on vagina and perineum	kŏl - pō - pĕr - ĭ - NĒ - ō - plăs - tē kŏl - pō - pĕr - ĭ - nē - ŎR - ăh - fē
conization	excision of a cone of tissue (usually infected), as of the mucous membrane to promote healing of the cervix	kŏn - ĭ - ZĀ - shŭn
dilatation and curettage (D&C)	a widening of the cervical canal with a dilator and the scraping of the uterine endometrium with a curette. It is performed to secure endometrial or endocervical tissue for cytologic examination, to control abnormal uterine bleeding, and as a therapeutic measure for incomplete abortion. Since this procedure usually	dĭl - ă - TĀ - shŭn/kū - rĕ - TĂHZH

Continued on following page

SURGICAL PROCEDURES RELATED TO THE FEMALE REPRODUCTIVE SYSTEM—*Continued*

TERM	DESCRIPTION	PRONUNCIATION
	is performed under anesthesia and requires surgical asepsis, it is performed in the operating room	
episiotomy	incision of perineum from the vaginal orifice, usually done to facilitate childbirth	ĕ - pĭz - ē - ŎT - ō - mē
episiorrhaphy	suturing of a lacerated perineum	ĕ - pĭz - ĕ - ŎR - ăh - fē
hymenotomy	incision of the hymen	hī - mĕn - ŎT - ō - mē
myomectomy	excision of a myomatous tumor, generally uterine	mī - ō - MĔK - tō - mē
panhysterectomy	removal of the entire uterus, including the cervix	păn - hĭs - tĕr - ĔK - tō - mē
salpingo-oophorectomy	excision of an ovary and fallopian tube, usually identified as right (R), left (L), or bilateral	săl - pĭng - gō - ō - ŏf - ō - RĔK - tō - mē
tubal ligation	ligating (tying) the uterine tubes to prevent pregnancy; sterilization surgery	TŪ - băl/lī - GĀ - shŭn

SURGICAL PROCEDURES RELATED TO OBSTETRICS

TERM	DESCRIPTION	PRONUNCIATION
amniocentesis	transabdominal puncture of the amniotic sac, using a needle and syringe, in order to remove amniotic fluid. The material obtained may be studied chemically or cytologically to detect genetic and biochemical disorders or maternal-fetal blood incompatibility. This procedure is performed no earlier than at 14 weeks' gestation	ăm - nē - ō - sĕn - TĒ - sĭs

Continued on following page

SURGICAL PROCEDURES RELATED TO OBSTETRICS—*Continued*

TERM	DESCRIPTION	PRONUNCIATION
chorion villus biopsy	guided by an ultrasound display, the doctor inserts an aspirator into the uterus to obtain a sample of the chorionic villi (one of the placental layers composed of fetal cells). This new technique is advantageous because it can be performed earlier than amniocentesis and does not require puncturing the abdominal wall	KŌ - rē - ăn VĬL - ŭs BĪ - ŏp - sē
therapeutic abortion	abortion induced legally by a qualified physician for medical or other reasons	

LABORATORY PROCEDURES

TERM	DESCRIPTION
Pap test, Papanicolaou smear	a smear examined microscopically to detect cancer cells from body excretions, secretions, or tissue scrapings. Cervical scrapings are most commonly performed to detect cancerous cells in the mucus of the uterus and cervix
pregnancy test	one of the most common laboratory tests performed to determine if a pregnancy exists. This tests for the presence of the human chorionic gonadotropin hormone produced by the placenta. It is found in the urine or blood of pregnant women. With its identification, a pregnancy can be diagnosed 4 to 5 days after the patient misses her monthly menstrual period
endometrial biopsy, endometrial smear	used in screening high-risk patients for endometrial cancer. This test is done as an office procedure during the gynecologic examination. Following the administration of a small amount of anesthetic, a thin, hollow curette is used to remove endometrial tissue for laboratory analysis

PHARMACOLOGY RELATED TO THE FEMALE REPRODUCTIVE SYSTEM

MEDICATION	ACTION
estrogens	female sex hormones used for replacement in women who complain of various menstrual disturbances, or during menopause to ease discomforts that may occur as natural estrogen decreases
oral contraceptives "the pill"	the most effective form of birth control, which offers almost 100 percent effective protection. However, this form of contraception has many undesirable side effects. Although some of them can be minimized through low dosages and appropriate estrogen/progesterone combinations, nausea, breakthrough bleeding, water retention, vaginal infections, and headaches are still evident

Continued on following page

PHARMACOLOGY RELATED TO THE FEMALE REPRODUCTIVE SYSTEM—*Continued*

MEDICATION	ACTION
	with pill users. More serious, however, are its links to blood clotting (embolism, thrombophlebitis, and so forth) and cancer. The long-term side effects of the "pill" are presently under study
oxytocin	medication used to cause contraction of the uterus. It is used to induce labor, or to rid the uterus of an unexpelled placenta or a fetus that has died
spermicide (jellies, creams, foam)	no prescription is needed, and studies show this method is 85 percent effective for birth control. An aerosol spray or applicator containing the spermicide is inserted into the vagina, providing a chemical barrier that inhibits the sperm's passage to the ovum. They also destroy sperm. It is recommended that a condom and/or diaphragm be used in conjunction with the spermicide

ABBREVIATIONS RELATED TO THE FEMALE REPRODUCTIVE SYSTEM

ABBREVIATION	MEANING
Maternal/Gynecologic	
AB	abortion
CPD	cephalopelvic disproportion
D&C	dilatation and curettage
DUB	dysfunctional uterine bleeding
EDC	estimated or expected date of confinement
FSH	follicle-stimulating hormone
GC	gonorrhea
Gyn	gynecology
IUD	intrauterine device
LH	luteinizing hormone
LMP	last menstrual period
MH	marital history
Path	pathology
PID	pelvic inflammatory disease
PMP	previous menstrual period
Fetal/Obstetric	
CS, C-section	cesarean section

Continued on following page

ABBREVIATIONS RELATED TO THE FEMALE
REPRODUCTIVE SYSTEM—Continued

ABBREVIATION	MEANING
Fetal/Obstetric	
CWP	childbirth without pain
Maternal/Gynecologic	
DOB	date of birth
FEKG	fetal electrocardiogram
FHR	fetal heart rate
FHT	fetal heart tone
FTND	full-term normal delivery
HSG	hysterosalpingography
HCG	human chorionic gonadotropin
NB	newborn
OB	obstetrics
UC	uterine contractions

WORKSHEET 1

A. Using the word root/combining form *gynec/o* (woman, female), build medical words to mean:

1. _____gynecomastia_____ abnormally large mammary glands in the male (some-times may secrete milk)

2. _____ study of the diseases of the female

3. _____ physician who specializes in diseases peculiar to women

4. _____ pertaining to women

B. Using the word root/combining form *cervic/o* (neck), build medical words to mean:

1. _____ pertaining to the cervix of an organ, as the cervix uteri

2. _____ inflammation of the cervix uteri and vagina

3. _____ inflammation of the cervix uteri

4. _____ pertaining to the cervix uteri and bladder

C. Using the word root/combining form *colp/o* (vagina), build medical words to mean:

1. _____ suture of the vagina

2. _____ instrument used to examine the vagina (and cervix)

3. _____ visual examination of the vagina (and cervix using a colposcope)

D. Using the word root/combining form *vagin/o* (vagina), build medical terms to mean:

1. _____ inflammation of the vagina

2. _____ relating to the vagina

3. _____ pertaining to development or origin in the vagina

4. _____ vaginal hernia

5. _____ roentgenography of the vagina

6. _____ a fungus infection (mycosis) of the vagina

7. _____ relating to the vagina and perineum

8. _____ an instrument to cut the vaginal walls

9. _____ related to the vagina and bladder

10. _____ related to the vagina and the labia

E. Using the word root/combining form hyster/o (uterus), build medical terms to mean:

1. _____ myoma of the uterus

2. _____ uterine disease

3. _____ uterine spasm

4. _____ rupture of the uterus (especially when pregnant)

5. _____ radiography of the uterus and oviducts (after injection of radiopaque material into those organs)

6. _____ pertaining to or relating to the uterus and vagina

F. Using the word root/combining form metr/o (uterus), build medical words to mean:

1. _____ condition of uterine hemorrhage (bleeding)

2. _____ inflammation near the uterus

3. _____ abnormal condition within the uterus

G. Using the word root/combining form uter/o (uterus), build medical words to mean:

1. _____ hernia of the uterus

2. _____ relating to the uterus and cervix

3. _____ pertaining to the uterus and rectum

4. _____ pertaining to the uterus and bladder

H. Using the word root/combining form oophor/o (ovary), build medical words to mean:

1. _____ inflammation of an ovary

2. _____ pain in an ovary

3. _____ ovarian tumor (carcinoma)

4. _____ inflammation of an ovary and oviduct

I. Using the word root/combining form salping/o (fallopian tube), build medical words to mean:

1. _____ hernial protrusion of a fallopian tube

2. _____ inflammation of the fallopian tube

3. _____ radiography of the uterine tubes (after intrauterine injection of a radiopaque medium)

4. _____ inflammation of a fallopian tube and ovary

J. Word building with suffixes

1. Using the suffix -cyesis, build a word to mean false pregnancy _____ _____

2. Using the suffix -tocia, build a word to mean difficult or painful labor (childbirth) _____

3. Using the suffix -salpinx, build a word to mean blood in the oviducts _____ _____

4. Using the suffix -gravida, build a word to mean many pregnancies _____ _____

5. Using the suffix -arche, build a word that means beginning of the menses _____ _____

290   ## WORKSHEET 2

Fill in the correct word from the right hand column that matches the definition in the statements below.

1. _____ an accumulation of pus in a uterine tube

Atresia

2. _____ a woman who has had one pregnancy that has resulted in a viable offspring

Corpus luteum

3. _____ pregnancy; 40 weeks in human beings

Down's syndrome

4. _____ last menstrual period

Dystocia

5. _____ enlargement of the cranium caused by abnormal accumulation of cerebrospinal fluid within the ventricles of the brain

Gestation

6. _____ a yellow glandular mass in the ovary formed by an ovarian follicle that has matured and discharged its ovum; an endocrine structure that secretes progesterone

Hydrocephalus

7. _____ abnormal labor or childbirth

LMP

8. _____ congenital absence or closure of a normal body opening

Primipara

9. _____ mongolism

Pruritus vulvae

10. _____ intense itching of the external genitalia in the female

Pyosalpinx

WORKSHEET 3

Build a surgical term for the following:

1. _____ excision or removal of the vagina

2. _____ fixation of a displaced ovary

3. _____ suture of a displaced ovary (to the pelvic wall)

4. _____ surgical repair of the vagina

5. _____ excision or removal of the uterus and one or both ovaries

6. _____ surgical repair of the vagina and perineum

7. _____ excision of the entire uterus, including the cervix uteri

8. _____ suturing of (a lacerated) perineum

9. _____ excision of the uterus, oviducts, and ovaries

10. _____ puncture of the amniotic sac

292 WORKSHEET 4

Define the following medical terms. Use the dictionary as a reference.

1. condyloma _____

2. dysmenorrhea _____

3. fibromyoma _____

4. gonorrhea _____

5. herpes simplex II _____

6. graafian follicle _____

7. PID _____

8. peritonitis _____

9. trichomoniasis _____

10. syphilis _____

WORKSHEET 5

Grammar Review—Female Reproductive System

Write the plural form for the words listed. Then, cover up the words in column one and rewrite the singular form in the last section.

SINGULAR	PLURAL	SINGULAR
1. cervix	cervices	cervix
2. ovum		
3. uterus		
4. spermatozoon		
5. pelvis		
6. labium		

7. Using the word root/combining form gynec/o/log (study of women), form a word with a noun ending that means one who specializes in women's diseases.

8. Form a word with an adjective ending from vaginitis.

9. Form a word with an adjective ending from the noun hydrocephalus.

10. Form another word with an adjective ending from the adjective vulval.

294   WORKSHEET 6

Label the figure below, and compare your answers with Figures 12-2 and 12-3.

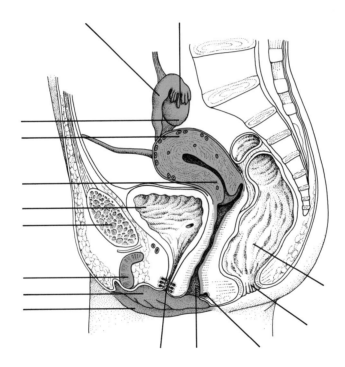

Uterine (fallopian) tube

Ovary

Uterus

Cervix

Bladder

Symphysis
pubis

Clitoris

Labia minor

Labia major

Urethra

Vagina

Bartholin's gland

Anus

Rectum

Fimbriae

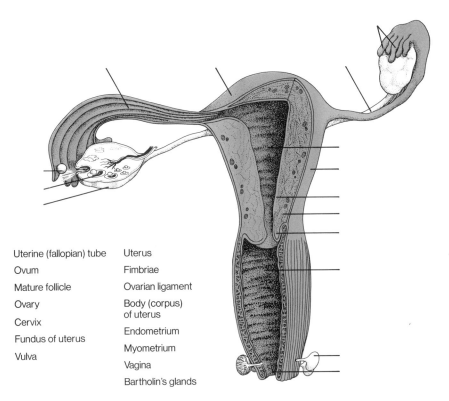

Uterine (fallopian) tube

Ovum

Mature follicle

Ovary

Cervix

Fundus of uterus

Vulva

Uterus

Fimbriae

Ovarian ligament

Body (corpus)
of uterus

Endometrium

Myometrium

Vagina

Bartholin's glands

296   WORKSHEET 7

Special Procedures, Pharmacology, and Abbreviations

Choose the word(s) that best describes the following statements:

abortion	laparoscopy
amniocentesis	LMP
chorion villus biopsy	miscarriage
colpocleisis	oxytocin
conization	panhysterectomy
contraceptives	Pap test
CPD	spermicide
cryosurgery	therapeutic abortion
D&C	tubal ligation
estrogens	ultrasonography

1. _____ cervical scrapings to detect cancerous cells in the mucus of the uterus and cervix

2. _____ a natural, spontaneous termination of pregnancy before the fetus is able to survive outside the uterus

3. _____ transabdominal puncture of the amniotic sac, using a needle and syringe, in order to remove amniotic fluid. The sample is then analyzed to determine congenital disorders

4. _____ destroying cells by the process of freezing tissue

5. _____ closure of the vaginal canal

6. _____ a widening of the cervical canal with a dilator and scraping of the uterine endometrium with a curette

7. _____ excision of the entire uterus, including the cervix

8. _____ tying the uterine tubes to prevent pregnancy; sterilization surgery

9. _____ cephalopelvic disproportion

10. _____ last menstrual period

11. _____ a deliberate termination of pregnancy before the fetus is capable of surviving outside the uterus

12. _____ a small incision in the abdominal wall that permits examination of the abdominal cavity to determine abnormalities

13. _____ a noninvasive ultrasound technique used to evaluate the female genital tract and fetus in the obstetric patient

14. _____ a new test to detect chromosomal abnormalities that does not require puncturing the uterine wall

15. _____ replacement hormones used during menopause to ease discomforts as the production of natural hormones decreases

CHAPTER 13

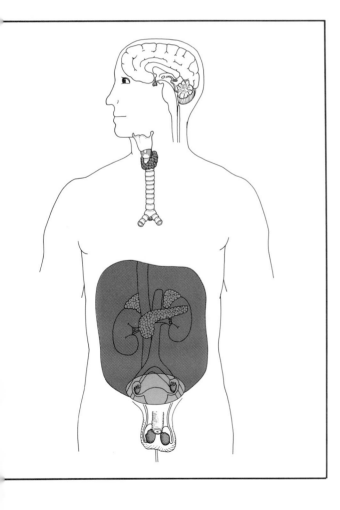

CHAPTER OUTLINE

Endocrine System

STUDENT OBJECTIVES

Upon completion of this chapter, you will be able to do the following:

List the glands of the endocrine system.

Describe the function of each gland.

Differentiate between endocrine glands and exocrine glands.

Identify principal hormones secreted by the endocrine glands and briefly explain their function.

Identify the word roots/combining forms and suffixes of the endocrine system.

Identify and discuss associated pathology related to the endocrine system.

Identify radiographic, surgical, and laboratory procedures and abbreviations related to the endocrine system.

Explain the pharmacology related to the treatment of endocrine disorders.

Build and analyze diagnostic, symptomatic, and surgical terms related to the endocrine system by completing the worksheets.

300   ANATOMY AND PHYSIOLOGY OF THE ENDOCRINE SYSTEM

Both the endocrine system and the nervous system regulate the basic metabolic activities of the body. Their functions are closely related because they work together to maintain homeostasis (the state of equilibrium in the internal environment of the body). The endocrine system is essentially a chemical communication system and is composed of endocrine glands, which are responsible for secretions of hormones (Table 13-1). Included in the endocrine system are a number of ductless glands located in various parts of the body (Fig. 13-1). These glands are called endocrine glands because they release their secretions di-

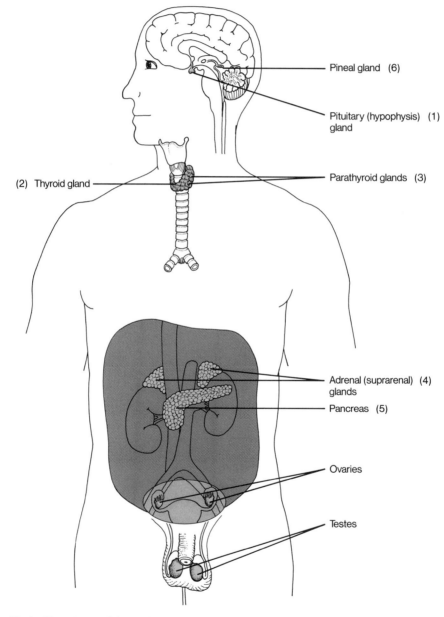

Figure 13–1. The glands of the endocrine system (ductless, internally secreting) are located in various parts of the body.

Table 13–1. DEFINITION, CHARACTERISTICS, STRUCTURE
OF HORMONES

DEFINITION

A chemical substance produced by cells of the body and transported by the bloodstream to
the cells and organs on which it has a specific regulatory effect.

COMMON CHARACTERISTICS

The rate of physiological response is altered by the action of the hormones.
All hormones circulate in the blood.
Most hormones are inactivated or excreted by the liver and kidneys.
Hormones are secreted in minute but effective amounts.

STRUCTURE OF HORMONES

They are either steroids or proteins.
Steroid hormones are synthesized from cholesterol, are lipid (fat) soluble, and are able to
penetrate into the cell, where specific receptors exist. Steroid hormones are secreted by
the adrenal cortices, ovaries, and testes.
Because of their large size and lipid insolubility, protein hormones are unable to penetrate
cell membranes. Instead, they act at receptor sites on the cell membrane which, in turn,
activate intracellular processes.

rectly into blood vessels that run through the glands. They are not to be confused with
exocrine glands, such as the sweat and oil glands of the skin, which release their secretions
externally through ducts. This chapter includes the function of the **pituitary**, **thyroid**,
parathyroid, **adrenals**, **pancreas**, and **pineal glands**. The functions of the other endocrine
glands are discussed in the following chapters: Chapter 9, Hematic and Lymphatic System
(thymus); Chapter 11, Urogenital System (testes); and Chapter 12, Female Reproductive
System (ovaries).
Refer to Figure 13-1 as you read the following material.

Pituitary Gland

The (1) **pituitary gland**, or **hypophysis**, is no larger than a pea and is located at the base of
the brain. It is known as the "master gland" because it regulates many body activities and
stimulates other glands to secrete their own specific hormone.
The gland consists of two distinct portions—an anterior lobe (adenohypophysis) and a
posterior lobe (neurohypophysis). Both lobes secrete a number of hormones, which are
summarized in Table 13-2.

Thyroid Gland

The (2) **thyroid gland** is the largest gland of the endocrine system. It is an H-shaped organ
located in the neck just below the larynx. This gland is composed of two fairly large lobes
that are separated by a strip of tissue called an isthmus.

Table 13–2. HORMONES OF THE PITUITARY GLAND

GLAND	HORMONE	MAJOR EFFECTS
adenohypophysis (anterior lobe)	growth hormone (GH), or somatotropin	stimulates bone and body growth
	thyroid-stimulating hormone (TSH), or thyrotropin	controls secretions of hormones from the thyroid gland
	prolactin	promotes growth of breast tissue stimulates milk production after birth
	adrenocorticotropic hormone (ACTH)	stimulates secretions by the adrenal cortex, especially cortisol
	gonadotropin: follicle-stimulating hormone (FSH)	stimulates development of eggs in the ovaries stimulates secretions of estrogen in females stimulates production of sperm cells in the testes
	luteinizing hormone (LH), or interstitial cell–stimulating hormone (ICSH) in males	promotes the secretion of sex hormones in both males and females plays a role in the release of the egg cell in females
neurohypophysis (posterior lobe)	antidiuretic hormone (ADH), or vasopressin	decreases volume of urine excreted increases volume of water reabsorbed in kidney
	oxytocin	causes contraction of the uterus during labor and childbirth stimulates milk secretion

The function of the thyroid gland is to produce, store, and release **thyroxine** (T_4) and triiodothyronine (T_3), the major thyroid hormones.

Both T_3 and T_4 regulate metabolism and are responsible for a person's energy level. They increase the rate of oxygen consumption and thus the rate at which carbohydrates are used and proteins are broken down. They also increase the rate at which fats are utilized. In addition, both hormones work with the growth hormone (GH) and stimulate activity in the nervous system. Refer to Table 13-3 for a summary of hormones of the thyroid gland.

Table 13–3.   SUMMARY OF HORMONES OF THE THYROID GLAND

HORMONE	MAJOR EFFECTS
thyroxine (T₄), triiodothyronine (T₃)	increase oxygen consumption and metabolism of all cells
calcitonin	lowers calcium level in blood by inhibiting the release of calcium from bones

Parathyroid Glands

The (3) **parathyroid glands** consist of at least four separate glands located on the posterior surface of the lobes of the thyroid gland. The only hormone known to be secreted by the parathyroid glands is a protein called parathyroid hormone (PTH), or parathormone (Fig. 13-2). PTH helps to regulate the metabolism of calcium by influencing three types of organs—the bones, the intestine, and the kidneys. PTH seems to stimulate the formation of new bone cells (osteoblasts). As a result of this increased activity, calcium and phosphates are released from the bones, and the blood concentrations of these substances increase. Thus, the calcium that is necessary for the proper functioning of body tissues is present in the bloodstream. At the same time, PTH enhances the absorption of calcium and phosphates from foods in the intestine, and this action also produces a rise in the blood levels of calcium and phosphates. PTH causes the kidneys to conserve blood calcium and to increase the excretion of phosphates in the urine.

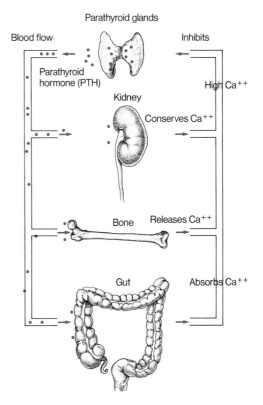

Figure 13-2. Parathyroid hormone stimulates the resorption of calcium from bone, the conservation of calcium by the kidneys, and the absorption of calcium by the intestine. The resulting increase in blood calcium level inhibits the secretion of this hormone.

Adrenal Glands

The (4) **adrenal glands** are paired structures located superior to the kidneys. Because of their location atop the kidneys, the adrenal glands are also known as **suprarenal glands**. Each adrenal gland is structurally and functionally differentiated into two sections: the outer **adrenal cortex**, which makes up the bulk of the gland, and the inner **adrenal medulla**. Although these regions are not sharply divided, they represent distinct glands that secrete different hormones. Steroids (see Table 13-1) are secreted by the **cortex**. Cells of the **adrenal medulla** secrete two closely related hormones, epinephrine (adrenaline) and norepinephrine (noradrenaline).

The hormones of the adrenal cortex are all steroids (corticosteroids) and are essential to life. In fact, in the absence of cortical secretions, a person usually dies within a week unless extensive electrolyte therapy (sodium, potassium, and calcium levels are carefully controlled) is provided.

Histologically, the cortex is subdivided into three zones. Each zone has a different cellular arrangement and secretes different groups of hormones. The three groups are as follows:

1. **Mineralocorticoids**, which help to regulate water and mineral salts (also called electrolytes) that are retained in the body. One of the mineralocorticoids of major importance in humans is **aldosterone**. Like all of the hormones of the adrenal cortex, aldosterone is a steroid. This hormone acts mainly through the kidneys to maintain the homeostasis of sodium and potassium. More specifically, aldosterone causes the kidneys to conserve sodium and to excrete potassium. At the same time, it promotes water conservation and reduces urine output.

2. **Glucocorticoids**, which influence the metabolism of carbohydrates, fats, and proteins. The glucocorticoid with the greatest activity is **cortisol**. It helps to regulate the concentration of glucose in the blood, protecting against low blood sugar between meals. Another effect of cortisol is to stimulate the breakdown of fats in adipose tissue and release fatty acids into the blood. The increase in fatty acids causes many cells to use relatively less glucose.

3. **Gonadocorticoids** (sex hormones), which affect sexual characteristics. Although the sex hormones are primarily male type (adrenal androgens), small quantities of female hormones (adrenal estrogens and progesterone) are also present. The normal functions of these hormones are not clear, but they may supplement the supply of

Table 13-4. SUMMARY OF THE HORMONES OF THE ADRENAL CORTEX

HORMONE	MAJOR EFFECTS
mineralocorticoids (aldosterone)	regulates the amount of salts in the body
glucocorticoids (cortisol)	regulates the metabolism of carbohydrates, proteins, and fats
gonadocorticoids (adrenal sex hormones: androgens, estrogens, and progestins)	maintain secondary sex characteristics

Table 13–5.   SUMMARY OF PANCREATIC HORMONES

HORMONE	MAJOR EFFECTS
insulin	promotes the movement of glucose through cell membranes, causing the blood glucose level to fall
glucagon	stimulates the liver to convert glycogen to glucose, causing the blood glucose level to rise

sex hormones from the gonads and stimulate early development of the reproductive organs. Also, there is some evidence that the adrenal androgens play a role in controlling the female sex drive. Refer to Table 13-4 for a summary of the hormones of the adrenal cortex.

Epinephrine (adrenaline) and norepinephrine (noradrenaline) are two closely related hormones secreted by the adrenal medulla. The effects of the medullary hormones resemble those of the sympathetic nervous system. The adrenal medulla, like the rest of the sympathetic nervous system, is not essential to life, but it is important to the ability of the organism to meet emergencies.

Pancreas (Islets of Langerhans)

The (5) **pancreas** lies inferior to the stomach in a bend of the duodenum. It functions both as an exocrine and endocrine gland. A large pancreatic duct runs through the gland carrying enzymes and other exocrine digestive secretions from the pancreas to the small intestine. (This is discussed in Chapter 6, Gastrointestinal System.) The pancreas has groups of cells called islets of Langerhans, which produce endocrine secretions. There are two kinds of main cells in the islets: A-cells (alpha cells) produce glucagon and constitute about 25 percent of the islet cells; B-cells (beta cells) produce insulin and constitute about 75 percent of the islet cells. Both of these hormones, glucagon and insulin, play an important role in the proper metabolism of sugars and starches in the body. Refer to Table 13-5 for a summary of pancreatic hormones.

Pineal Gland

The (6) **pineal gland** is shaped like a pine cone and is attached to the posterior part of the third ventricle of the brain. Although the exact functions of this gland have not been established, there is evidence that it secretes melatonin hormone. It is believed that melatonin may inhibit the activities of the ovaries. When melatonin production is high, ovulation is blocked, and there may be a delay in puberty development. The pineal gland starts to degenerate at about 7 years of age; in the adult, it consists mostly of fibrous tissue.

WORD ROOTS/COMBINING FORMS RELATED TO THE ENDOCRINE SYSTEM

WORD ROOT/ COMBINING FORM	MEANING	EXAMPLE	PRONUNCIATION
acr/o	extremity	acr/o/megaly enlargement	ăk - rō - MĔG - ă - lē

Continued on following page

**WORD ROOTS/COMBINING FORMS RELATED TO THE
ENDOCRINE SYSTEM**—*Continued*

WORD ROOT/ COMBINING FORM	MEANING	EXAMPLE	PRONUNCIATION

adren/o ⎫
 	
 adrenal/o ⎭
	adrenal glands	adren/al
		     relating to,
		     adjective ending
		 adrenal/ism
		       condition
			ăd - RĒ - năl
			
			 ă - DRĔN - ăl - ĭzm

andr/o	male	andr/o/gen produce	ĂN - drō - jĕn
calc/o	calcium	hypo/calc/em/ ia under, blood condi- below tion (of)	hĭ - pō - kăl - SĒ - mē - ăh
gluc/o ⎫ glyc/o ⎭	sugar, sweetness	gluc/o/genesis to produce hyper/glyc/em/ ia exces- blood condi- sive tion (of)	gloo - kō - JĔN - ĕ - sĭs hĭ - pĕr - glĭ - SĒ - mē - ăh

gonad/o	sex glands (testes in the male; ovaries in the female)	hypo/gonad/ism
		 below condition,
		        state of
		        being
			hĭ - pō - GŌ - năd - ĭzm

home/o	likeness, resemblance	home/o/stasis
		     standing still
		     (state of
		     equilibrium)
			hō - mē - ō - STĀ - sĭs

parathyroid/o	parathyroid glands	parathyroid/ectomy excision	păr - ăh - thĭ - roi - DĔK - tō - mē
pancreat/o	pancreas	pancreat/itis inflammation	păn - krē - ă - TĪ - tĭs
somat/o	body	somat/ic pertaining to	sō - MĂT - ĭk
thym/o	thymus	thym/o/lysis destroy	thĭ - MŎL - ĭ - sĭs

thyr/o ⎫
 	
 thyroid/o ⎭
	thyroid	thyr/o/toxic/osis
		     poi- abnormal
		     son condition
		        (of)
		 thyroid/ectomy
		     excision
			thĭ - rō - tŏks - ĭ - KŌ - sĭs
			
			 thĭ - roid - ĔK - tō - mē

SUFFIXES RELATED TO THE ENDOCRINE SYSTEM

SUFFIX	MEANING	EXAMPLE	PRONUNCIATION
-crine	to secrete	end/o/<u>crine</u> within	ĔN - dō - krĭn or krĭn
-dipsia	thirst	poly/<u>dips</u>/ia many, noun much ending	pŏl - ē - DĬP - sē - ăh
-phagia	eating	poly/<u>phagia</u> much	pŏl - ē - FĀ - jē - ăh
-trophy	nourishment, development	a/<u>trophy</u> with- out	ĂT - rō - fē
-toxic	poison	thyr/o/<u>toxic</u> thyroid	thī - rō - TŎKS - ĭk
-uria	urine	poly/<u>uria</u> much	pŏl - ē - Ū - rē - ăh
-phylaxis	protection	ana/<u>phylaxis</u> with- out	ăn - ăh - fĭ - LĂX - sĭs
-physis	growth	adeno/hypo/<u>physis</u> gland under	ăd - ĕ - nō - hī - PŎF - ĭ - sĭs
-tropin	stimulate	somat/o/<u>tropin</u> body	sō - măt - ō - TRŌ - pĭn

PATHOLOGY OF THE ENDOCRINE SYSTEM

Disorders of the endocrine system are based on underproduction (**hyposecretion**) or over-production (**hypersecretion**) of hormones. In general, hyposecretion is treated by the use of hormones in drug therapy replacement. Hypersecretion is generally treated by surgery. Most hormone deficiencies result from genetic defects in the glands, surgical removal of the glands, or production of poor-quality hormones.

Pituitary

Hypersecretion or hyposecretion of growth hormone (GH) leads to abnormalities of body size, while abnormal variations of antidiuretic hormone (ADH) secretions lead to disorders in the composition of the blood. Some pituitary disorders are summarized in Table 13-6.

Thyroid

Thyroid gland disorders are not uncommon and may develop at any time during a person's life as a result of a developmental problem, an injury, a disease, or a dietary deficiency. One

Table 13–6. PITUITARY DISORDERS

DISORDER	HORMONE	HYPOSECRETION OR HYPERSECRETION	POSSIBLE CAUSE	EFFECTS
acromegaly	GH	hypersecretion as an adult	primary tumor after puberty	disproportionate increase in size of bones of face, hands, and feet
diabetes insipidus	ADH	hyposecretion	damage to the hypothalamus	failure of kidneys to reabsorb needed salts and water
giantism	GH	hypersecretion during childhood	pituitary tumor before puberty	abnormal overgrowth of the body
high blood level of ADH	ADH	hypersecretion	pituitary tumor, head injury	excessive sodium, water retention in the body
pituitary dwarfism, hypopituitary dwarfism	GH	hyposecretion during childhood	congenital deficiency or destruction of GH-producing cells	small but well-proportioned body; sexual immaturity

form of hypothyroidism that develops in an infant is called **cretinism**. If not treated, it leads to mental retardation, impaired growth, low body temperatures, and abnormal bone formation. Usually, these symptoms do not appear at birth because the infant has received a supply of thyroid hormones from the mother's blood during development.

When hypothyroidism develops after growth and development, it is known as **myxedema**. The characteristics of this disease are edema, low levels of T_3 and T_4 in the blood, mental retardation, weight gain, and sluggishness.

Hyperthyroidism results from excessive secretions of T_3, T_4, or both. Two of the most common disorders of hyperthyroidism are **Graves' disease** and **toxic goiter**. Grave's disease is considerably more prevalent and is characterized by an elevated metabolic rate, abnormal weight loss, excessive perspiration, muscular weakness, and emotional instability. Also, the eyes are likely to protrude **(exophthalmos)** because of edematous swelling in the tissues behind them. At the same time, the thyroid gland is likely to enlarge, producing goiter.

It is believed that toxic goiter may occur because of an excessive release of thyroid-stimulating hormone (TSH) from the anterior lobe of the pituitary gland. Overstimulation by TSH causes the thyroid cells to enlarge and secrete extra amounts of hormones. Treatment for this condition may involve drug therapy to block the production of thyroid hormones or surgical removal of all or part of the thyroid gland. Another method for treating this disorder is to administer a sufficient amount of radioactive iodine to destroy the thyroid secretory cells.

As with the thyroid gland, dysfunction of the parathyroids is usually characterized by excessive hormone secretion **(hyperparathyroidism)** or inadequate hormone secretion **(hypoparathyroidism)**.

Hypoparathyroidism can result from an injury or from surgical removal of these glands, sometimes in conjunction with thyroid surgery. The primary effect of hypoparathyroidism is the lowering of the blood calcium level. The decreased calcium **(hypocalcemia)** lowers the threshold and causes neurons to depolarize more easily and the number of nerve impulses to increase. This condition results in muscle twitches and spasms, producing the clinical picture of **tetany**.

Hyperparathyroidism is most often caused by a benign tumor. The resulting increase in parathyroid hormone (PTH) secretion results in demineralization of bones **(osteitis fibrosa cystica)**, making them porous **(osteoporosis)** and highly susceptible to fracture and deformity. When this condition is the result of a benign tumor of the parathyroid gland **(adenoma)**, the tumor is removed. Treatment may also include orthopedic surgery to correct severe bone deformities. An excess of PTH also causes calcium to be deposited in the kidneys. When the disease is generalized, all the bones are affected, and this disorder is then known as **von Recklinghausen's disease**. Renal symptoms are the most common effects seen. Nephrolithiasis due to hypercalcemia is a frequent condition.

Adrenals

ADRENAL MEDULLA

There are no specific diseases that can be traced directly to a deficiency of hormones from the medulla. However, medullary tumors sometimes cause excess secretions. The most common disorder is in the form of a neoplasm known as pheochromocytoma, which produces excessive amounts of epinephrine and norepinephrine. Most of these tumors are encapsulated and benign. These hypersecretions produce stress, fear, palpitations, headaches, visual blurring, muscle spasms, and sweating. The usual form of treatment consists of administration of antihypertensive drugs and surgery.

ADRENAL CORTEX

Addison's disease, a relatively uncommon chronic disorder caused by a deficiency of cortical hormones, results when the adrenal cortex is destroyed. It is caused by atrophy of the adrenals, probably the result of some autoimmune process in which circulating adrenal antibodies slowly destroy the gland. Ninety percent of the gland is usually destroyed before clinical signs of adrenal insufficiency appear. Hypofunction of the adrenal cortex interferes with the body's ability to handle internal and external stress. In severe cases, the disturbance of sodium and potassium metabolism may be marked by depletion of the sodium and water through the urine, resulting in severe chronic dehydration. Other clinical manifestations include muscular weakness, anorexia, gastrointestinal symptoms, fatigue, hypoglycemia, hypotension, low blood sodium **(hyponatremia)**, and high serum potassium **(hyperkalemia)**. If treatment for this condition begins early, usually with adrenocortical hormone therapy, the prognosis is excellent. If untreated, the disease will continue a chronic course with progressive but relatively slow deterioration. In some patients, the deterioration may be rapid.

Cushing's syndrome is caused by hypersecretion of the adrenal cortex and results in excessive production of glucocorticoids. This overactivity is commonly due to an abnormal growth of the adrenal cortices. It may also be caused by a tumor arising in the cortex of one of the adrenal glands, a pituitary tumor, or excessive administration of cortisone. Symptoms include rapidly developing adiposity of the face (moon-face) and neck, purple striae on the skin, fatigue, high blood pressure, and excessive hair growth in unusual places **(hirsutism)**, especially in females. Treatment is partial removal of the adrenal gland **(adrenalectomy)** or removal of the tumor. The symptoms of this syndrome are mimicked by the use of prolonged cortisone therapy for the treatment of inflammatory conditions.

Pancreas

Diabetes mellitus (DM) is by far the most common pancreatic disorder. DM is now recognized to exist in two forms: the insulin-dependent form, caused by a failure of the B-cells to produce an adequate amount of insulin; and the non–insulin-dependent form, caused by a failure of insulin to facilitate the movement of glucose. In both forms, the blood glucose is elevated above the normal range. Clinical manifestations of both forms are summarized in Tables 13-7 and 13-8.

There are a number of complications associated with diabetes. It is characterized by severe upsets in carbohydrate metabolism as well as disturbances in protein and fat metabolism. There is a rise in the concentration of blood sugar **(hyperglycemia)**. Some of the glucose, along with electrolytes (particularly sodium), is excreted in the urine **(glycosuria)**, causing excessive urination **(diuresis)**, dehydration, and thirst **(polydipsia)**. Sodium and potassium losses cause muscle weakness and fatigue. Since glucose cannot enter the cell, cellular starvation results. This leads to hunger and an increased appetite **(polyphagia)**. Unless treatment is initiated, ketoacidosis, which is an advanced stage of hyperglycemia, will develop.

Ketoacidosis, also referred to as diabetic acidosis or diabetic coma, may develop quickly over several days or weeks. It can be caused by too little insulin, failure to follow a diet, physical or emotional stress, or undiagnosed diabetes. Low blood sugar **(hypoglycemia)** occurs when there is proportionately too much insulin in the blood for the available glucose. Hyperinsulinism may also be due to a tumor involving the islet cells, but similar symptoms occur if a diabetic receives too large a dosage of insulin. In either case, the condition is referred to as insulin shock. Treatment includes administering glucose intravenously, which usually brings the patient out of shock within a few minutes.

Table 13–7. CLINICAL MANIFESTATIONS OF INSULIN-DEPENDENT DIABETES*

Insulin-dependent diabetes is characterized by the sudden appearance of:

Constant urination (polyuria) and glycosuria
Abnormal thirst (polydipsia)
Unusual hunger (polyphagia)
The rapid loss of weight
Irritability
Obvious weakness and fatigue
Nausea and vomiting

Any one of these signals can indicate diabetes. Children usually exhibit dramatic, sudden symptoms and must receive prompt treatment.

*From American Diabetes Association, New York.

Table 13–8. CLINICAL MANIFESTATIONS OF NON–INSULIN-DEPENDENT DIABETES*

311

Non–insulin-dependent diabetes may include any of the signs of insulin-dependent diabetes or:

Drowsiness
Itching
A family history of diabetes
Blurred vision
Excessive weight
Tingling, numbness, pain in the extremities
Easily fatigued
Skin infections and slow healing of cuts and scratches, especially of the feet

Many adults may have diabetes with none of these symptoms. The disease is often discovered during a routine physical examination.

*From American Diabetes Association, New York.

OTHER TERMS RELATED TO THE ENDOCRINE SYSTEM

TERM	MEANING	PRONUNCIATION
acromegaly	disease characterized by enlarged features, particularly the face and hands. This is the result of oversecretion of the pituitary growth hormone	ăk - rō - MĔG - ă - lē
diuresis	increased excretion of urine. This occurs in diabetes mellitus. It can also be an early sign of chronic interstitial nephritis	dĭ - ū - RĒ - sĭs
glucagon	a hormone secreted by the pancreatic alpha cells that increases blood glucose concentration	GLOO - kă - gŏn
glucose	a simple sugar	GLOO - kōs
glucosuria, glycosuria	presence of glucose in the urine; an abnormal amount of sugar in the urine	gloo - kō - SŪ - rē - ăh GLĪ - kō - sū - rē - ăh
hirsutism	abnormal hairiness, especially in women	hĕr - SOOT - ĭzm
homeostasis	state of equilibrium in the internal environment of the body	hō - mē - ō - STĀ - sĭs
hypercalcemia	excessive amount of calcium in the blood	hĭ - pĕr - kăl - SĒ - mē - ăh
hyperkalemia	excessive amount of potassium in the blood, most often due to defective renal excretion	hĭ - pĕr - kă - LĒ - mē - ăh

Continued on following page

OTHER TERMS RELATED TO THE ENDOCRINE SYSTEM—*Continued*

TERM	MEANING	PRONUNCIATION
hyponatremia	abnormal condition of low sodium in the blood	hĭ - pō - nă - TRĒ - mē - ăh
obesity	excessive accumulation of fat in the body	ō - BĒ - sĭ - tē
pheochromocytoma	a small chromaffin cell tumor, usually located in the adrenal medulla	fē - ō - krō - mō - sĭ - TŌ - măh
virile	masculine; having the characteristics of an adult male, especially copulative powers	VĬR - ĭl
virilism	masculinization in a woman; development of male secondary sex characteristics in the female	VĬR - ĭl - ĭzm

SPECIAL PROCEDURES RELATED TO THE ENDOCRINE SYSTEM

RADIOGRAPHIC PROCEDURES

TERM	DESCRIPTION
thyroid echogram (ultrasound examination of the thyroid)	valuable for distinguishing cystic from solid nodules. If the nodule is found to be purely cystic and fluid filled, it is aspirated. Thus, surgery is avoided. However, if the nodule has a mixed or solid appearance, carcinoma is a likely possibility and surgery is usually necessary. A nonfunctioning thyroid nodule can be evaluated with the use of reflected sound waves
CT scan of the adrenals (computerized tomographic study of the adrenal glands)	a noninvasive and yet very accurate method of detecting very small tumors such as adenomas, carcinomas, and pheochromocytomas of the adrenal glands. Adrenal hemorrhage can also be detected with this procedure
thyroid scan	useful for determining location, size, shape, and anatomical function of the thyroid gland. Scanner passes over the thyroid and makes a graphic recording of radiation emitted. Abnormal scans usually exhibit a change in thyroidal shape, size, and position, as well as function. The scan is helpful in the evaluation of thyroid nodules, carcinomas, and masses in the tongue, neck, and mediastinum

SURGICAL PROCEDURES

TERM	DESCRIPTION	PRONUNCIATION
adrenalectomy	excision of an adrenal gland	ăd - rē - năl - ĔK - tō - mē
microneurosurgery of pituitary gland	magnification using a binocular surgical microscope for microdissection of a tumor	mī - krō - nū - rō - SĔR - jĕr - ē pǐ - TŪ - ǐ - tār - ē
parathyroidectomy	excision of one or more of the parathyroid glands, usually done to control hyperparathyroidism	păr - ăh - thī - roi - DĔK - tō - mē
pinealectomy	removal of the pineal body	pǐn - ē - ăl - ĔK - tō - mē
thymectomy	excision of the thymus gland	thī - MĔK - tō - mē
thyroid surgery, lobectomy of thyroid	usually the removal of the isthmus and involved lobe for solitary thyroid nodule	lō - BĔK - tō - mē/THĪ - roid
partial thyroidectomy	method of choice for removal of fibrous nodular thyroid	thī - roi - DĔK - tō - mē
subtotal thyroidectomy	the removal of most of the thyroid to relieve hyperthyroidism	thī - roi - DĔK - tō - mē

LABORATORY PROCEDURES

TERM	DESCRIPTION
radioactive iodine uptake test (RAIU)	this test is based on the ability of the thyroid gland to trap and retain iodine, and provides an indirect measure of thyroid activity. A designated quantity of radioactive iodine is administered orally or intravenously (IV). Then a gamma-ray detector (as is used in most nuclear scanning) determines the quantity or percentage of radioactive iodine taken up by the gland over a specific period of time. A 24-hour urine specimen may also be analyzed

Serum Studies

serum glucose tests	are helpful in diagnosing insulin deficiency or adjusting insulin dosages. In general, true glucose elevations may indicate diabetes mellitus. But there are also many other possible causes of hyperglycemia
fasting blood sugar (FBS)	measures circulating glucose level after a 12-hour fast
glucose tolerance test (GTT)	evaluates insulin response to a glucose load after a 12-hour fast. The oral GTT is the most sensitive test for diabetes. Elevated levels strongly suggest diabetes mellitus. Three days prior to the test, the patient's diet should be high in carbohydrates. After a

Continued on following page

LABORATORY PROCEDURES—*Continued*

TERM	DESCRIPTION
Serum Studies	
	12-hour overnight fast, blood samples are drawn at 30 minutes, 1-hour, 2-hours, and 3-hours. The test is performed after glucose ingestion
insulin tolerance test	evaluates patients suspected of having hypopituitarism. It tests GH secreting capacity. Intravenous (IV) injection of regular insulin is administered based on body weight. Blood samples are drawn 0, 30, 45, 60, and 90 minutes after injection. GH should rise twofold to threefold over baseline levels. If there is GH deficiency, the response is subnormal or absent
protein-bound iodine (PBI)	measures the concentration of PBI in a blood sample. The results of this test furnish an index of the thyroid gland's activity
thyroxine iodine test (T_4)	evaluates thyroid function. The amount of iodine associated with the thyroxine in the sample is measured using several laboratory procedures. The value obtained is then compared with the normal range of thyroxine iodine concentrations
triiodothyronine uptake (T_3)	determines how much thyroid hormone is bound to the protein in a blood sample
total calcium	measures calcium to detect bone and parathyroid disorders. Hypercalcemia can indicate primary hyperparathyroidism. Hypocalcemia can indicate hypoparathyroidism
two-hour postprandial glucose tolerance test	screening test used to evaluate glucose metabolism. An overnight fast and a 3-day high-carbohydrate diet precedes collection of a 2-hour postprandial (after a meal) blood sample

PHARMACOLOGY RELATED TO THE ENDOCRINE SYSTEM

MEDICATION	ACTION
antihyperlipidemics	lower cholesterol levels in the bloodstream; help prevent atherosclerosis (fatty build-up in the blood vessels)
corticosteroids	replacement hormones for adrenal insufficiency (Addison's disease). Corticosteroids are widely used for suppressing inflammation, controlling allergic reactions, reducing the rejection process in transplantation, and in the treatment of some cancers
insulin	major drug for diabetes. Lowers glucose level and is obtained from pork or beef pancreas. Administered by injection
oral hypoglycemics	can be used only with certain types of diabetes mellitus patients, mainly those who have developed the condition as adults and often are overweight. These drugs are unrelated to insulin and they are used in cases where the pancreas is already producing

Continued on following page

MEDICATION	ACTION
	some insulin. Their effect is to stimulate the pancreas to secrete more insulin and make the body cells more receptive to the action of insulin
vasopressin	controls diabetes insipidus and subsequent polyuria due to antidiuretic hormone (ADH) deficiency. It replaces ADH of pituitary; promotes reabsorption of water in the kidneys

ABBREVIATIONS RELATED TO THE ENDOCRINE SYSTEM

ABBREVIATION	MEANING
ACTH	adrenocorticotropic hormone
ADH	antidiuretic hormone (vasopressin)
DI	diabetes insipidus; diagnostic imaging
DM	diabetes mellitus
ECF	extracellular fluid
FBS	fasting blood sugar
FSH	follicle-stimulating hormone
GH	growth hormone
GTT	glucose tolerance test
HDL	high-density lipoproteins
ICF	intracellular fluid
LDL	low-density lipoproteins
MSH	melanocyte-stimulating hormone
NPH	neutral protamine Hagedorn (insulin)
PGH	pituitary growth hormone
PTH	parathyroid hormone
RAI	radioactive iodine
T_3	triiodothyronine
T_4	thyroxine
TSH	thyroid-stimulating hormone
VLDL	very-low-density lipoproteins
XX	female sex chromosomes
XY	male sex chromosomes

WORKSHEET 1

A. Using the word root/combining form adren/o (adrenal glands), build medical words to mean:

1. _____ inflammation of the adrenal glands

2. _____ pertaining to the adrenal glands and the genitalia

3. _____ excision of an adrenal gland

4. _____ pertaining to the adrenal cortex

B. Using the word root/combining form glyc/o (sugar), build medical words to mean:

1. _____ pertaining to the formation of glycogen

2. _____ condition of excessive sugar in the blood

3. _____ condition of deficiency of sugar in the blood

4. _____ formation of glycogen (from glucose)

C. Using the word root/combining form pancreat/o (pancreas), build medical words to mean:

1. _____ inflammation of the pancreas

2. _____ produced in or originating in the pancreas

3. _____ destruction of the pancreatic substance

4. _____ any pancreatic disease

D. Using the word root/combining form thyr/o (thyroid), build medical words to mean:

1. _____ pertaining to the thyroid gland and the tongue

2. _____ inflammation of the thyroid gland

3. _____ excision of the thyroid gland

4. _____ enlarged condition (swelling) of the thyroid

WORKSHEET 2

Fill in the correct word from the right hand column that matches the definition in the statements below.

1. _____ a hormone that helps maintain the pressure in blood vessels and that works as a diuretic — Adenohypophysis

2. _____ hypothyroidism that develops after puberty — Addison's disease

3. _____ a glandlike structure which is the anterior lobe of the pituitary — Cretinism

4. _____ excessive growth of hair or the presence of hair in unusual places, especially in women — Exophthalmic goiter

5. _____ hypothyroidism that develops in an infant — Hirsutism

6. _____ B-cells (beta cells) of the pancreas produce — Hyperparathyroidism

7. _____ disease resulting from deficiency in the secretion of adrenocortical hormones — Insulin

8. _____ a condition marked by protrusion of the eyeballs, increased heart action, enlargement of the thyroid gland, weight loss, and nervousness — Myxedema

9. _____ condition due to increased activity of the parathyroid glands; also known as osteitis fibrosa cystica — Neurohypophysis

10. _____ posterior lobe of the pancreas — Vasopressin

318   WORKSHEET 3

Build a surgical term for the following:

1. _____ excision of the thyroid

2. _____ surgical incision of thyroid cartilage

3. _____ excision of a parathyroid gland

4. _____ excision of the head of the pancreas and the adjacent portion of the duodenum

5. _____ removal of the adrenal

6. _____ removal of the adrenal glands on both sides

WORKSHEET 4

Define the following diagnostic and symptomatic terms. Use the dictionary as a reference.

1. Cushing's disease _____

2. dwarfism _____

3. hyperinsulinism _____

4. hypothyroidism _____

5. goiter _____

6. hyperglycemia _____

7. diabetes insipidus _____

8. Addison's disease _____

9. ketoacidosis _____

10. diabetes mellitus _____

WORKSHEET 5

Grammar Review—Endocrine System

Write the plural form for the following words.

1. gonad   1. _____

2. ovum   2. _____

3. stria   3. _____

4. atrophy   4. _____

5. myxoadenoma   5. _____

Form noun endings that mean abnormal condition or state of being.

6. cretin   6. _____

7. dwarf   7. _____

8. hirsute   8. _____

9. giant   9. _____

10. Using the word root/combining form endocrin/o (pertaining to a gland that secretes directly into the bloodstream), form a word with a noun ending that means one who specializes in endocrinology _____

WORKSHEET 6

Label the figure below, and compare your answers with Figure 13-1.

Pineal gland

Pituitary (hypophysis) gland

Thyroid gland

Parathyroid glands

Adrenal (suprarenal) glands

Pancreas

Ovaries

Testes

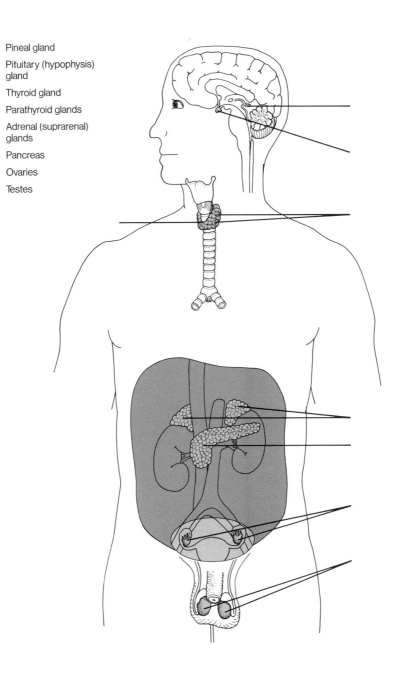

322   ## WORKSHEET 7

Special Procedures, Pharmacology, and Abbreviations

Choose the word(s) that best describes the following statements:

antihyperlipidemics	T_3
corticosteroids	T_4
FBS	thyroid echogram
HDL	vasopressin
insulin	VLDL
RAI	XX
RAIU	XY
serum glucose test	

1. _____ measures circulating glucose level after a 12-hour fast

2. _____ this test is based on the ability of the thyroid gland to trap and retain iodine, and provides an indirect measure of thyroid activity

3. _____ replacement hormones for adrenal insufficiency. Also, widely used for suppressing inflammation, controlling allergic reactions, reducing the rejection process in transplantation, and treatment of some cancers

4. _____ controls diabetes insipidus and subsequent polyuria due to ADH deficiency

5. _____ ultrasound examination of the thyroid

6. _____ thyroxine

7. _____ female sex chromosomes

8. _____ major drug for diabetics. Lowers glucose level and is administered by injection

9. _____ helpful for diagnosing insulin deficiency or adjusting dosages

10. _____ lowers cholesterol levels in the bloodstream, and helps prevent atherosclerosis

11. _____ radioactive iodine

12. _____ high-density lipoproteins

13. _____ triiodothyronine

14. _____ male sex chromosomes

15. _____ very-low-density lipoproteins

CHAPTER 14

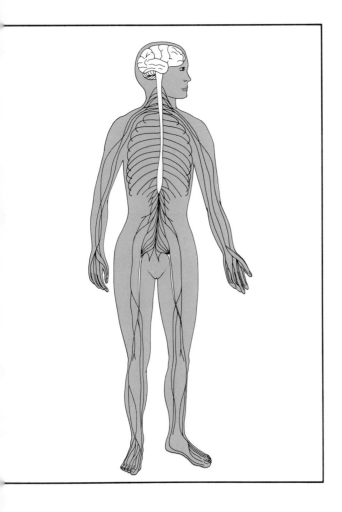

Nervous System

STUDENT OBJECTIVES

Upon completion of this chapter, you will be able to do the following:

Identify the divisions of the nervous system according to location and function.

Describe the two types of nervous tissue.

List and identify the major structures and functions of the brain and spinal cord.

Identify the word roots/combining forms and suffixes associated with the nervous system.

Identify and discuss the pathology associated with the nervous system.

Identify radiographic, clinical, surgical, and laboratory procedures and abbreviations related to the nervous system.

Explain the pharmacology related to the treatment of nervous disorders.

Build and analyze diagnostic, symptomatic, and surgical terms related to the nervous system by completing the worksheets.

326   ANATOMY AND PHYSIOLOGY OF THE NERVOUS SYSTEM

The nervous system is one of the most complicated systems of the body (Fig. 14-1). Along with the endocrine system, it controls many bodily activities. The nervous system senses changes in both the internal and external environments, interprets these changes, and then coordinates appropriate responses that are designed to maintain homeostasis, which is a state of equilibrium in the internal environment. Figure 14-2 illustrates the divisions of the nervous system. Refer to this figure as you read the following paragraphs.

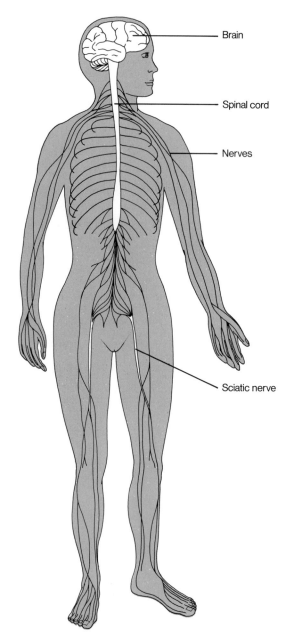

Brain

Spinal cord

Nerves

Sciatic nerve

Figure 14–1. The nervous system.

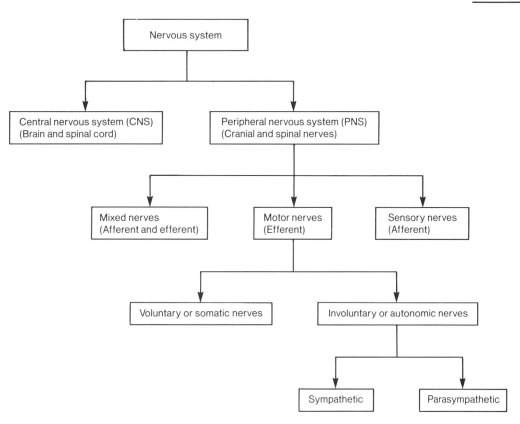

Figure 14–2. Subdivisions of the nervous system.

Divisions of the Nervous System

The brain, spinal cord, and nerves all interact in relaying information. The nervous system has two major divisions: the **central nervous system (CNS)**, which is composed of the brain and spinal cord; and the **peripheral nervous system (PNS)**, which includes all other nervous tissue of the body found outside of the CNS.

The PNS includes 12 pairs of cranial nerves, which emerge from the base of the skull, and 31 pairs of spinal nerves, which emerge from the spinal cord. All of these nerves consist of fibers that may be either sensory or motor, or a mixture of both sensory and motor fibers.

Sensory nerves receive impulses from the sense organs, such as the eyes, ears, nose, tongue, and skin, and then transmit the impulses to the CNS. Because they conduct impulses toward a specific site—the central nervous system—they are also known as **afferent nerves**.

Motor nerves conduct impulses away from the CNS; thus, they are known as **efferent nerves**. These impulses travel to muscles and other body organs, causing them to respond in some manner.

Nerves composed of both sensory and motor fibers are called **mixed nerves**. An example of a mixed nerve is the facial nerve. When it supplies the facial muscles with impulses for smiling or frowning, the facial nerve is functioning as a motor nerve. But when the tongue transmits a taste impulse to the brain through this nerve, it is responding in a sensory capacity.

Functionally, the PNS is divided into two specialized systems: the **somatic nervous system (SNS)** and the **autonomic nervous system (ANS)**. The somatic component is under the direct control of the individual. It innervates (supplies with nerves) the extremities and the body wall, including the skeletal muscles and the skin. Since the somatic nervous system produces movement only in the skeletal muscles, it is under conscious control of the organism and is therefore voluntary. Examples of voluntary activity include walking, talking, and playing tennis. In contrast, the autonomic component conveys impulses to glands, smooth muscles, and cardiac muscles. This division is therefore considered involuntary since it operates without conscious control. Examples of autonomic activity include digestion, heart contraction, and vasoconstriction.

The autonomic nervous system is further specialized into two subdivisions: the **sympathetic** and **parasympathetic** divisions. To a large extent, these subdivisions function in opposing the action of each other, although in certain instances, they may exhibit independent action. In general, sympathetic nerve fibers produce vasoconstriction, increased heart rate, elevated blood pressure, and depressed gastrointestinal activity, while the parasympathetic system generally conveys impulses to bring about vasodilation, a slower heart rate, a decrease in blood pressure, and a return to normal gastrointestinal activity. These autonomic functions are evident in "fight or flight" situations. Blood flow increases in skeletal muscles to prepare the individual to either fight or run away from a threatening situation. When the danger passes, more blood is directed to the internal organs.

Nervous Tissue

In spite of its complexity, the nervous system is composed of only two principal types of nerve cells, **neurons** and **neuroglia**. Neurons, the functional cells of the nervous system, are responsible for impulse conduction. All neural circuits are composed of neuron chains. In contrast to neurons, neuroglia do not transmit impulses. Neuroglia is specialized nervous tissue that functions as connective tissue supporting and binding neurons. During infection, neuroglia is capable of performing certain phagocytic activities.

NEURONS

Neurons consist of three major structures:
1. Dendrites, which are branching cytoplasmic projections that receive impulses and transmit them to the cell body.
2. Cell body, which contains the cell nucleus.
3. Axon, which is a long single projection that transmits the impulse from the cell body.

Refer to Figure 14-3 as you read the following material.

Many axons in both the PNS and CNS are covered with a white, lipoid sheath called **myelin**. This wrapping acts as an electrical insulator that reduces the possibility of an impulse stimulating adjacent nerves. In addition, myelin accelerates impulses through the axon. The presence of myelin on axons in the brain and spinal cord gives a white appearance to these structures, and they make up what is called the white matter of the CNS. Unmyelinated fibers, dendrites, and nerve cell bodies make up the gray matter.

On peripheral nerves, a thin cellular membrane called **neurolemma**, or **neurolemmal sheath**, wraps around the myelin sheath. The neurolemmal sheath permits a damaged axon to regenerate. Since neurolemma is not found in the CNS, severed nerves in the CNS cannot regenerate; therefore, nerve function is permanently lost unless alternate pathways are established.

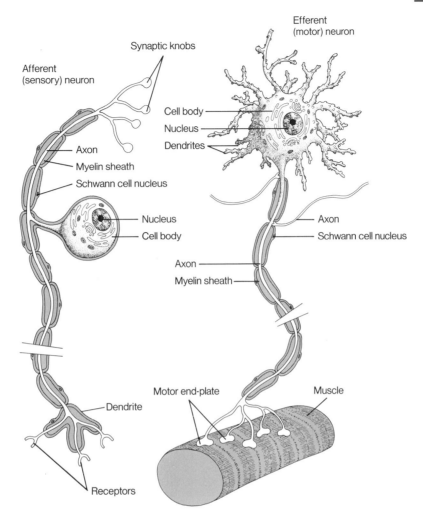

Figure 14–3. *Illustration shows sensory neuron transmitting an impulse to the central nervous system, and a motor neuron transmitting an impulse from the central nervous system.*

Neurons are not continuous with one another. Instead, a small space, known as a **synapse**, is found between the axon of one neuron and the dendrite or cell body of another. In order for the impulse to travel along a nerve path, it must be transmitted at the synapse. This transmission is facilitated by certain chemical substances called **neurotransmitters**.

NEUROGLIA

The term neuroglia literally means nerve glue. It was once believed that neuroglia served only a supporting role for neurons. But it is now known that different shaped neuroglia cells, as shown in Figure 14-4, perform many other functions. **Astrocytes**, as their name suggests, are star-shaped neuroglia and are believed to be involved in the transfer of substances from the blood to the brain. **Oligodendrocytes** are cells with only a few processes. They are believed to help in the development of myelin on neurons of the CNS. **Microglia**, the smallest of the neuroglia, possess phagocytic properties and may become very active during times of infection.

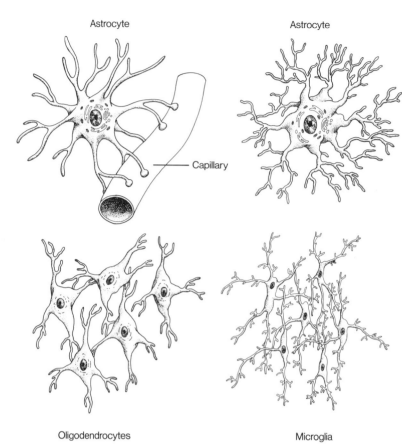

Figure 14–4. Neuroglia.

Brain

In addition to being one of the largest organs of the body, the brain is also the most complex in structure and function. It integrates almost every physical and mental activity of the body. This organ is also the center for memory, emotion, thought, judgment, reasoning, and consciousness.

The brain is composed of four major sections: the cerebrum, cerebellum, diencephalon (interbrain), and brain stem. In order to develop a better understanding of the anatomy of the brain, refer to Figure 14-5 as you read the following material.

The (1) **cerebrum** is the largest and uppermost portion of the brain. It consists of two hemispheres divided by a deep longitudinal fissure, or groove. The fissure does not completely separate the hemispheres. A structure called the corpus callosum joins them medially on their inferior surfaces. Each hemisphere is further divided into five lobes. Four of these lobes are named for the bones that lie directly above them. The fifth lobe of the cerebrum is hidden from view and can only be seen upon dissection.

Numerous folds, or convolutions, called gyri are found on the cerebral surface. These are separated by furrows or fissures called sulci. A thin layer of gray matter, the cerebral cortex, which is composed of millions of cell bodies, covers the entire cerebrum and is responsible for its gray color

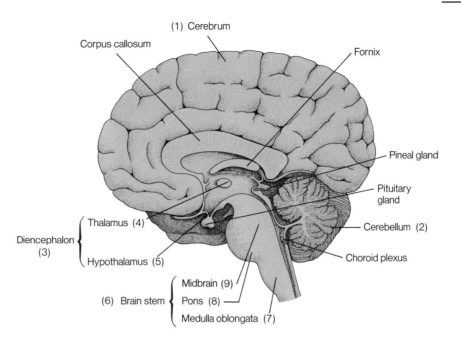

Figure 14–5. *Sections of the brain.*

The remainder of the cerebrum is composed primarily of white matter (myelinated axons). Major functions of the cerebrum include sensory perception and interpretation, muscular movement, and the emotional aspects of behavior and memory.

The second largest part of the brain, the (2) **cerebellum**, occupies the back portion of the brain. It is attached to the brain stem. When the cerebrum initiates muscular movement, the cerebellum coordinates and refines the movement. The cerebellum also aids in maintaining equilibrium and balance of the body.

The (3) **diencephalon**, or interbrain, is composed of many smaller structures, two of which are the (4) **thalamus** and the (5) **hypothalamus**. All sensory stimuli, except olfactory, are received by the thalamus. Here they are processed and transmitted to the proper area of the cerebral cortex. In addition, impulses from the cerebrum are received by the thalamus and relayed to efferent nerves. Beneath the thalamus is a small structure called the hypothalamus. Its chief function is the integration of autonomic nerve impulses and the regulation of certain endocrine functions.

The (6) **brain stem** completes the last major section of the brain. It is composed of three structures: the (7) **medulla oblongata**, the (8) **pons**, and the (9) **midbrain** (mesencephalon). In general, the brain stem serves as a pathway for impulse conduction between the brain and the spinal cord. The brain stem also serves as the origin for 10 of the 12 pairs of cranial nerves. The brain stem is the center that controls respiration, blood pressure, and heart rate.

Spinal Cord

The spinal cord conveys to the brain sensory impulses from different parts of the body and also transmits motor impulses from the brain to all muscles and organs. The sensory nerve tracts are also called ascending tracts, since the direction of the impulse is upward. Conversely, motor nerve tracts that relay motor impulses to muscles and organs are called

332

descending tracts, since they carry impulses in a downward direction. A cross-section of the spinal cord reveals an inner gray area composed of cell bodies and dendrites, with a white outer area composed of myelinated tissue of the ascending and descending tracts.

The entire spinal cord is located within the spinal cavity of the vertebral column. Thirty-one pairs of spinal nerves exit from between the intervertebral spaces almost throughout the entire length of the spinal column. Unlike the cranial nerves, which have specific names, the spinal nerves are known by the region of the vertebral column from which they exit. Refer to Chapter 10, Musculoskeletal System, for the divisions of the vertebral column.

Meninges

Bones protect both the brain and the spinal cord against injury. The brain is enclosed within the skull, and the spinal cord is enclosed within the vertebral column. In addition, both the brain and the spinal cord receive limited protection from a set of three coverings called **meninges**. The outermost coat, the **dura mater**, is tough and fibrous. Immediately beneath the dura mater is a cavity called the **subdural space**. It is filled with serous fluid. The next layer of the meninges is the **arachnoid**. As its name suggests, the arachnoid has a spider-web appearance. A **subarachnoid space**, which is filled with cerebrospinal fluid, provides additional protection for the brain and spinal cord by acting as a shock absorber. Finally, the innermost layer, the **pia mater**, contains numerous blood vessels and lymphatics, which provide nourishment for the underlying tissues.

Cerebrospinal fluid circulates around the spinal cord and the brain and through spaces called **ventricles**. These ventricles are located within the inner portion of the brain. This clear, colorless fluid contains proteins, glucose, urea, salts, and some white blood cells. As it circulates, this fluid provides nutritive substances to the central nervous system. It also acts as a shock absorber for the delicate structures of the central nervous system. Normally, cerebrospinal fluid is absorbed as rapidly as it is formed. Any interference with absorption results in hydrocephalus.

WORD ROOTS/COMBINING FORMS RELATED TO THE NERVOUS SYSTEM

WORD ROOT/ COMBINING FORM	MEANING	EXAMPLE		PRONUNCIATION
cerebell/o	cerebellum	cerebell/ar pertaining to		sĕr - ĕ - BĔL - ăr
cerebr/o	cerebrum	cerebr/o/spin/ spine	al pertaining to	sĕr - ĕ - brō - SPĪ - năl
crani/o	skull	crani/o/tomy incision		krā - nē - ŎT - ō - mē
encephal/o	brain	encephal/itis inflammation		ĕn - SĔF - ăh - LĪ - tĭs

Continued on following page

WORD ROOTS/COMBINING FORMS RELATED TO THE
NERVOUS SYSTEM—*Continued*

WORD ROOT/ COMBINING FORM	MEANING	EXAMPLE	PRONUNCIATION

gangli/o
 ganglion/o
	ganglion (knot)	gangli/oma
		     tumor
		 ganglion/ectomy
		     excision
			găng - glē - Ō - măh
			
			 găng - glē - ō - NĚK - tō - mē

gli/o	glue	neur/o/gli/a nerve noun ending	nū - RŎG - lē - ăh
kinesi/o	movement	kinesi/o/therapy treatment	kĭ - nē - sē - ō - THĚR - ăh - pē
medull/o	medulla	medull/ary pertaining to	MĚD - ū - lār - ē

mening/o
 meningi/o
	meninges, brain covering	mening/o/cele
		     hernia
		 meningi/oma
		     tumor
			mě - NĬNG - gō - sēl
			
			 měn - ĭn - jē - Ō - măh

myel/o	spinal cord, bone marrow	myel/algia pain	mĭ - ě - LĂL - jē - ăh
narc/o	sleep	narc/o/lepsy seizure	NĂR - kō - lěp - sē
neur/o	nerve, neuron	neur/o/tripsy crush	nū - rō - TRĬP - sē
thalam/o	thalamus, chamber	thalam/o/tomy incision	thăl - ăh - MŎT - ō - mē
ton/o	tone	cata/ton/ic below pertaining to	kăt - ăh - TŎN - ĭk
ventricul/o	ventricles, little belly	ventricul/o/gram record	věn - TRĬK - ū - lō - grăm

SUFFIXES RELATED TO THE NERVOUS SYSTEM

SUFFIX	MEANING	EXAMPLE	PRONUNCIATION
-algesia	pain	an/algesia with- out	ăn - ăl - JĒ - zē - ăh
-esthesia	feeling, sensation	an/esthesia with- out	ăn - ěs - THĒ - zē - ăh
-kinesia	movement	hyper/kinesia excessive	hĭ - pěr - kĭ - NĒ - zē - ăh

Continued on following page

SUFFIXES RELATED TO THE NERVOUS SYSTEM—Continued

SUFFIX	MEANING	EXAMPLE	PRONUNCIATION
-lepsy	seizure	epi/lepsy above	ĔP - ĭ - lĕp - sē
-paresis	partial or incomplete paralysis	hemi/paresis half	hĕm - ē - PĂR - ē - sĭs
-phasia	speech	a/phasia lack of	ăh - FĀ - zē - ăh
-plegia	paralysis	hemi/plegia half	hĕm - ē - PLĒ - jē - ăh
-asthenia	without strength	my/asthenia muscle	mĭ - ăs - THĒ - nē - ăh
-taxia	muscular coordination	a/taxia lack of	ăh - TĂK - sē - ăh
-trophy	nourishment, development	dys/trophy poor	DĬS - trō - fē

PATHOLOGY OF THE NERVOUS SYSTEM

Bell's Palsy

Bell's palsy is a facial paralysis due to a functional disorder of the seventh cranial nerve. It produces asthenia and numbness of the face. The cornea becomes dry owing to the lack of the blink reflex, which often leads to corneal infections **(keratitis)**. The patient may also experience speech difficulties **(dysphasia)** and pain behind the ear or in the face. There may also be an overflow of tears down the cheek **(epiphora)** due to keratitis.

Bell's palsy often produces grotesque facial disfigurement and facial spasms. In some instances, it may result in unilateral paralysis of facial muscles and distortion of taste perception.

Treatment for this condition involves the use of anti-inflammatory drugs and the application of heat to promote circulation. Spontaneous recovery can be expected in most patients in about 3 to 5 weeks.

Cerebrovascular Disease

Cerebrovascular disease refers to any functional abnormality of the cerebrum caused by disorders of the blood vessels that supply the brain. These disorders include hemorrhage from a vessel or an impairment of cerebral circulation owing to hardening of blood vessels **(arteriosclerosis)**, cerebral thromboses, or emboli. Both hemorrhage and occlusion may lead to stroke **(cerebral vascular accident, CVA, apoplexy)**. During a CVA, blood supply to the neurons of the brain is diminished or absent. This leads to destruction of brain tissue

(infarction). If the CVA is mild, the individual may experience a brief "blackout," blurred vision, or dizziness, and may not even realize that anything serious has happened. In more serious cases, the clinical manifestations may include weakness in one half of the body **(hemiparesis)**, paralysis in one half of the body **(hemiplegia)**, inability to speak **(aphasia)**, lack of muscular coordination **(ataxia)**, stupor, or coma. Treatment involves speech, physical, or occupational therapy, depending on the severity.

Epilepsies

Epilepsies are transient seizure disorders that involve several brain malfunctions, especially electrical disturbances **(dysrhythmias)** in the brain. These dysrhythmias result in abnormal, recurrent, and uncontrolled electrical discharges. Many structural, chemical, or physiological disorders may cause epilepsy. These include brain injury, congenital anomalies, metabolic disorders, brain tumors, vascular disturbances, and genetic disorders. Three types of seizures are identified: petit mal, grand mal, and psychomotor.

Clinical manifestations of petit mal epilepsy are brief episodes (10 to 30 seconds) of unconsciousness, eye or muscle flutterings, and occasionally, loss of muscle tone. In grand mal seizures, there is a loss of consciousness, with tonic (firm or violent) then clonic (alternation of rigidity and then relaxation) contraction of the muscles, involuntary convulsive movements, disturbances of autonomic function, and disorders of sensation of special senses. Psychomotor seizures are focal seizures characterized by a 1- to 2-minute loss of association with the surroundings. The patient appears confused, often mumbling incoherently.

Epilepsy can be effectively controlled, in many instances, by the use of anti-epileptic medications.

Parkinson's Disease

Parkinson's disease is a progressive neurological disorder affecting the portion of the brain responsible for control of movement. A degeneration of the neurons in this area of the brain leads to slowness of movement **(bradykinesia, hypokinesia)**, tremor, stiffness of large joints, and unblinking eyes.

Treatment is based on a combination of drug therapy, physical therapy, and rehabilitation techniques.

Multiple Sclerosis (MS)

Multiple sclerosis is a progressive degenerative disease in which there is an inflammation and subsequent hardening of myelin in many areas of the spinal cord and brain; hence the name, multiple sclerosis. The destruction of myelin interferes with the transmission of electrical impulses from one neuron to another. In effect, it short-circuits the conduction pathway. This disease generally strikes young adults between the ages of 20 and 40. It is believed that MS is an autoimmune disease or a result of an infection by a slow virus.

This chronic disease is characterized by tremors, weakness of muscles, and slowness of movement. Occasionally, there are visual disturbances. During remissions, symptoms temporarily disappear, but progressive hardening of myelin areas leads to other attacks.

Ultimately, most voluntary motor control is lost and the patient becomes bedridden. Death occurs anywhere from 7 to 30 years after the onset of the disease.

336   Tay-Sachs Disease

Tay-Sachs disease is a genetic disorder resulting from an enzyme deficiency at birth. The lack of the enzyme hexosaminidase causes an accumulation of lipid substances in CNS cells, which distends and destroys them.

The Tay-Sachs gene is found mostly in descendants from the Ashkenazic Jews of Eastern Europe. The afflicted child develops normally until the age of 4 to 8 months. After this time, a progressive deterioration of the infant is imminent. Paralysis, blindness, inability to eat, and, inevitably, death is the final outcome. There is no known cure; therefore, treatment is only supportive in nature. A simple blood test can identify carriers of this gene.

OTHER TERMS RELATED TO THE NERVOUS SYSTEM

TERM	MEANING	PRONUNCIATION
Alzheimer's disease	progressive neurologic disorder of unknown etiology. The symptoms include memory loss and impaired judgment, orientation, and intellectual function. In addition, patients often exhibit emotional instability	ĂLTS - hī - mĕrz
aura	a premonitory awareness of an approaching physical or mental disorder; the peculiar sensation that precedes an epileptic seizure	ĂW - răh
Babinski's reflex	dorsiflexion of the great toe upon stimulating the sole of the foot	bă - BĬN - skēz
cerebrospinal otorrhea	escape of cerebrospinal fluid through the ear as a result of trauma to the head	sĕr - ē - brō - SPĪ - năl ō - tō - RĒ - ăh
coma	abnormally deep unconsciousness with the absence of voluntary response to stimuli	KŌ - măh
concussion	an injury (usually to the brain) resulting from impact with an object	kŏn - KŬSH - ŭn
convulsion	paroxysms of involuntary muscle contractions and relaxations	kŏn - VŬL - shŭn
grand mal	a serious form of epileptic seizure with or without coma	grăn/măl
Huntington's chorea	an inherited disease of the CNS that usually has its onset between 30 and 50 years of age. This condition is characterized by quick, involuntary movements, speech disturbances, and mental deterioration owing to	HŬNT - ing - tŭnz/kō - RĒ - ăh

Continued on following page

OTHER TERMS RELATED TO THE NERVOUS SYSTEM—*Continued*

TERM	MEANING	PRONUNCIATION
	degenerative changes in the cerebral cortex and basal ganglia	
hydrocephalus	increase of cerebrospinal fluid within the ventricles of the brain due to interference with normal circulation and absorption	hĭ - drō - SĔF - ă - lŭs
idiopathic	self-originated or occurring without a known cause	ĭd - ē - ō - PĂTH - ĭk
lethargy, torpor	a condition of sluggishness; abnormal inactivity or a lack of response to normal stimuli	LĔTH - ăr - jē
meningitis	an inflammatory disease of the meninges, usually of bacterial or viral origin	mĕn - ĭn - JĪ - tĭs
meningocele	protrusion of the meninges through the skull or spinal column	mĕn - NĬNG - gō - sēl
meningomyelocele	protrusion of the meninges and spinal cord through a defect in the vertebral column	mĕn - ĭn - gō - mĭ - ĔL - ō - sēl
microcephaly	abnormally small head	mĭ - krō - SĔF - ăh - lē
myelopathy	disease of the spinal cord	mĭ - ĕ - LŎP - ăh - thē
nerve block	a loss of sensation in a localized region, such as the anesthetic administered by a dentist	
paraplegia	paralysis of the lower spine; paralysis of the lower portion of the trunk and both legs	păr - ăh - PLĒ - jē - ăh
petit mal	mild form of epileptic seizure lasting 10 to 30 seconds	pĕt - Ē/măl
quadriplegia	paralysis of upper spine; paralysis of all four extremities and usually the trunk	kwŏd - rĭ - PLĒ - jē - ăh
Romberg's sign	inability to maintain body balance when the eyes are shut and the feet are close together	RŎM - bĕrgs
spina bifida	an abnormality of one or more vertebrae characterized by a failure of the arch to fuse during embryonic development. This leads to an exposed spinal cord. (See p. 219.)	SPĪ - năh/BĪ - fĭ - dah

Continued on following page

OTHER TERMS RELATED TO THE NERVOUS SYSTEM—*Continued*

TERM	MEANING	PRONUNCIATION
syncope	fainting	SĬN - kō - pē
tic	spasmodic muscular contraction, most commonly involving the face, head, and neck	
transient ischemic attack (TIA)	temporary interference with blood supply to the brain	
tremor	involuntary shaking or trembling	TRĔM - or or TRĒ - mor

SPECIAL PROCEDURES RELATED TO THE NERVOUS SYSTEM

RADIOGRAPHIC AND CLINICAL PROCEDURES

TERM	DESCRIPTION
cerebral angiography (cerebral arteriography)	provides visualization of the cerebral vascular system after an intra-arterial injection of a radiopaque dye. The dye is usually introduced into the carotid or vertebral artery. Abnormalities of the cerebrovascular circulation, such as vascular tumors, aneurysms, and occlusions, are visualized. In addition, non-vascular tumors, abscesses, and hematomas are often identified since they distort the normal vascular image. This test is an invasive diagnostic technique with associated risks of anaphylaxis, hemorrhage, and emboli
computerized tomography scan (cranial)	provides a 3-dimensional view of the cranial contents. Tissue density affects the amount of radiation that is absorbed. Bone, which is the densest tissue, appears white; brain matter appears as shades of gray. Structures are evaluated according to density, size, shape, and position. The test is relatively safe and helps in differentiating intracranial pathologies such as tumors, cysts, edema, hemorrhage, and cerebral aneurysms
echoencephalography (echogram, ultrasound)	a noninvasive test that employs harmless, high-frequency sound waves. These sounds (echos) are reflected by the brain back to a device known as a transducer. The reflected echos are then amplified and displayed on an electronic receiving device, the oscilloscope. The echogram provides information about the position of the structures within the brain. Most notably, it detects shifts of the cerebral midline, which often occur in subdural hematoma, intracerebral hemorrhage, and cerebral infarction or tumor
electroencephalography (EEG)	a graphic recording of the electrical activities of the brain. Like the heart, the brain also generates weak electrical impulses that may be detected and graphically represented. In the EEG, elec-

Continued on following page

TERM	DESCRIPTION
	trodes are placed on the scalp over multiple areas of the brain to detect and record brain impulses. EEGs are used to investigate epileptic states, to determine cerebral lesions (hemorrhage, abscess, neoplasm, and infarction), and to determine cerebral death in comatose patients
myelography	examination of the spinal cord after injection of a radiopaque dye in the spinal canal
pneumoencephalograph	assessment of the ventricles and subarachnoid spaces of the brain following withdrawal of cerebrospinal fluid and injection of air or gas via a lumbar puncture

SURGICAL PROCEDURES

TERM	DESCRIPTION	PRONUNCIATION
cisternal puncture	a spinal puncture through the dura mater, at the base of the brain, to extract spinal fluid or inject medications	sĭs - TĔR - năl
cordectomy	removal of part of the spinal cord	kŏr - DĔK - tō - mē
craniectomy	excision of part of the skull bone	krā - nē - ĔK - tō - mē
craniotomy	surgical opening of the skull to remove a tumor or repair head injury	krā - nē - ŎT - ō - mē
cryosurgery	technique of exposing tissue to extreme cold, sometimes used to destroy portions of the brain (e.g., the thalamus)	krī - ō - SĔR - jĕr - ē
encephalopuncture	puncture into brain substance	ĕn - sĕf - ăh - lō - PŬNK - tūr
ganglionectomy	removal of a ganglion	găng - glē - ō - NĔK - tō - mē
laminectomy	excision of vertebral posterior arch to relieve pressure on spinal nerves due to a slipped disk	lăm - ĭ - NĔK - tō - mē
neurolysis	freeing of a nerve from an adhesion	nū - RŎL - ĭ - sĭs
stereotaxic neurosurgery	method of precisely locating areas in the brain using a 3-dimensional measurement; essential for certain neurologic procedures	stĕr - ē - ō - TĂK - sĭk
thalamotomy	partial destruction of the thalamus in order to treat psychosis or intractable pain	thăl - ăh - MŎT - ō - mē

Continued on following page

SURGICAL PROCEDURES—Continued

TERM	DESCRIPTION	PRONUNCIATION
tractotomy	transection of a fiber tract of the CNS, sometimes resorted to for relief of intractable pain	trăk - TŎT - ō - mē
trephination	cutting a circular opening into the skull to reveal brain tissue and decrease intracranial pressure	trĕf - ĭ - NĀ - shŭn
sympathectomy	excision or resection of part of the sympathetic nervous pathways	sĭm - păh - THĔK - tō - mē
vagotomy	interruption of the function of the vagus nerve to relieve peptic ulcer	vā - GŎT - ō - mē

LABORATORY PROCEDURE

TERM	DESCRIPTION
lumbar puncture (spinal tap, spinal puncture)	insertion of a needle into the subarachnoid space of the spinal column at the level of the fourth intervertebral space. This test is performed in order to determine subarachnoid pressure as well as to remove cerebrospinal fluid (CSF) for evaluation. CSF is checked for blood, bacteria, glucose, cytology, and serology for syphilis

PHARMACOLOGY RELATED TO THE NERVOUS SYSTEM

MEDICATION	ACTION
analgesics (painkillers)	inhibit the passage of pain impulses. A major non-narcotic painkiller is aspirin. An intermediate analgesic is codeine. Morphine is an example of a very potent analgesic with a high addiction potential
anticonvulsants	suppress seizures by changing the permeability of the neuron cell membrane so that it does not depolarize so readily. Anticonvulsants are used to treat both petit mal and grand mal epilepsies
antidepressants	used to treat depressive psychological illness. They function by causing an elevation of norepinephrine and/or serotonin in the central nervous system
opiates	sedative narcotics that contain opium or its derivatives
psychotropic drugs	these drugs are capable of modifying mental activity and mental state. They are often employed in the management of psychotic disorders, especially schizophrenia. Included in this broad classification of drugs are stimulants, such as caffeine, amphetamines,

Continued on following page

PHARMACOLOGY RELATED TO THE NERVOUS SYSTEM—*Continued*

MEDICATION	ACTION
	and cocaine; opiates, such as morphine, heroin, and methadone; and hallucinogens, such as marijuana, mescaline, LSD, and PCP
sedative/hypnotics	medications that calm nervousness, irritability, and excitement. They also induce sleep. Most frequently, these drugs are employed for treatment of anxiety or for sedation
tranquilizers	medications that act to reduce mental tension and anxiety without interfering with normal mental activity

ABBREVIATIONS RELATED TO THE NERVOUS SYSTEM

ABBREVIATION	MEANING
ANS	autonomic nervous system
CT scan	computerized tomography scan
CNS	central nervous system
CP	cerebral palsy
CSF	cerebrospinal fluid
CVA	cerebrovascular accident
EEG	electroencephalogram
EST	electric shock therapy
HNP	herniated nucleus pulposus (herniated disk)
LP	lumbar puncture
MS	multiple sclerosis
PNS	peripheral nervous system
TIA	transient ischemic attack

WORKSHEET 1

A. Using the word root/combining form encephal/o (brain), build medical words to mean:

1. _____ disease of the brain

2. _____ inflammation of the brain

B. Using the word roots/combining forms cerebell/o (cerebellum), cerebr/o (cerebrum), and crani/o (skull), build medical words to mean:

1. _____ pertaining to the cerebellum

2. _____ pertaining to the cerebrum

3. _____ pertaining to the cerebrum and spine

4. _____ pertaining to the skull

C. Using the word root/combining form neur/o (nerve), build medical words to mean:

1. _____ nerve cell

2. _____ embryonic nerve cell

3. _____ inflammation of a nerve

4. _____ pain in a nerve

5. _____ nerve poison

D. Using the word root/combining form ventricul/o (ventricles), build medical words to mean:

1. _____ radiography of the ventricles

2. _____ measurement of the ventricles

3. _____ visual examination of the ventricles

WORKSHEET 2

Fill in the correct word from the right hand column that matches the definitions in the statements below.

1. _____ lack of feeling or sensation   Anesthesia

2. _____ muscular incoordination   Aphasia

3. _____ loss of strength, weakness, debility   Apoplexy

4. _____ inability to speak   Asthenia

5. _____ paralysis of half of the body   Ataxia

6. _____ stroke, cerebral vascular accident   Bradykinesia

7. _____ irregular electrical waves of the brain   Clonic spasm

8. _____ rapid alternate involuntary muscle contraction and relaxation   Dysrhythmias

9. _____ slowness of movement   Hemiplegia

10. _____ trembling   Tremor

WORKSHEET 3

Build a surgical term for the following:

1. _____ incision of the skull

2. _____ incision of the cerebrum

3. _____ excision of part of the skull

4. _____ surgical repair of the skull

5. _____ excision of a ganglion

6. _____ surgical repair of the nerves

7. _____ suturing (of ends) of nerves

8. _____ cutting of a nerve

9. _____ surgical crushing of a nerve

10. _____ incision of the thalamus

WORKSHEET 4

Define the following diagnostic and symptomatic terms. Use the dictionary for reference.

1. encephalocele _____

2. encephalogram _____

3. encephalopyosis _____

4. cerebromalacia _____

5. cerebrosclerosis _____

6. craniomalacia _____

7. craniocele _____

8. myeloplegia _____

9. myelorrhagia _____

10. neuralgia _____

11. neuromalacia _____

12. synkinesia _____

13. meningioma _____

14. meningocele _____

WORKSHEET 5

Special Procedures, Pharmacology, and Abbreviations

Choose the word(s) that best describes the following statements:

analgesics	MS
ANS	myelography
anticonvulsant	opiate
antidepressants	pneumoencephalography
computerized tomography	psychotropic drugs
echoencephalography	TIA
electroencephalography	tranquilizer
lumbar puncture	

1. _____ examination of spinal cord after injection of a radiopaque dye into the spinal canal

2. _____ assessment of ventricles and subarachnoid space following the injection of air or gas

3. _____ used to treat depressive psychological illness

4. _____ procedure that determines subarachnoid pressure as well as removes cerebrospinal fluid for evaluation

5. _____ drugs capable of modifying mental state, often used in psychotic disorders, especially schizophrenia

6. _____ transient ischemic attack

7. _____ sedative narcotic containing opium or its derivatives

8. _____ medication that acts to reduce mental tension and anxiety without interfering with normal mental activity

9. _____ procedure that uses ultrasound to assess structures of the brain

10. _____ inhibit the passage of pain impulses

11. _____ suppresses seizures by altering neuron permeability; used in treating epilepsies

12. _____ provides a 3-dimensional view of the cranial contents

348

WORKSHEET 6

Grammar Review—Nervous System

Build plural words for the singular forms listed.

SINGULAR	PLURAL
1. meningococcus	1. _____
2. cranium	2. _____
3. cerebellum	3. _____
4. nucleus	4. _____

Build adjectives for the nouns listed below.

NOUN	ADJECTIVE
5. sense	5. _____
6. periphery	6. _____
7. nucleus	7. _____
8. neuroglia	8. _____
9. spine	9. _____

WORKSHEET 7

Label the following diagram, and compare your answers with Figure 14-5.

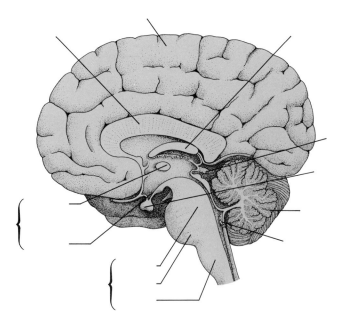

Corpus callosum

Cerebrum

Fornix

Pineal gland

Cerebellum

Choroid plexus

Diencephalon

Thalamus

Hypothalamus

Pituitary
gland

Brain stem

Midbrain

Pons

Medulla oblongata

CHAPTER 15

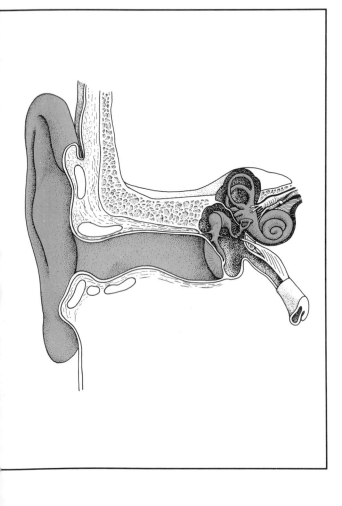

CHAPTER OUTLINE

Special Senses

STUDENT OBJECTIVES

Upon completion of this chapter, you will be able to do the following:

List and briefly describe each of the special senses of the body.

Identify the major structures and functions of the eye.

Identify the major structures and functions of the ear.

Identify the word roots/combining forms and suffixes associated with the special senses.

Identify and discuss associated pathology related to the special senses.

Identify endoscopic, clinical, and surgical procedures and abbreviations related to the special senses.

Explain the pharmacology related to the treatment of eye and ear disorders.

Build and analyze diagnostic, symptomatic, and surgical terms related to the special senses by completing the worksheets.

ANATOMY AND PHYSIOLOGY OF THE SPECIAL SENSES

The special senses of the body include the senses of taste, smell, equilibrium, sight, and hearing. These senses allow us to detect changes in our environment, and each of them has a structurally complex receptor organ.

Taste

The ability to taste is accomplished by numerous structures located on the tongue, the taste buds. In order for the taste buds to be stimulated, substances must be dissolved in saliva. When this occurs, the solution containing the dissolved substance enters the taste bud and stimulates the particular receptor, producing taste. Despite the fact that we believe that we taste many flavors, the taste buds of the tongue respond to only four sensations: sour, salty, bitter, and sweet. All other "tastes" are actually odors that are stimulating the olfactory bulb in the nose.

Smell

Olfactory sensation, or the sensation of smell, is accomplished by a highly specialized collection of nervous tissue, the olfactory bulb. Odors emitted from substances enter the nasal passageways and stimulate the olfactory bulb, producing the sensation of smell. The "taste" of pizza and coffee are actually the sensation of smell, not taste.

Equilibrium

The ability to maintain equilibrium is accomplished, to a large extent, by a complex structure located in the inner portion of the ear, the semicircular canals. The posture and orientation of the body is sensed by this structure, which transmits impulses to the brain. As the brain integrates these impulses, it makes the necessary physiologic adjustments that are required to maintain equilibrium.

The Eye

The eye functions in a manner similar to that of a camera. Light rays pass through a small opening and are focused by a lens upon a photoreceptive surface. In a camera, this surface is a photographic film; in the eye, it is the retina.

Refer to Figure 15-1 as you read the following paragraphs.

The eye is a globe-shaped organ that is composed of three distinct layers. Its outermost layer is the (1) **sclera**. As the name suggests, it is a tough fibrous tissue that serves as a protective shield for the more sensitive structures beneath. The sclera is also known as the white of the eye. A highly vascular middle layer, the (2) **choroid**, provides the blood supply for the entire eye. The innermost layer of the eye, the (3) **retina**, is composed of nerve endings that are responsible for the reception and transmission of light impulses.

A specialized portion of the sclera, the (4) **cornea**, passes in front of the lens. Rather than being opaque, it is transparent and thus permits the entrance of light into the interior of the eye.

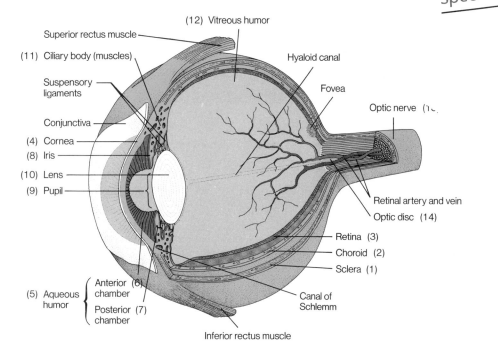

Figure 15–1. Components of the eye.

One of the two major humors, or fluids, of the eye is the (5) **aqueous humor**. The iris divides the aqueous humor into two small chambers, the (6) **anterior chamber** and the (7) **posterior chamber**. A colored, contractile membrane, the (8) **iris**, functions as a sphincter. Its perforated center is the (9) **pupil**. The amount of light entering the eye is regulated by the size of the pupil. As the environmental light increases, the pupil constricts; as the light decreases, the pupil dilates.

Located behind the posterior chamber is the (10) **lens**. This crystalline structure is suspended between the (11) **ciliary muscles**. As these muscles relax or contract, they alter the shape of the lens, making it thicker or thinner, respectively, thus enabling the light rays to focus upon the retina. This process is called **accommodation**.

The second major humor of the eye is the (12) **vitreous humor**. This clear, jellylike fluid occupies the entire orbit of the eye behind the lens. The vitreous humor, the lens, and the aqueous humor are the refractive structures of the eye. They are responsible for the bending of light rays so that they focus sharply on the retina. If any one of these structures does not function properly, vision is impaired.

The retina is an extremely delicate eye membrane. It is continuous with the optic nerve and has two types of light receptors upon its surface, rods and cones. **Rods** function in dim light and provide black-and-white vision. **Cones** function in bright light and provide color vision.

Rods and cones contain chemicals called **photopigments**. As light strikes the pigments, a chemical change occurs that produces a nerve impulse. These impulses are then transmitted to the brain through the (13) **optic nerve**. The brain interprets them as vision.

Both the optic nerve and the blood vessels of the eye enter the eyeball at the (14) **optic disc**. Its center is referred to as the **blind spot** because the area has neither rods nor cones.

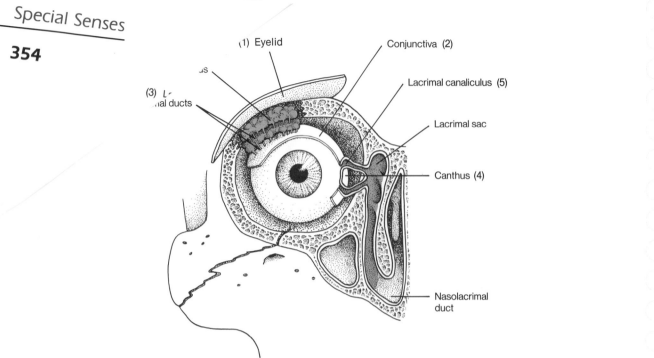

Figure 15–2. The front of the eye

Six muscles control the movement of the eye: the superior, inferior, lateral, and medial rectus muscles, and the superior and inferior oblique muscles. These muscles are coordinated to move both eyes in a synchronized manner.

Refer to Figure 15-2 as you read the following paragraphs.

The front of the eye is protected by two movable folds of skin, the (1) **eyelids**. Their edges are lined with two or three rows of **eyelashes**, which protect the surface of the eye.

A thin mucous membrane called the (2) **conjunctiva** lines the inner surface of the eyelids and passes over the cornea. Lying superior and to the outer edges of each eye are the (3) **lacrimal glands**. They produce tears to bathe and lubricate the eyes. The tears collect at the inner edges of the eyes, the (4) **canthi** (singular, canthus), and pass through pinpoint openings, the (5) **lacrimal canaliculi**, to the nose.

The Ear

The ear is the sense organ of hearing. It consists of three major sections: the **external**, or **outer**, ear; the **middle ear**, or **tympanic cavity**; and the **inner ear**, or **labyrinth**. Although each of these sections transmits sound waves, each accomplishes the task in a different way. The external ear conducts sound waves through air; the middle ear, through bone; and the inner ear, through fluid. As will be subsequently explained, this series of transmissions plays an integral part in hearing.

Refer to Figure 15-3 to facilitate coverage of the following material.

The external ear is designed to channel sound waves from the environment to the middle and inner ears. An (1) **auricle**, or **pinna**, is the external structure designed to collect waves traveling through air. The auricle channels the waves through the (2) **ear canal**, which is a slender tube that leads to the middle ear. The canal is lined with glands that produce a waxy secretion called **cerumen**. Cerumen prevents foreign particles from enter-

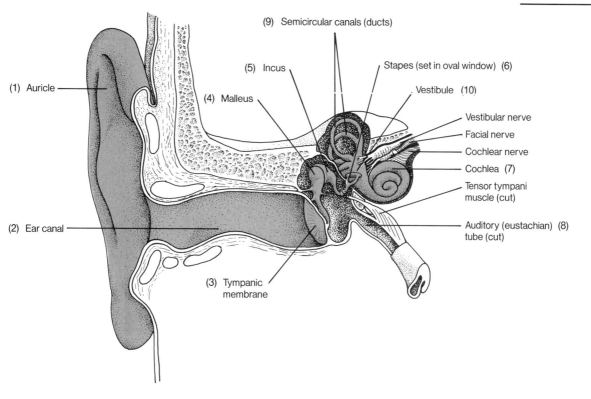

(9) Semicircular canals (ducts)

(5) Incus

Stapes (set in oval window) (6)

(4) Malleus

Vestibule (10)

(1) Auricle

Vestibular nerve

Facial nerve

Cochlear nerve

Cochlea (7)

Tensor tympani
muscle (cut)

(2) Ear canal

Auditory (eustachian) (8)
tube (cut)

(3) Tympanic
membrane

Figure 15–3. *Structures of the external, middle, and inner ear.*

ing the ear. A flat membranous structure, the (3) **tympanum (tympanic membrane,** or **eardrum)** is drawn over the end of the canal. Sound waves that enter the ear canal strike against the tympanum.

In the middle ear, vibrations of the tympanum are picked up by three tiny articulating bones called **ossicles.** These bones are responsible for the transmission of sound waves through the middle ear. The three bones are the (4) **malleus** (hammer), the (5) **incus** (anvil), and the (6) **stapes** (stirrups). These bones form a chain that stretches from the inner surface of the tympanum to an inner ear structure called the (7) **cochlea.**

A tube, called the (8) **eustachian tube,** connects the nose and the throat with the cavity of the middle ear. Its purpose is to equalize pressure on the outer and inner surfaces of the eardrum. In situations in which sudden pressure changes occur, equalization of pressure is achieved by deliberate swallowing.

The inner ear, sometimes referred to as the labyrinth because of its complicated maze-like design, is composed of three structures: a snail-shaped (7) **cochlea,** the (9) **semicircular canals,** and the (10) **vestibule,** which is a chamber that joins the cochlea and the semicircular canals.

The cochlea is filled with fluid. Lining its inner surface are tiny nerve endings called the hairs of Corti. There is a membrane-covered opening on the external surface of the cochlea, called the **oval window.** It is on this membrane that the stapes is attached to the cochlea. Transmission of sound along the ossicles in the middle ear causes the stapes to exert a gentle pumping action against the oval window. The pumping action forces the cochlear fluid to move. Disturbance of the fluid stimulates the hairs of Corti, causing them to generate a series of nerve impulses. The impulses are transmitted to the brain by way of the auditory nerve, where they are interpreted as sound.

WORD ROOTS/COMBINING FORMS RELATED TO THE SPECIAL SENSES

WORD ROOT/ COMBINING FORM	MEANING	EXAMPLE	PRONUNCIATION
Eye			
ambly/o	dull, dim	ambly/opia vision	ăm - blē - Ō - pē - ăh
aque/o	water	aque/ous pertaining to	Ā - kwē - ŭs
blephar/o	eyelid	blephar/o/ptosis prolapse	blĕf - ă - rō - TŌ - sĭs
choroid/o	choroid	choroid/itis inflammation	kō - rŏid - Ī - tĭs
corne/o	cornea	corne/al pertaining to	KŎR - nē - ăl
cycl/o	ciliary body	cycl/o/plegia paralysis	sĭ - klŏ - PLĒ - jē - ăh
dacry/o	tear	dacry/o/rrhea flow	dăk - rē - ō - RĒ - ăh
dacryoaden/o	tear gland	dacryoaden/ectomy excision	dăk - rē - ō - ăd - ĕ - NĔK - tō - mē
emmetr/o	correct measure	emmetr/opia vision	ĕm - ĕ - TRŌ - pē - ăh
irid/o ⎫		irid/ectomy excision	ĭr - ĭ - DĔK - tō - mē
ir/o ⎭ iris	iris	ir/itis inflammation	ĭ - RĬ - tĭs
kerat/o	hard, horny, cornea	kerat/itis inflammation	kĕr - ă - TĪ - tĭs
lacrim/o	tear	lacrim/al pertaining to	LĂK - rĭm - ăl
ophthalm/o ⎫		ophthalm/o/plegia paralysis	ŏf - thăl - mō - PLĒ - jē - ăh
ocul/o ⎬ eye	eye	ocul/ar pertaining to	ŎK - ū - lăr
opt/o ⎭		opt/o/metr/ ist mea- one who sure specializes	ŏp - TŎM - ĕ - trĭst

Continued on following page

WORD ROOTS/COMBINING FORMS RELATED TO THE SPECIAL SENSES—*Continued*

WORD ROOT/ COMBINING FORM	MEANING	EXAMPLE	PRONUNCIATION
Eye			
phak/o	lens	a/phak/ia with- noun ending out	ă - FĀ - kĕ - ăh
presby/o	old age, elderly	presby/opia vision	prĕz - bē - Ō - pē - ăh
pupill/o	} pupil	pupill/o/meter instrument for measuring	pū - pĭ - LŎM - ĕ - tĕr
core/o	} pupil	core/lysis separate	kor - ĔL - ĭ - sĭs
cor/e	}	cor/ectasis dilation	kor - ĔK - tā - sĭs
retin/o	retina	retin/o/pathy disease	rĕt - ĭn - ŎP - ă - thē
scler/o	sclera, hard	scler/o/corne/al cor- pertaining nea to	sklē - rō - KŎR - nē - ăl
Ear			
audi/o	hearing	audi/o/logy study of	aw - dē - ŎL - ō - jē
labyrinth/o	labyrinth, inner ear, maze	labyrinth/itis inflammation	lăb - ĭ - rĭn - THĪ - tĭs
mastoid/o	mastoid process	mastoid/o/tomy incision	măs - toyd - ŎT - ō - mē
ot/o	ear	ot/algia pain	ō - TĂL - jē - ăh
salping/o	eustachian tube, oviduct	salping/itis inflammation	săl - pĭn - JĪ - tĭs
staped/o	stapes	staped/ectomy excision	stā - pĕ - DĔK - tō - mē
tympan/o	} tympanic membrane, eardrum	tympan/o/plasty surgical repair	tĭm - păh - nō - PLĂS - tē
myring/o	}	myring/o/tomy incision	mĭr - ĭn - GŎT - ō - mē

SUFFIXES RELATED TO THE SPECIAL SENSES

SUFFIX	MEANING	EXAMPLE	PRONUNCIATION
Eye			
-opia	vision	emmetr/opia correct measure	ĕm - ĕ - TRŌ - pē - ăh
-tropia	turning	ex/o/tropia out- ward	ĕk - sō - TRŌ - pē - ăh
-opsia	vision	heter/opsia different	hĕt - ĕr - ŎP - sē - ăh
Ear			
-cusis	hearing	ana/cusis with- out	ăn - ăh - KŪ - sĭs
-mycosis	fungal infection	ot/o/mycosis ear	ō - tō - mĭ - KŌ - sĭs
-pyorrhea	discharge of pus, purulent discharge	ot/o/pyorrhea ear	ō - tō - pĭ - ō - RĒ - ăh

PATHOLOGY OF THE SPECIAL SENSES

The Eye

ERRORS OF REFRACTION

An error of refraction **(ametropia)** is caused when light rays are not brought into proper focus on the retina. This may be due to a defect in the lens, cornea, or the shape of the eyeball. If the eyeball is too long, the image falls in front of the retina. This condition is called nearsightedness **(myopia)** (Fig. 15-4). Correction is made by employing a concave lens. Farsightedness **(hyperopia, hypermetropia)** is the opposite of myopia. In farsighted-

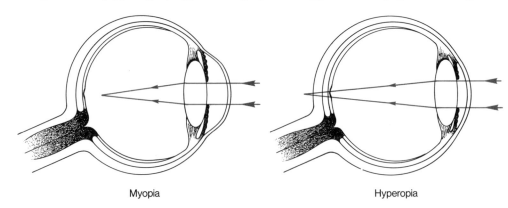

Myopia   Hyperopia

Figure 15-4. Myopia and hyperopia.

ness, the eyeball is too short and causes the image to fall behind the retina (see Fig. 15-4). Correction involves the use of a convex lens.

Another form of ametropia is a condition in which the cornea or lens has a defective curvature. This causes the light rays to diffuse over a large area of the retina, rather than being sharply focused on a given point. This gives rise to a condition known as **astigmatism**. Lenses that compensate for the imperfect curvature of the cornea or lens are used to correct astigmatism.

CATARACTS

Cataracts are opacities that form on the lens or the capsule that encloses the lens. These opacities are produced by a build-up of protein, layer by layer, until there is a loss of vision. The only effective treatment is removal of the lens or capsule.

Several techniques may be employed for cataract removal. In one method, a super-cooled metal probe **(cryoprobe)** is placed on the cataract. The cataract bonds to the cold probe, and the cataract and lens are gently lifted from the eye. This method of treatment is known as **intracapsular extraction**. It is usually the method of choice when the cataract develops as a result of old age **(senescent** or **senile cataract)**.

Cataracts found in children are usually a result of genetic defects or maternal rubella during the first trimester of pregnancy. In children and young adults, the surgery of choice is **extracapsular extraction**. Both the cortex and lens are removed, but the posterior lens capsule is retained.

GLAUCOMA

Glaucoma is an eye disease characterized by increased pressure within the eyeball **(intraocular pressure)**. This pressure leads to a degeneration of the optic nerve. Glaucoma may result in blindness if not successfully treated.

The increased intraocular pressure is due to the failure of the aqueous humor to drain from the eye through a tiny duct called the canal of Schlemm. Treatment involves the use of medications that cause the pupils to constrict, permitting this fluid to escape from the eye. If this treatment proves ineffective, surgery may be necessary. Three possible kinds of surgery for glaucoma include puncturing the cornea **(paracentesis of the cornea)**; the excision of a small portion of the iris **(partial iridectomy)**; or separating the iris from its attachment **(iridodialysis, coredialysis)**.

Glaucoma is diagnosed by using an instrument that measures the internal pressure of the eye **(tonometer)**. This procedure is a simple, painless technique and should be performed on all patients over the age of 35 during routine eye examinations.

STRABISMUS

Strabismus is a condition in which the eyes turn from the normal position so that they are not aimed in the same direction. If the eyes deviate outward **(exotropia)**, causing a divergent squint, the individual is said to be wall-eyed. If the eyes turn toward each other **(esotropia)**, causing a convergent squint, the individual is said to be cross-eyed. Strabismus may be due to poor vision **(decreased visual acuity)**, unequal ocular muscle tone, or an oculomotor nerve lesion.

In children, strabismus is associated with "lazy eye syndrome" **(amblyopia)**. Vision is suppressed in one eye so that the child uses only the other eye for vision. The suppression of vision in the "lazy eye" is generally due to extreme nearsightedness (**unilateral myopia**) or from double vision that develops because of strabismus.

Methods of treatment include eye testing (**refraction**), prescribing corrective lenses, eye exercises (**orthoptic training**), and surgery (**strabotomy**) in which the ocular tendons are cut.

RETINITIS PIGMENTOSA

Retinitis pigmentosa is a chronic progressive disease that results in degeneration of the retina and atrophy of the optic nerve. In all forms of this disease, the retinal rods deteriorate and the pigmented layer of the retina undergoes irreversible change. This genetic disorder usually occurs before adulthood, beginning with night blindness and loss of peripheral vision. In some cases, cataracts form, in addition to choroidal sclerosis and glaucoma. Ultimately, this disorder leads to complete blindness, usually before age 50. There is no known cure for retinitis pigmentosa.

The Ear

OTITIS MEDIA

Otitis media is an inflammation of the middle ear. It is found most commonly in infants and young children and is frequently associated with an upper respiratory infection (**URI**). Symptoms may include earache, draining of pus from the ear (**otopyorrhea**), or rupturing of the eardrum (**tympanorrhexis, myringorrhexis**). Treatment consists of bed rest, medications to relieve pain (**analgesics**), and antibiotics. Occasionally, an incision of the eardrum (**myringotomy, tympanotomy**) may be necessary to relieve pressure and promote draining of pus from the middle ear.

Recurrent episodes of otitis media may cause scarring of the tympanic membrane with associated hearing loss. If left untreated, otitis media may lead to infection of the mastoid process (**mastoiditis**) or inflammation of the brain tissue near the middle ear (**otoencephalitis**).

OTOSCLEROSIS

Otosclerosis is characterized by the hardening of spongy bone around the oval window. This decreases the ability of the stapes to move the oval window (**ankylosis**). Consequently, there is a hearing loss. Occasionally, the individual perceives a ringing sound (**tinnitus**) within the ear. Surgical correction involves the removal of the stapes (**stapedectomy**) and reconstruction of the oval window. Sometimes, insertion of an artificial stapes is necessary to restore hearing.

OTHER TERMS RELATED TO THE SPECIAL SENSES

TERM	MEANING	PRONUNCIATION
Eye		
achromatopsia	color blindness	ăh - krō - măh - TŎP - sē - ăh

Continued on following page

OTHER TERMS RELATED TO THE SPECIAL SENSES—*Continued*

TERM	MEANING	PRONUNCIATION
Eye		
aphakia	absence of the crystalline lens of the eye. It may occur congenitally or from trauma, but is more commonly caused by extraction of a cataract	ăh - FĀ - kē - ăh
conjunctivitis, pink eye	inflammation of the conjunctiva caused by bacteria, virus, allergy, or chemical or physical factors. When caused by virus or bacteria, it becomes highly contagious	kŏn - jŭnk - tĭ - VĪ - tĭs
diabetic retinopathy	appearance of small aneurysms on retinal capillaries due to diabetes	dī - ăh - BĚT - ĭk rĕt - ĭ - NŎP - ăh - thē
ectopia lentis	displacement of the crystalline lens of the eye	ĕk - TŌ - pē - ăh/LĔN - tĭs
ectropion	eversion of the edge of the eyelid	ĕk - TRŌ - pē - ŏn
entropion	inversion of the edge of the eyelid	ĕn - TRŌ - pē - ŏn
exophthalmos, exophthalmus	abnormal protrusion of the eyeball, which results in a marked stare. It is usually due to hyperthyroidism	ĕk - sŏf - THĂL - mŏs ĕk - sŏf - THĂL - mŭs
nyctalopia	a condition in which the individual cannot see well in faint light or at night	nĭk - tăh - LŌ - pē - ăh
nystagmus	involuntary eye movement that appears jerky	nĭs - TĂG - mŭs
papilledema, choked disc	edema and hyperemia of the optic disc. It is usually associated with increased ocular pressure resulting from intracranial pressure	păp - ĭl - ĕ - DĒ - măh
presbyopia	gradual decrease of visual acuity due to old age, resulting in the inability of the eyes to focus for near vision (e.g., when reading or sewing)	prĕs - bē - Ō - pē - ăh
sty(e)	a localized circumscribed inflammatory swelling of one of the several sebaceous glands of the eyelid, generally caused by a bacterial infection	stī
trachoma	a chronic infectious disease of the conjunctiva and cornea, fairly com-	trā - KŌ - măh

Continued on following page

OTHER TERMS RELATED TO THE SPECIAL SENSES—Continued

TERM	MEANING	
Eye		
	mon in the southwestern states but chiefly found in Africa and Asia. Without treatment, it may lead to blindness	
visual field	the area within which objects may be seen when the eye is fixed	
Ear		
anacusis	total hearing loss; deafness	ăn - ăh - KŪ - sĭs
labyrinthitis	inflammation of the inner ear that usually results from an acute febrile process. It may cause progressive vertigo	lăb - ĭ - rĭn - THĪ - tĭs
Meniere's disease	disorder of the labyrinth that leads to progressive loss of hearing, characterized by vertigo, sensorineural hearing loss, and tinnitus	měn - ē - ĀRZ/dĭ - ZĒZ
mastoid	process of the temporal bone, consisting of loosely arranged osseous material, with numerous small, air-filled cavities	MĂS - toid
presbyacusis, presbycusis	impairment of hearing due to old age	prěs - bě - ăh - KŪ - sĭs prěs - bě - KŪ - sĭs
vertigo	feeling of dizziness or spinning in space	VĚR - tĭ - gō
vestibulocochlear nerve	the combined portions of the eighth cranial nerve, one branch being cochlear (hearing) and the other, vestibular (balance)	věs - tĭb - ū - lō - KŎK - lē - ěr něrv

SPECIAL PROCEDURES RELATED TO THE SPECIAL SENSES

ENDOSCOPIC PROCEDURES

TERM	DESCRIPTION
gonioscopy	a specialized ophthalmoscopic procedure that permits the physician to examine the angle of the anterior chamber of the eye. This angle contains the opening through which aqueous humor drains from the eye. When the angle is excessive, aqueous humor cannot drain from the eye and may lead to glaucoma

Continued on following page

ENDOSCOPIC PROCEDURES—*Continued*

TERM	DESCRIPTION
otoscopy	an examination and inspection of the ear canal and eardrum. Using this test, foreign material in the ear canal or pathological changes of the eardrum are diagnosed
retinoscopy	a technique that employs the use of a beam of light that is reflected from the retina. The path in which it emerges from the eye determines whether the eye is nearsighted or farsighted

CLINICAL PROCEDURES

TERM	DESCRIPTION
audiometry	assesses the patient's ability to hear various frequencies of sound waves at different intensities. A graph that indicates the type and extent of hearing loss is plotted
ophthalmodynamometry	determination of pressure in the ophthalmic artery by use of an instrument that produces pressure in the eyeball until pulsations in the ophthalmic artery are seen through an ophthalmoscope
tonometry	determines the intraocular pressure. When intraocular pressure is elevated, damage to the optic nerve results, often leading to blindness
visual acuity test	most commonly employs the Snellen chart. This chart is imprinted with lines of block letters graduating in size from smallest on the bottom to largest on the top

SURGICAL PROCEDURES

TERM	DESCRIPTION	PRONUNCIATION
Eye		
blepharectomy	excision of a lesion of the eyelid	blĕf - ăh - RĔK - tō - mē
blepharorrhaphy	suturing of an eyelid	blĕf - ăh - RŎR - ăh - fē
cyclodialysis	formation of an opening between the anterior chamber and the suprachoroidal space for the draining of aqueous humor in glaucoma	sĭ - klō - dĭ - ĂL - ĭ - sis
dacryocysto-rhinostomy	creation of an opening into the nose for drainage of tears	dăk - rē - ō - sĭs - tō - rĭ - NŎS - tō - mē
enucleation	removal of an organ or other mass intact from its supporting tissues. Removal of the eyeball from the orbit	ē - nū - klē - Ā - shŭn

Continued on following page

364

SURGICAL PROCEDURES—*Continued*

TERM	DESCRIPTION	PRONUNCIATION
Eye		
evisceration	removal of the contents of the eye but leaving the sclera and cornea	ē - vĭs - ĕr - Ā - shŭn
keratocentesis	surgical puncture of the cornea	kĕr - ăh - tō - sĕn - TĒ - sĭs
phacoemulsification	a method of treating cataracts by using ultrasonic waves to disintegrate the cataract, which is then aspirated and removed	făk - ō - ē - MŬL - sĭ - fĭ - kā - shŭn
sclerostomy	surgical formation of an opening in the sclera	sklē - RŎS - tō - mē
Ear		
mastoid antrotomy	surgical opening of a cavity within the mastoid process	MĂS - toid/ăn - TRŎT - ō - mē
myringoplasty, tympanoplasty	reconstruction of the eardrum	mĭ - RĬNG - gō - plăs - tē tĭm - păh - nō - PLĂS - tē
otoplasty	corrective surgery for a deformed or excessively large or small pinna (macrotia, or microtia)	Ō - tō - plăs - tē
paracentesis tympani, myringotomy	puncture of the eardrum with evacuation of fluids from the middle ear	păr - ăh - sĕn - TĒ - sĭs TĬM - păh - nē mĭr - ĭn - GŎT - ō - mē

PHARMACOLOGY RELATED TO THE SPECIAL SENSES

MEDICATION	ACTION
antibiotics	substances, produced by microorganisms, that have the ability to kill or inhibit the growth of bacteria. These chemicals are used to treat infectious diseases
beta-adrenergic blocking agents (ophthalmic)	used in the treatment of glaucoma. These drugs lower intraocular pressure by reducing the production of aqueous humor
cycloplegic agents	paralyze the ciliary muscles and result in dilation of the pupils. Since these drugs cause a loss of accommodation, they are used by ophthalmologists to facilitate certain eye examinations
miotics/cholinergics	constrict the pupil by contracting the sphincter and ciliary muscles of the eye. This enables the aqueous humor to flow from the anterior chamber, thereby decreasing intraocular pressure. Miotics are very effective in the treatment of glaucoma
mydriatics	drugs that cause the dilation of the pupils

ABBREVIATION	MEANING
Acc	accommodation
AC	air conduction
AD	right ear (auris dextra)
AS	left ear (auris sinistra)
Astigm	astigmatism
D	diopter (lens strength)
Em	emmetropia
ENT	ear, nose, and throat
EOM	extraocular movement
IOP	intraocular pressure
mix. astig.	mixed astigmatism
OD	right eye (oculus dexter)
OS	left eye (oculus sinister)
OU	both eyes (oculi unitas) each eye (oculus uterque)
REM	rapid eye movement
ST	esotropia
VA	visual acuity
VF	visual field
XT	exotropia

366   WORKSHEET 1

A. Using the word root/combining form ophthalm/o (eye), build medical words to mean:

1. _____ pertaining to the eye

2. _____ inflammation of the eye

3. _____ paralysis of the eye

4. _____ instrument to visually examine the eye

5. _____ study of the eye

B. Using the word root/combining form cor/e (pupil), build medical words to mean:

1. _____ dilation of the pupil

2. _____ pupil out of the normal position

C. Using the word root/combining form pupill/o (pupil), build medical words to mean:

1. _____ visual examination of the pupil

2. _____ pertaining to the pupil

3. _____ instrument to measure (the diameter of) the pupil

D. Using the word root/combining form kerat/o (cornea), build medical words to mean:

1. _____ instrument for examination of the cornea

2. _____ instrument for measuring (the curvature of) the cornea

3. _____ instrument to cut the cornea

4. _____ inflammation of the cornea

E. Using the word root/combining form scler/o (sclera), build medical words to mean:

1. _____ inflammation of the sclera

2. _____ softening of the sclera

3. _____ inflammation of the sclera and iris

4. _____ inflammation of the sclera and cornea

F. Using the word root/combining form retin/o (retina), build medical words to mean:

1. _____ pertaining to the retina

2. _____ inflammation of the retina

3. _____ instrument to examine the retina (refractive errors)

4. _____ inflammation of the retina and choroid

G. Using the word root/combining form irid/o (iris), build medical words to mean:

1. _____ pertaining to the iris

2. _____ paralysis of the iris

3. _____ inflammation of the iris and the ciliary body

4. _____ protrusion of the iris (through a defective cornea)

5. _____ softening of the iris

6. _____ pain (felt) in the iris

H. Using the word root/combining form cycl/o (ciliary body), build medical words to mean:

1. _____ inflammation of the ciliary body and cornea

2. _____ paralysis of the ciliary body

3. _____ inflammation of the ciliary body and the choroid

I. Using the word root/combining form blephar/o (eyelid), build medical words to mean:

1. _____ collection of fluid in the eyelid

2. _____ pain in the eyelid

3. _____ paralysis of the eyelid

4. _____ prolapse of the eyelid

5. _____ spasm of the eyelid

J. Using the word root/combining form dacryocyst/o (tear sac), build medical words to mean:

1. _____ pain in the tear sac

2. _____ prolapse of the tear sac

3. _____ protrusion of the tear sac

4. _____ inflammation of the tear sac

K. Using the suffix -opia (vision), build medical words to mean:

1. _____ correct (measure) vision

2. _____ dim, dull vision

3. _____ farsightedness (far vision)

4. _____ green vision (vision defect in which all things appear green)

5. _____ night vision (night blindness)

L. Using the suffix -opsia (vision), build medical words to mean:

1. _____ lack of one half of (the visual field) vision

2. _____ lack of color vision (color blindness)

3. _____ different vision (in each of the two eyes)

M. Using the word root/combining form ot/o (ear), build medical words to mean:

1. _____ pain in the ear (earache)

2. _____ instrument to visually examine the ear

3. _____ hemorrhage from the ear

4. _____ purulent discharge from the ear

5. _____ inflammation of the ear

N. Using the word root/combining form audi/o (hearing), build medical words to mean:

1. _____ recording of an audiometer

2. _____ instrument to measure hearing

3. _____ study of hearing (disorders)

O. Using the word root/combining form myring/o (eardrum, tympanic membrane, tympanum), build medical words to mean:

1. _____ inflammation of the tympanum and mastoid cells

2. _____ inflammation of the eardrum

3. _____ instrument for cutting the eardrum

4. _____ fungal infection of the eardrum

P. Using the suffixes -cusia, -cusis (hearing), build medical words to mean:

1. _____ lack of hearing (deafness)

2. _____ poor hearing due to old age

WORKSHEET 2

Fill in the correct word from the right hand column that matches the definitions in the statements below.

1. _____	swelling due to fluid at the optic disc	Achromatopsia
2. _____	eversion of the edge of the eyelid	Anacusis
3. _____	turning outward of the eyes (wall-eyes)	Aphakia
4. _____	lack of a lens	Cerumen
5. _____	color blindness	Ectopia lentis
6. _____	displacement of lens	Ectropion
7. _____	earwax	Exotropia
8. _____	located near the ear	Papilledema
9. _____	ringing in the ear	Parotid
10. _____	feeling of spinning in space	Tinnitus
11. _____	deafness	Vertigo

370   ## WORKSHEET 3

Build surgical terms for the following:

1. _____ incision of the eye

2. _____ incision into the vein of the eye (to relieve congestion of the conjunctival veins)

3. _____ incision of the iris (to establish a new pupil)

4. _____ excision of a portion of the ciliary body

5. _____ surgical connection formed between the tear sac and the nose (nasal cavity)

6. _____ incision (or dissection) of the ear

7. _____ surgical repair of an ear deformity

8. _____ surgical repair of the eardrum

9. _____ incision into the tympanic membrane

10. _____ removal of the stapes

11. _____ incision of the tendon of the stapes muscle (stapedius)

12. _____ surgical puncture of the mastoid process

13. _____ removal of the mastoid process

14. _____ incision of the labyrinth

WORKSHEET 4

Define the following diagnostic and symptomatic terms. Use the dictionary as reference.

1. leukoma _____

2. hypertensive retinopathy _____

3. hypermetropia _____

4. photophobia _____

5. nystagmus _____

6. anisometropia _____

7. salpingoscopy _____

8. audiometry _____

9. meatal atresia _____

10. otogenic _____

11. perimetry _____

12. lacrimation _____

372 **WORKSHEET 5**

Special Procedures, Pharmacology, and Abbreviations

Choose the word(s) that best describes the following statements:

AD
AS
audiometry
beta-adrenergic blocking agents
cycloplegic agents
enucleation
evisceration
gonioscopy
miotics/cholinergics
mydriatics

OD
ophthalmodynamometry
OS
otoscopy
OU
retinoscopy
test
tonometry
visual acuity test

1. _____ used to determine the intraocular pressure of the eye

2. _____ medications that paralyze the ciliary muscles, causing loss of accommodation

3. _____ test that assesses the type and extent of hearing loss

4. _____ medication that constricts pupils, enabling aqueous humor to drain from the eye

5. _____ determines the pressure in the ophthalmic artery

6. _____ permits an assessment of the angle of the anterior chamber to monitor glaucoma

7. _____ lowers intraocular pressure by reducing the production of aqueous humor

8. _____ drugs that cause the dilation of pupils

9. _____ right eye

10. _____ right ear

11. _____ left eye

12. _____ left ear

13. _____ both eyes; each eye

14. _____ visualization of the ear canal and eardrum, using an endoscope

15. _____ technique that employs the use of a beam of light that is reflected from the retina to determine whether the eye is nearsighted or farsighted

WORKSHEET 6

Grammar Review—Special Senses

Provide the adjective for the nouns listed below.

NOUNS

ADJECTIVES

1. tympanum   _____tympanic_____

2. meatus   _____

3. antrum   _____

4. auricle   _____

5. auditus   _____

Provide the plural form for the singular words listed below.

SINGULAR

PLURAL

6. pinna   _____

7. antrum   _____

374   WORKSHEET 7

Label the following diagrams, and check your answers with Figures 15-1 and 15-2.

Suspensory ligaments

Ciliary body (muscles)

Lens

Cornea

Conjunctiva

Iris

Pupil

Anterior chamber

Posterior chamber

Aqueous humor

Canal of Schlemm

Inferior rectus muscle

Superior rectus muscle

Vitreous humor

Hyaloid canal

Fovea

Optic nerve

Retinal artery and vein

Choroid

Sclera

Optic disc

Retina

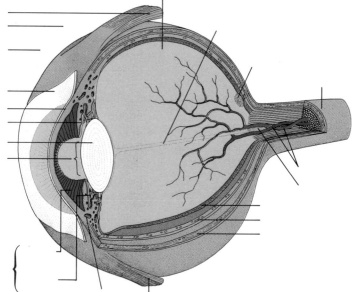

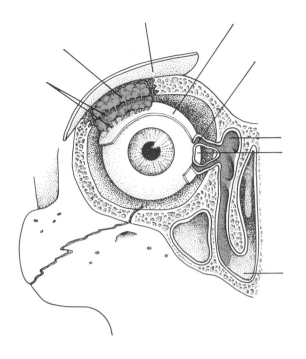

Eyelid

Lacrimal glands

Lacrimal ducts

Conjunctiva

Lacrimal canaliculus

Lacrimal sac

Canthus

Nasolacrimal duct

WORKSHEET 8

Label the following diagram, and check your answers with Figure 15-3.

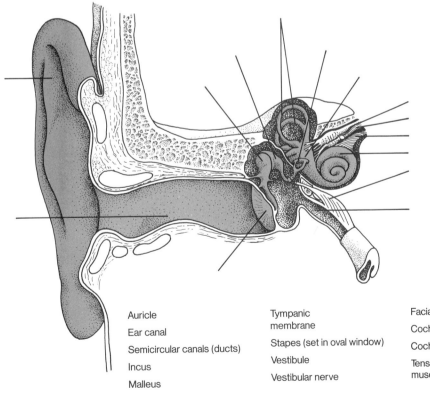

Auricle

Ear canal

Semicircular canals (ducts)

Incus

Malleus

Tympanic membrane

Stapes (set in oval window)

Vestibule

Vestibular nerve

Facial nerve

Cochlear nerve

Cochlea

Tensor tympani muscle (cut)

C H A P T E R 16

Oncology

STUDENT OBJECTIVES

Upon completion of this chapter, you will be able to do the following:

Differentiate benign and malignant neoplasms.

Give examples of four tissue types used in tumor identification.

Name tumors based upon tissue of origin (histogenesis).

Explain the difference between carcinoma and sarcoma.

Explain staging and define four oncologic stages.

Define the four grades used in evaluating the degree of malignancy of a neoplasm.

Identify the word roots/combining forms and suffixes related to oncology.

Relate information on the pathology discussed in the chapter.

Identify radiographic, laboratory, and surgical procedures and abbreviations related to oncology.

Explain the pharmacology related to the treatment of malignancies.

Build and analyze diagnostic, symptomatic, and surgical terms related to oncology by completing the worksheets.

Oncology is the study of tumors. It includes both malignant and nonmalignant growths. The purpose of this chapter is to provide a better understanding of the specialized terminology related to oncology.

CHARACTERISTICS OF NEOPLASMS

In healthy individuals, cell division is an orderly process in which body cells are produced for growth of the individual or for replacement of cells that are destroyed or worn out. In some instances, however, cell division is without purpose. The newly formed cells increase at an uncontrolled rate, producing a lump or swelling known as a **tumor** or **neoplasm**. These neoplasms may be either benign or malignant.

Benign Neoplasms

Benign neoplasms are new growths that develop in body tissues. They are composed of the same type of cells as the tissue in which they are growing. For example, a benign tumor of a gland is composed of the glandular tissue from which it is developing. Benign neoplasms are contained within a capsule and do not invade the surrounding tissue. They harm the individual only insofar as they place pressure on surrounding structures. If the benign neoplasm remains small and places no pressure on adjacent structures, it often is not removed. When it becomes excessively large or places pressure on other organs or structures, excision is necessary. Benign brain tumors are always very serious since the cranial cavity is enclosed and pressure on other parts of the brain inevitably results. As a general rule, however, benign tumors are not life-threatening. Once they are removed, they usually do not regrow.

Malignant Neoplasms

The cells that compose a **malignant neoplasm** often do not resemble the tissue in which they are growing. That is, the tumor cells lack specialization in both structure and function. In such cases, the tumor is said to be dedifferentiated. In dedifferentiation, cells lose their ability for specialized function and revert to an immature or embryonic form. More significantly, however, the cells of the malignant neoplasm are not encapsulated and are thus able

CHARACTERISTICS OF NEOPLASMS

BENIGN	MALIGNANT
1. Encapsulated	1. Non-encapsulated, having projections infiltrating surrounding tissues
2. Composed of tissue that closely resembles the tissue in which the neoplasm arises	2. Composed of tissue that does not resemble the tissue in which the neoplasm arises
3. Does not spread to remote areas of the body	3. If left untreated, the cells of the neoplasm metastasize to remote regions of the body
4. Generally poses little risk, if any, to the patient	4. If left untreated, poses a risk to the patient

to spread to normal tissues. This invasive growth develops by either direct extension or metastasis. In direct extension, the tumor grows directly into normal tissue. This phenomenon is called proliferation. With metastasis, the malignant cells from the primary tumor site find their way into lymph channels or blood vessels and are carried to remote body structures in which secondary malignant neoplasms then develop.

NOMENCLATURE OF TUMORS

Tumor nomenclature is based, in part, upon the type of tissue in which the tumor originates. This is referred to as **histogenesis**.

For purposes of tumor nomenclature, four tissue types are identified: epithelial, connective (including muscle), hematopoietic (blood and lymph), and nervous tissue.* The following chart is provided in order to organize the material presented hereafter.

TISSUE TYPE	EXAMPLES OF COMBINING FORMS
Epithelial Tissue	
External skin	
nipple-like protuberance	papill/o
Internal linings	
gland	aden/o
Connective Tissue	
Fibrous	fibr/o
Cartilage	chondr/o
Bone	oste/o
Fat	lip/o
Blood vessel	hem/angi/o
Lymph vessel	lymph/angi/o
Smooth muscle	lei/o/my/o
Striated muscle	rhabd/o/my/o
Hematopoietic Tissue	
Leukocytes	leuk/o
lymphocytes	lymph/o
granulocytes	granulo/cyt/o
Erythrocytes	erythr/o
Nervous Tissue	
nerve	neur/o
glial (neuroglia) cells	gli/o
meninges	meningi/o

To indicate a **benign** tumor that arises from epithelial or connective tissue, add the suffix -oma to the word root. An exception to this rule is **melanoma**, which is a malignant tumor of epithelial origin.

---

*Medical word-building for neoplasms of nervous tissue origin does not follow well-defined rules. Only through association with these terms can you gain an understanding of this complex area of oncology.

380

EXAMPLES OF BENIGN TUMORS OF EPITHELIAL AND CONNECTIVE TISSUE ORIGIN

Medical Term	Benign Tumor of
papilloma (epithelial)	epithelial tissue
adenoma (epithelial)	gland tissue
hemangioma (connective)	blood vessel
osteoma (connective)	bone
rhabdomyoma (connective)	striated muscle

To indicate a **malignant** tumor of epithelial origin, add the suffix -carcinoma to the word root, or include the word carcinoma with the affected structure. Remember that glandular (epithelial) tissue covers many structures of the body (e.g., organs and mucous membranes).

EXAMPLES OF MALIGNANT TUMORS OF EPITHELIAL TISSUE ORIGIN

Medical Term	Malignant Tumor of
adenocarcinoma	gland
pancreatic carcinoma	pancreas
papillocarcinoma	epithelial tissue
gastric adenocarcinoma	stomach glandular epithelium
adenocarcinoma of the lung	lung glandular tissue

To indicate malignant tumors of connective tissue origin, add the suffix -sarcoma to the word root or include the word sarcoma with the affected structure.

EXAMPLES OF MALIGNANT TUMORS OF CONNECTIVE TISSUE ORIGIN

Medical Term	Malignant Tumor of
fibrosarcoma	fibrous tissue
hemangiosarcoma	blood vessels
chondrosarcoma	cartilage
synovial sarcoma	synovial tissue
leiomyosarcoma	smooth muscle

HEMATOPOIETIC TISSUE

Leukemias

Leukemias are one of the malignant neoplasms of hematopoietic cells. Both maturation and functional ability of the leukocytes are impaired. Leukemias are classified according to duration and cellular involvement.

EXAMPLES OF LEUKEMIAS

Medical Term	Cellular Involvement
acute/chronic lymphocytic	lymphocytes
acute/chronic myelogenous	bone marrow
plasma cell	plasma cells

EXAMPLES OF LYMPHOMAS

Medical Term	Cellular Involvement
malignant granuloma (lymphogranuloma, Hodgkin's disease)	lymph nodes
multiple myeloma	plasma cells, bone marrow

Erythroleukemia

Erythroleukemia is a malignancy that affects both the erythropoietic and leukopoietic tissues. The patient often exhibits extreme anemia along with the appearance of neoplastic white blood cells.

HISTOGENESIS OF NEOPLASMS

Table 16-1 lists benign and malignant neoplasms based on histogenesis.

In addition to the general rules of neoplastic classification based on histogenesis, other classifications are employed to further describe or evaluate neoplastic growth. These classifications include **staging, grading,** and **gross appearance**.

Table 16–1.   HISTOGENESIS OF BENIGN AND MALIGNANT NEOPLASMS*

HISTOGENESIS	BEHAVIOR	
(Tissue or Origin)	**(Benign)**	**(Malignant)**
1. Epithelial Tumors:		
surface epithelium	papilloma	carcinoma
glandular epithelium	adenoma	adenocarcinoma
2. Connective Tissue Tumor:		
fibrous tissue	fibroma	fibrosarcoma
cartilage	chondroma	chondrosarcoma
bone	osteoma	osteosarcoma
fat	lipoma	liposarcoma
blood vessels	hemangioma	hemangiosarcoma
lymph vessels	lymphangioma	lymphangiosarcoma
smooth muscle	leiomyoma	leiomyosarcoma
striated muscle	rhabdomyoma	rhabdomyosarcoma
3. Hematopoietic Tumors:		
lymphoid tissue		

Continued on following page

Table 16–1.   HISTOGENESIS OF BENIGN AND MALIGNANT NEOPLASMS*—*Continued*

HISTOGENESIS	BEHAVIOR	
(Tissue or Origin)	**(Benign)**	**(Malignant)**
granulocytic tissue		myelocytic leukemia
erythrocytic tissue		erythroleukemia
plasma cells		multiple myeloma
4. Nerve Tissue Tumors:		
glial tissue		glioma
meninges	meningioma	meningeal sarcoma
nerve cells	neuroma ganglioneuroma	
		melanoma
neuroectoderm	nevus (nevocytoma)	neuroblastoma neurolymphoma
retina		retinoblastoma
adrenal medulla	pheochromocytoma	
		pheochromocytoma
nerve sheaths	neurilemoma	neurilemmic sarcoma
5. Tumors of More than One Tissue:		
breast	fibroadenoma	cystosarcoma phyllodes
embryonic kidney		nephroblastoma
multipotent cells	teratoma	teratoma choriocarcinoma
uterus		mixed mesodermal
6. Tumors that Do Not Fit Easily into One of the Above Groups:		
melanoblasts	pigmented nevus	melanoma
placenta	hydatidiform mole	choriocarcinoma
ovary	granulosa-theca cell tumors	carcinoma dysgerminoma
	Brenner tumor arrhenoblastoma gynandroblastoma hilar cell tumor sex cord mesenchyme	

Continued on following page

Table 16–1. HISTOGENESIS OF BENIGN AND MALIGNANT NEOPLASMS—*Continued*

HISTOGENESIS	BEHAVIOR	
(Tissue or Origin)	(Benign)	(Malignant)
testis	interstitial cell tumor	seminoma carcinoma choriocarcinoma yolk-sac
thymus	thymoma	thymoma

*Adapted from Fisher and Fisher: *Biological Aspects of Cancer Cell Spread*. Fifth National Cancer Conference Proceedings. JB Lippincott, Philadelphia, 1964.

Staging

Staging is an attempt to define the extent of cancer by classifying it into three categories: T, N, and M. T represents the primary tumor site or place of origin; N represents local or regional node involvement; and M indicates whether or not there is metastasis. When the primary site contains classifications of T1, T2, T3, or T4, the higher numbers indicate progressive increases in tumor size and involvement. Similarly, N0, N1, N2, or N3 represents progressively advancing nodular involvement. Finally, M0 or M+ defines absence or presence of metastasis, respectively. Table 16-2 illustrates staging categories in greater detail.

Table 16–2. STAGING*

Three capital letters are used:	
T	PRIMARY TUMOR
N	REGIONAL LYMPH NODES
M	DISTANT METASTASIS
This classification is extended by the following designations:	
tumor	
T0	No evidence of primary tumor
TIS	Carcinoma in-situ
T1 T2 T3 T4	Progressive increase in tumor size and involvement
TX	Tumor cannot be assessed

Continued on following page

Table 16–2. STAGING*—*Continued*

	nodes	
	N0	Regional lymph nodes not demonstrably abnormal
	N1 N2 N3 etc	Increasing degrees of demonstrable abnormality of regional lymph nodes
		(For many primary sites the subscript "a," eg $N1_a$, may be used to indicate that metastasis to the node is not suspected; and the subscript "b," eg $N1_b$, may be used to indicate that metastasis to the node is suspected or proved.)
	NX	Regional lymph nodes cannot be assessed clinically
	metastasis	
	M0	No evidence of distant metastasis
	M1 M2 M3	Ascending degrees of distant metastasis, including metastasis to distant lymph nodes
		TNM assignments may be grouped into a small number of stages.

*From *Classification and Staging of Cancer by Site: A Preliminary Handbook.* American Joint Committee for Cancer Staging and End Results Reporting, 1976.

Grading

Histologically, mature cells are referred to as differentiated, that is, they carry on specialized activities. When differentiated cells revert to their primitive or embryonic state, this phenomenon is referred to as **anaplasia**, or **dedifferentiation**. Grading of a malignant tumor is an evaluation of the histologic makeup, that is, the extent of differentiation or dedifferentiation, of the neoplasm. Generally, four grades are employed, 1 through 4. Neoplasms that are composed of cells that closely resemble the tissue from which they arise are given a grade 1 rating. The tissue demonstrates a minimum amount of anaplasia.

At the other extreme is grade 4, in which there is a great deal of anaplasia within the tumor. Such tumors are more serious and the prognosis is very poor. Grades 2 and 3 are intermediate grades between these two extremes.

Gross Appearance

Neoplasms may be classified according to their gross appearance. The following terms are used to designate the neoplasm upon visual examination.

BENIGN:
papilloma—epithelial tissue having a velvety appearance
polyp—a protuberance from mucous membranes that is generally attached to a thin stalk
encapsulation—being enclosed within a sheath or membrane

MALIGNANT:
infiltrating—penetrating the spaces within tissue
annular—ring-shaped or circular
fungating—growing rapidly, like a fungus
ulcerative—forming or causing ulcers

WORD ROOTS/COMBINING FORMS RELATED TO ONCOLOGY

WORD ROOT/ COMBINING FORM	MEANING	EXAMPLE	PRONUNCIATION
blast/o	embryonic	neur/o/blast/oma nerve tumor	nū - rō - blăs - TŌ - măh

carcin/o	cancer	carcin/o/gen/ ic
		     pro- pertain-
		     duc- ing to
		     ing
			kăr - sĭn - ō - JĔN - ĭk

chem/o	chemical, drug	chem/o/therapy treatment	kē - mō - THĔR - ăh - pē
cry/o	cold	cry/o/gen to produce	KRĪ - ō - jĕn

cyst/o	bladder, sac of fluid	cyst/o/scope
		     instrument to ex-
		     amine the blad-
		     der and ureter
			SĬS - tĭk

kerat/o	horny or hornlike	dys/kerat/osis
		bad abnormal
		     condition
		     (of)
			dĭs - kĕr - ăh - TŌ - sĭs

leiomy/o	smooth (visceral) muscle	leiomy/oma tumor	lĭ - ō - mĭ - Ō - măh
ne/o	new	neo/plasm growth	NĒ - ō - plăzm
onc/o	tumor, mass	onc/o/logy study of	ŏng - KŎL - ō - jē
papill/o	nipple-like protuberance or elevation	papill/oma tumor	păp - ĭ - LŌ - măh
rhabdomy/o	striated (skeletal) muscle	rhabdomy/oma tumor	răb - dō - mĭ - Ō - măh
sarc/o	flesh	sarc/oma tumor	săr - KŌ - măh
scirrh/o	hard	scirrh/ous pertaining to	SKĬR - rŭs
therm/o	heat	therm/o/gram record	THĔR - mō - grăm
tox/o	poison	tox/ic pertaining to	TŎKS - ĭk

SUFFIXES RELATED TO ONCOLOGY

SUFFIX	MEANING	EXAMPLE	PRONUNCIATION
-plakia	plate	leuk/o/plakia white	loo - kō - PLĂK - ē - ăh
-plasia } -plasm }	formation, growth, development	hyper/plasia excessive neo/plasm new	hī - pĕr - PLĀ - sē - ăh NĒ - ō - plăzm
-stasis	control, stop, standing	meta/stasis beyond	mĕ - tăs - TĂ - sĭs
-therapy	treatment	chem/o/therapy chemical	kē - mō - THĔR - ăh - pē

NEOPLASTIC PATHOLOGY

Hodgkin's Disease (Lymphogranuloma)

Hodgkin's disease is a malignancy of lymphatic tissue that primarily affects the lymph nodes but may also involve the spleen, gastrointestinal tract, liver, or bone marrow. It usually begins with a painless enlargement of lymph nodes, generally on one side of the neck, but spreading later progresses to lymphoid tissue throughout the body. When lymph nodes enlarge, they may cause pressure on other structures, resulting in pain or dysfunction. For instance, when the nodes in the neck become excessively large and exert pressure on the trachea or esophagus, the patient may experience dyspnea and/or dysphagia. Other symptoms include itching **(pruritus)**, weight loss, progressive anemia, and fever.

Radiation and chemotherapy are important methods in the management of the disease, and impressive advances have been made in treating the affected areas.

Leukemia

Leukemias are malignant diseases of the blood-forming organs (spleen, lymphatic system, and bone marrow). Numerous embryonic (blastic) leukocytes spread and proliferate throughout the bone marrow. These cells are unable to function in a normal manner. Since the leukemic process drastically reduces the body's ability to produce normal blood cells, anemia and increased susceptibility to infections are also noted in the leukemic patient.

There are many clinical manifestations of leukemia, including fatigue, bleeding from the gums, nose **(epistaxis)**, and rectum, rapid heart beat **(tachycardia)**, difficulty in breathing **(dyspnea)**, and weight loss. The prognosis has improved, especially in children. The major method of treatment is chemotherapy.

OTHER TERMS RELATED TO ONCOLOGY

TERM	MEANING	PRONUNCIATION
anaplasia, dedifferentiation	the reverting of a specialized cell to its primitive or embryonic state	ăn - ă - PLĀ - zē - ăh

Continued on following page

OTHER TERMS RELATED TO ONCOLOGY—Continued

TERM	MEANING	PRONUNCIATION
carcinogenic	pertaining to an agent that produces cancer	kăr - sĭ - nō - JĔN - ĭk
differentiation	the ability of a cell to carry on specialized activities	
disseminated	scattered or distributed over a considerable part of the body	dĭs - SĔM - ĭ - nāt - ĕd
dormant	time period when cancer cells remain inactive	DŎR - mănt
dysplasia	abnormal development in number, size, or organization of cells or tissue	dĭs - PLĀ - sē - ăh
hyperplasia	excessive development of normal cells in the tIssue arrangement of an organ	hĭ - pĕr - PLĀ - zē - ăh
in situ	in a localized site; confined to one place	in/SĪ - tū
latent period	a time during which a disease is in existence but does not manifest itself; a period of dormancy	LĀ - tĕnt/PĒ - rē - od
multicentric	occurrence of neoplasms at several sites of the same type of tissue	mŭl - tĭ - SĔN - trĭk
remission	lessening in severity or abatement of symptoms of a disease	rē - MĬSH - ŭn
scirrhous	hard, densely packed tumor caused by an overgrowth of connective tissue	SKĬR - ŭs
spontaneous regression	the phenomenon in which cancer cells revert back to normal; very few cancers regress spontaneously	spŏn - TĀ - nē - ŭs rē - GRĔSH - ŭn

SPECIAL PROCEDURES RELATED TO ONCOLOGY

RADIOGRAPHIC PROCEDURE

TERM	DESCRIPTION
radiation therapy	ionizing radiation is used in cancer therapy in an attempt to destroy malignant cells. The application of the radiation may be either internal or external. Internal radiation therapy involves the implantation of the sealed radiation source in or near the malignant tissue, or the direct administration of radiation into the bloodstream. External radiation employs high-energy x-rays and gamma rays. These are directed at the malignant tissue from an external x-ray machine

LABORATORY PROCEDURES

TERM	DESCRIPTION
cytologic examination	the study of cells—their origin, structure, and function. There are two major types of cytologic studies: aspiration biopsy and exfoliative cytology. In the first technique, cells for study are obtained from superficial or internal lesions by suction through a fine needle. In the second technique, desquamated cells from body surfaces or lesions are examined (e.g., Pap smears). Specimens for cytologic studies are usually composed of many different cells. Abnormalities may include the number of cells present, the cell distribution, surface modification, inclusions, size, shape, and staining properties. Some of these abnormalities are indicative of malignancy.
carcinoembryonic antigen (CEA) test	a serologic study that assesses the amount of CEA in the blood. CEA blood levels may elevate as cancer invades normal tissue, especially the colon and gastrointestinal tract. These levels appear to be highest in patients with metastatic colon neoplasm. This test cannot be used as a screening test for cancer, but it can be used effectively to diagnose colon cancer and to manage patients with diagnosed colon cancer for signs of recurrent tumors
alpha-fetoprotein (AFP)	a plasma protein found normally in some embryonic tissue. It is also present in the blood of adults with hepatocellular carcinoma and germ cell neoplasms. The AFP levels are used to monitor the effectiveness of cancer therapy in patients with these types of malignancies

SURGICAL PROCEDURES

TERM	DESCRIPTION
bone marrow aspiration	surgical procedure in which bone marrow is aspirated from the sternum or the iliac crest of the pelvis for microscopic evaluation
cryosurgery	surgery using a super-cooled probe containing liquid nitrogen; used effectively in cancers of the oral cavity, brain, and prostate
endoscopic resection	surgical excision through a natural body opening or a small incision. Questionable polyps of the bowel may be removed through this technique
laparotomy	surgical opening of the abdomen that is often used to determine primary tumor and nodal extent
lumbar puncture	puncture made by placing an aspiration needle in the subarachnoid space for withdrawal of spinal fluid; often used for brain tumor diagnosis
needle biopsy	removal of body fluid for cytologic study

Continued on following page

SURGICAL PROCEDURES—*Continued*

TERM	DESCRIPTION
surgical exploration	operative procedure in which inspections and biopsies are performed. This procedure is used to remove tissue at the margin of a neoplasm to determine the presence of malignancy when indicated

PHARMACOLOGY RELATED TO ONCOLOGY

MEDICATION	ACTION
alkylating agents	a variety of drugs used in chemotherapy that destroy portions of the DNA molecule. Not only do these drugs destroy malignant cells, but they also may destroy rapidly proliferating non-malignant cells. Systemic toxic effects including nausea, vomiting, hemorrhaging, erythropenia, and leukopenia often result
antimetabolite	inhibits the formation of certain enzymes required for cell division
antibiotic	product of certain bacteria that act on DNA and RNA to prevent cell reproduction. These antibiotics often cause toxic effects such as alopecia and myelosuppression
cytotoxic agent	drug that is capable of destroying cells by inhibiting cellular division. Many cytotoxic drugs are alkylating agents

ABBREVIATIONS RELATED TO ONCOLOGY

ABBREVIATION	MEANING
ABC	aspiration biopsy cytology
adeno-CA	adenocarcinoma
AFP	alpha-fetoprotein
BCE	basal cell epithelioma
bx	biopsy
CA	cancer; carcinoma
CEA	carcinoembryonic antigen
DES	diethylstilbestrol
DNA	deoxyribonucleic acid
HD	Hodgkin's disease

Continued on following page

ABBREVIATIONS RELATED TO ONCOLOGY—Continued

ABBREVIATION	MEANING
mets	metastases
RATx	radiation therapy
RNA	ribonucleic acid
st	stage (i.e., staging of a disease)
TNM	(primary) tumor, (regional lymph) nodes, (remote) metastasis
Tx	tumor cannot be assessed

A. Using the word root/combining form onc/o (tumor), build medical words to mean:

1. _____ development of a tumor

2. _____ a specialist who studies tumors

3. _____ pertaining to a tumor

4. _____ abnormal condition of a tumor

5. _____ destruction of a tumor

B. Using the word root/combining form carcin/o (cancer), build medical words to mean:

1. _____ excision of a cancerous growth

2. _____ causing or producing cancer

3. _____ resembling cancer

4. _____ destruction of cancer

5. _____ morbid fear of cancer

6. _____ cancer containing sarcoma cells (mixed-cell cancer)

C. Using the suffix -oma (benign tumor), build medical words to mean:

1. _____ benign tumor of fat

2. _____ benign tumor of fibrocytes

3. _____ benign tumor of smooth muscle

4. _____ benign tumor of the meninges

5. _____ benign tumor of nervous tissue

6. _____ benign tumor of lymph vessels

7. _____ benign tumor of a gland

392   D. Using the suffix -sarcoma (malignant tumor), build medical words to mean:

1. _____ malignant tumor of cartilage

2. _____ malignant tumor of bone

3. _____ malignant tumor of blood vessels

4. _____ malignant tumor of lymph vessels

5. _____ malignant tumor of smooth muscles

6. _____ malignant tumor of skeletal muscles

Fill in the correct word from the right hand column that matches the definitions in the statements below.

1. _____ spread of malignant cells into the sur-   Carcinoma
                         rounding tissue

2. _____ a method of classifying malignant   Grading
                         spread

3. _____ malignancy of connective tissue origin   Lymphomas

4. _____ malignancy of epithelial origin   Metastasis

5. _____ a new growth of tissue   Neoplasm

6. _____ a method of evaluating the histological   Proliferation
                         makeup of a neoplasm

7. _____ neoplastic disorders of the lymphatic   Sarcoma
                         system

8. _____ spread of malignant cells from one site   Staging
                         of the body to another, generally through
                         blood and lymph channels

394   ## WORKSHEET 3

Define the following diagnostic and symptomatic terms. Use the dictionary as a reference.

1. polyp _____

2. malignant _____

3. fungating _____

4. fibromatoid _____

5. proliferation _____

6. metastasis _____

7. leukemia _____

8. melanoma _____

WORKSHEET 4

Build plural words for the singular forms listed.

SINGULAR   PLURAL

myxoma   1. _____

carcinoma   2. _____

sarcoma   3. _____

Build adjectives for the nouns listed below.

NOUNS   ADJECTIVES

carcinogen   4. _____

carcinolysis   5. _____

carcinoma   6. _____

carcinophobia   7. _____

fibroma   8. _____

lymphoma   9. _____

melanoma   10. _____

sarcoma   11. _____

APPENDIX A

INTRODUCTION

WORKSHEET 1

1. word roots
2. Greek and Latin
3. combining form
4. "o"
5. consonant

WORKSHEET 2

1. cardi = WR
2. cardi/o
3. gastr/o
4. cyt = WR
5. erythr/o
6. oste = WR
7. oste/o
8. gastr = WR
9. nephr = WR
10. erythr = WR

WORKSHEET 3

1. mast/o
2. hepat/o
3. arthr/o
4. cyst/o
5. phleb/o
6. thorac/o
7. abdomin/o
8. trache/o

WORKSHEET 4

1. rhin
2. splen
3. hyster
4. enter
5. neur

6. ot
7. dermat
8. hydr

WORKSHEET 5

1.	gastro/enteritis	gastr(o)
2.	entero/anastomosis	enter(o)
3.	nephro/sclerosis	nephr(o)
4.	ileo/colic	ile(o)
5.	gastro/intestinal	gastr(o)
6.	nephro/abdominal	nephr(o)
7.	micro/scope	micr(o)
8.	thermo/meter	therm(o)
9.	leuko/derma	leuk(o)
10.	hydro/chloride	hydr(o)

CHAPTER 1
Suffixes: Surgical, Diagnostic, Symptomatic

WORKSHEET 1

1. cystotomy
2. colectomy
3. arthrocentesis
4. splenectomy
5. colostomy
6. dermatome
7. myringotomy
8. tracheostomy
9. lithotomy
10. phlebotomy
11. mastectomy
12. hemorrhoidectomy
13. tracheotomy
14. mastectomy
15. colectomy
16. myringotomy
17. colostomy
18. tracheotomy

Answer Key

19. splenectomy
20. dermatome
21. tracheostomy
22. lithotomy
23. arthrocentesis
24. hemorrhoidectomy
25. phlebotomy

WORKSHEET 2

1. episiotomy
2. mastopexy
3. nephropexy
4. gastrorrhaphy
5. hysteropexy
6. rhinoplasty
7. arthrodesis
8. splenopexy
9. hysteropexy
10. gastropexy
11. rhinoplasty
12. arthrodesis
13. mastopexy
14. splenorrhaphy
15. arthrocentesis

WORKSHEET 3

1. osteoclasis
2. lithotripsy
3. hemolysis
4. neurotripsy
5. oste
6. neuro
7. nephr
8. gastro
9. hemolysis
10. osteoclasis
11. lithotripsy
12. neurotripsy
13. enterolysis

WORKSHEET 4

1. bronchiectasis
2. gastrodynia
3. neuralgia
4. gastritis
5. cephalalgia
6. leukemia
7. carcinogen
8. dermatosis
9. lipoid
10. carcinoid
11. cytopenia
12. leukopenia
13. otorrhea
14. leukorrhea
15. gastrospasm
16. blepharospasm
17. neurolysis
18. myolysis

WORKSHEET 5

1. cystocele
2. quadriplegia
3. myelocele
4. lithiasis
5. nephrolithiasis
6. hemiparesis
7. leukopoiesis
8. hepatomegaly
9. gastritis
10. osteomalacia
11. nephromalacia
12. nephromegaly
13. cardiomegaly
14. erythropenia
15. splenomegaly
16. nephroma
17. nephrosis
18. sclerosis

397

19. gastropathy
20. nephropathy
21. gastroptosis
22. nephroptosis
23. angiorrhexis
24. hysterorrhexis
25. dermatitis

WORKSHEET 6

1. inflammation
2. enlargement
3. disease
4. puncture
5. surgical repair, plastic repair, formation
6. separate, destroy, break down
7. suture
8. blood
9. pain
10. flow, discharge
11. twitching
12. softening
13. paralysis
14. rupture
15. hernia, swelling
16. expansion, dilation
17. presence of, formation of, condition
18. burst forth
19. prolapse, falling, dropping
20. tumor
21. to produce
22. standing still
23. decrease, lack of
24. mouth, forming a new opening
25. incision, cut into
26. speech
27. formation, production
28. ingesting, eating, swallowing
29. decrease, deficiency, lack of
30. constriction, narrowing

CHAPTER 2
Suffixes: Adjective, Noun,
Diminutive, Singular,
Plural

WORKSHEET 1

1. narcotic
2. gastric
3. hepatic
4. duodenal

5. bacterial
6. aqueous
7. ciliary
8. necrotic
9. nephrocardiac
   nephrocardial
10. fibrous, fibrotic, fibroid
11. ossiferous
12. thoracic
13. meningitic, meningeal
14. membranous, membranoid
15. prophylactic
16. mucous, mucoid

WORKSHEET 2

1. internist
2. leukemia
3. sigmoidoscopy
4. alcoholism
5. allergist
6. pubis
7. senilism
8. mania
9. orthopedist
10. pelvis

WORKSHEET 3

Plural	Rule
1. enemata	Retain ma and add ta.
2. aquae	Retain a and add e.
3. fornices	Drop ix and add ices.
4. apices	Drop ex and add ices.
5. bursae	Retain a and add e.
6. vertebrae	Retain a and add e.
7. calcanea	Drop um and add a.
8. keratoses	Drop is and add es.
9. bronchi	Drop us and add i.
10. urinalyses	Drop is and add es.
11. specula	Drop um and add a.
12. uteri	Drop us and add i.
13. deliveries	Drop y and add ies.
14. spermatozoa	Drop on and add a.
15. adenomata	Retain ma and add ta.

WORKSHEET 4

Plural	Rule
1. media	Drop um and add a.
2. septa	Drop um and add a.
3. cocci	Drop us and add i.

4. bursae — Retain a and add e.
5. ganglia — Drop on and add a.
6. prognoses — Drop is and add es.
7. thrombi — Drop us and add i.
8. appendices — Drop ix and add ices.
9. bacteria — Drop um and add a.
10. radii — Drop us and add i.
11. conjunctivae — Retain a and add e.
12. phenomena — Drop on and add a.
13. testes — Drop is and add es.
14. apices — Drop ex and add ices.
15. nevi — Drop us and add i.

13. median
14. midsternum
15. epigastric

CHAPTER 3
Prefixes

WORKSHEET 1

1. between
2. under, beneath
3. left side
4. above
5. back
6. after, behind
7. side
8. behind, back
9. right side
10. under, beneath
11. before
12. middle
13. beneath
14. blue
15. white
16. white protein
17. yellow
18. yellow
19. grey
20. black

WORKSHEET 2

1. sinistropedal
2. acrocyanosis
3. posteromedial
4. leukorrhea
5. retrocolic
6. erythema
7. ambilateral
8. prenatal
9. infra-axillary
10. dorsodynia
11. melanoma
12. intercostal

WORKSHEET 3

1. after
2. four
3. above, too much
4. first
5. small
6. three
7. many, more than
8. one
9. not
10. without
11. large
12. beyond
13. from
14. outside
15. within
16. above
17. through
18. around
19. toward, near
20. around

WORKSHEET 4

1. quadriplegia
2. macrocephaly
3. unilateral
4. multiglandular
5. polyphobia
6. hyperglycemia
7. hemiparesis
8. superlactation
9. intramuscular
10. intracranial
11. suprasternal
12. microbe
13. transverse
14. circumoral
15. primigravida

WORKSHEET 5

1. brady/cardia — slow
2. tachy/pnea — rapid, fast
3. dys/pnea — bad, painful, difficult
4. eu/pnea — good, normal
5. cyan/osis — blue

6. hidr/adenitis   sweat
7. hydro/phobia   water
8. mal/function   bad, poor
9. peri/osteum   around
10. scler/oma   hard

WORKSHEET 6

1. hydrophobia
2. bradypnea
3. tachypnea
4. dyspnea
5. sclerosis
6. malnutrition
7. panophobia
8. pseudoencephalitis
9. hidrosis
10. eupnea

CHAPTER 4
The Body as a Whole

WORKSHEET 1

1. organism
2. system
3. organ
4. tissue
5. cell
6. true
7. false
8. true
9. false
10. true
11. true

WORKSHEET 2

1. ventral cavities
2. thoracic cavity
3. abdominopelvic cavity
4. abdominal cavity
5. pelvic cavity
6. cranial cavity
7. spinal cavity
8. dorsal cavities

WORKSHEET 3

1. cranial cavity
2. thoracic cavity
3. abdominopelvic cavity
4. thoracic cavity
5. spinal cavity
6. abdominopelvic cavity
7. abdominopelvic cavity
8. abdominopelvic cavity
9. distal
10. superior
11. lateral
12. ventral
13. anterior
14. superficial
15. visceral
16. distal
17. superficial

WORKSHEET 4

1. right hypochondriac
2. epigastric
3. left hypochondriac
4. right lumbar
5. umbilical
6. left lumbar
7. right inguinal
8. hypogastric
9. left inguinal

WORKSHEET 5

1. superior aspect
2. saggital planes
3. midsaggital plane
4. anterior (ventral) aspect
5. frontal or coronal planes
6. transverse (horizontal) planes
7. posterior (dorsal) aspect

1. right upper quadrant, RUQ, liver
2. left upper quadrant, LUQ, stomach, spleen
3. right lower quadrant, RLQ, appendix, ascending colon
4. left lower quadrant, LLQ, descending colon, sigmoid colon

CHAPTER 5
Integumentary System

WORKSHEET 1

A
1. mastodynia, mastalgia
2. mastitis
3. mastopathy
4. mastorrhagia
5. mastoptosis
6. amastia

B
1. mammitis
2. mammary
3. mammalgia, mammodynia

C
1. adipoma, lipoma
2. adipocele, lipocele
3. adipoid, lipoid
4. adipogenous, lipogenous, lipogenesis

D
1. dermatitis
2. dermalgia or dermatodynia
3. dermatologist
4. dermoid or dermatoid
5. dermatoplasty

E
1. erythroderma, erythrodermia, erythema
2. erythematic

F
1. hidrosis
2. hidradenoma, hidroadenoma
3. anhidrosis

G
1. onychia, onychitis
2. onychoma
3. onychalgia
4. onychotrophy
5. onychoid
6. onychopathy
7. onychomycosis
8. onychomalacia
9. onychoptosis
10. onychocryptosis

H
1. trichoid
2. trichology
3. trichopathy
4. trichophobia
5. trichitis
6. trichomycosis

WORKSHEET 2

1. pediculosis
2. onychia
3. tinea
4. scabies
5. impetigo
6. urticaria
7. chloasma
8. ecchymosis
9. petechiae
10. alopecia

WORKSHEET 3

1. mastectomy, mammectomy
2. mastotomy
3. mastopexy
4. mammoplasty, mastoplasty
5. adipectomy, lipectomy
6. onychectomy
7. onychotomy
8. homograft
9. autograft
10. biopsy of the breast

WORKSHEET 4

1. any inflammatory condition of the sebaceous glands
2. inflammatory condition producing lesions, crusts, and scales
3. absence of a breast nipple
4. inflammation of a nipple
5. abnormally large mammary gland in the male; sometimes may create milk
6. seen in inflammatory breast cancer
7. blackhead
8. a scar left by a healed wound
9. congenital lack of normal skin pigment
10. a bedsore

WORKSHEET 5

1. keratoses
2. milia
3. capilli
4. bacilli
5. mammae
6. allergic
7. epithelial

8. ceruminous or ceruminal
9. keratotic
10. pilonidal
11. albinism
12. alopecia
13. dermatologist
14. dermis
15. dermatopathy
   dermatopathia

WORKSHEET 7

1. intradermal tests
2. mammography
3. negative
4. scratch tests
5. xerography
6. patch tests
7. positive
8. positive

WORKSHEET 8

1. anti-inflammatory drugs
2. antiseptics
3. keratolytics
4. antipruritics
5. anti-infectives
6. parasiticides
7. topical anesthetics
8. protectives
9. astringents
10. vasodilation

CHAPTER 6
Gastrointestinal System

WORKSHEET 1

A 1. esophagitis
2. esophagodynia or esophagalgia
3. esophagoplasty
4. esophagoscope
5. esophagectomy

B 1. gastrectomy
2. gastritis
3. gastrodynia or gastralgia
4. gastropathy
5. gastroplegia
6. gastromegaly

7. gastroptosis
8. gastrorrhaphy
9. gastroenterology
10. gastrostenosis

C 1. duodenal
2. duodenitis
3. jejunitis
4. jejunoileitis
5. ileocecal

D 1. enteral, enteric
2. enteritis
3. enteropathy
4. enteropexy
5. enteroplasty

E 1. colitis
2. colonoscopy
3. colopathy, colonopathy
4. colorectitis, coloproctitis
5. coloptosis

F 1. proctodynia or proctalgia
   rectodynia or rectalgia
2. rectitis or proctitis
3. rectostenosis
4. proctoptosis
5. proctoplegia

G 1. cholecyst
2. cholecystolith
3. cholecystolithiasis
4. cholelithotripsy
5. cholemesis
6. choledochal
7. choledocholithiasis
8. choledochitis
9. choledochectomy
10. choledochorrhaphy

H 1. hepatoma
2. hepatodynia or hepatalgia
3. hepatomegaly
4. hepatocirrhosis
5. pancreatitis
6. pancreatic
7. pancreatectomy

WORKSHEET 2

1. hematemesis
2. dysphagia
3. fecalith
4. halitosis
5. anorexia

6. dyspepsia
7. melena
8. cirrhosis
9. obstipation
10. bulimia

WORKSHEET 3

1. gingivectomy
2. glossectomy
3. esophagoplasty
4. gastrectomy
5. gastrojejunostomy
6. proctosigmoidoscopy
7. gastroenterocolostomy
8. enteroplasty
9. enteropexy
10. jejunostomy
11. colostomy
12. hepatopexy
13. proctoplasty
14. cholecystectomy
15. choledochoplasty

WORKSHEET 4

1. white plates or patches
2. dilatation of the stomach
3. inflammation of the lips
4. spasm of small intestine, painful peristalsis
5. swallowing of air
6. excessive secretion of saliva
7. backflow of gastric contents into the mouth
8. narrowing down of an orifice; stricture
9. a sac or pouch in the walls of a canal or an organ
10. a twisting of the bowel upon itself causing obstruction

WORKSHEET 5

1. duodenal
2. hepatic
3. gastroenterologist
4. rectal
5. bulimia
6. proctologist
7. rugae
8. omenta
9. stomata
10. diverticula

WORKSHEET 8

1. p.c.
2. occult blood
3. emetics
4. b.i.d.
5. choledochoplasty
6. lower GI
7. laparoscopy
8. stomatoplasty
9. cathartics
10. anastomosis
11. oral cholecystography
12. spleen scan
13. antiflatulants
14. antacids
15. FBS
16. intravenous cholecystography
17. q.i.d.
18. stat.
19. proctosigmoidoscopy
20. upper GI

CHAPTER 7
Respiratory System

WORKSHEET 1

A 1. rhinorrhagia
2. rhinitis
3. rhinorrhea
4. nasal, rhinal

B 1. laryngitis
2. laryngoscopy
3. laryngospasm
4. laryngostenosis
5. laryngotracheal
6. laryngopathy

C 1. bronchoscope
2. bronchitis
3. bronchiectasis
4. bronchogenic
5. bronchorrhagia
6. bronchiospasm bronchospasm
7. bronchopathy

D 1. pneumonitis
2. pneumothorax
3. pneumonectomy
4. pulmonary pneumonic

404

E 1. thoracentesis, thoracocentesis
2. thoracodynia
   thoracalgia
3. thoracic

F 1. eupnea
2. tachypnea
3. orthopnea
4. apnea
5. hyperpnea
6. bradypnea
7. hypopnea
8. dyspnea

WORKSHEET 2

1. sputum
2. rales, crackles
3. hemoptysis
4. percussion
5. auscultation
6. Cheyne-Stokes respiration
7. atelectasis
8. empyema
9. anosmia
10. anoxemia
11. apnea
12. coryza
13. epiglottis
14. epistaxis

WORKSHEET 3

1. laryngectomy
2. pneumonectomy
   pulmonectomy
3. lobectomy
   pneumonectomy
4. rhinoplasty
5. thoracocentesis
   thoracentesis
6. pneumonorrhaphy
7. pneumopexy
   pneumonopexy
8. bronchoplasty
9. tracheostomy
10. laryngotomy
11. laryngoplasty
12. pneumolithectomy

WORKSHEET 4

1. inflammation of the alveoli
2. fungal infection of the bronchi
3. condition of dust in the lungs
4. condition in which silicone is in the lungs
5. paralysis of the voice box
6. expansion of the bronchi with sputum production
7. blood in the chest cavity
8. seeping of fluids into the pleural cavity
9. listening to chest sounds

WORKSHEET 5

1. pulmonary function studies
2. bronchography
3. laminography
4. throat culture
5. AP
6. COLD
7. antitussive
8. antihistamine
9. decongestant
10. mucolytic
11. bronchodilator
12. IPPB
13. arterial blood gases
14. culture and sensitivity

WORKSHEET 6

1. hyperplasia
2. orthopnea
3. paroxysm
4. embolus
5. mucus
6. lumina
7. sputa
8. thoraces
9. bronchi
10. tracheae
11. nares

CHAPTER 8
Cardiovascular System

WORKSHEET 1

A 1. atheroma

2. atherogenesis
3. atherosclerosis

B
1. phlebitis
2. phlebosclerosis
3. phlebectasia, phlebectasis
4. phlebolith
5. phleboid
6. phleborrhexis
7. phlebothrombosis

C
1. venosclerosis
2. venospasm
3. venous
4. venostenosis

D
1. cardiomegaly, megalocardia
2. endocarditis
3. epicarditis
4. cardiopulmonary
5. cardiovascular
6. myocarditis
7. cardiomyopathy

E
1. arteriosclerosis
2. arteriospasm
3. arteriorrhexis
4. arterial

WORKSHEET 2

1. ventricles
2. S-A node
3. capillaries
4. epicardium
5. veins
6. pericardium
7. atria
8. aorta
9. arteries
10. septum

WORKSHEET 3

1. cardiotomy
2. cardiocentesis
3. phlebopexy
4. arteriorrhaphy
5. pericardiectomy
6. phlebotomy, venotomy
7. arterioplasty
8. aneurysmectomy
9. embolectomy
10. phlebocentesis, venipuncture

WORKSHEET 4

1. a condition of tissue death
2. local anemia of tissue or organ
3. high blood pressure
4. quivering or spontaneous contraction of individual muscle fibers
5. a tracing of a venous pulse
6. irregular heart action
7. a narrowing of the aorta
8. a record of electrical heart impulses
9. radiography of aorta after injection of contrast dye
10. process in which vessel lumen decreases
11. multiple angiomata of blood vessels
12. rapid heart action

WORKSHEET 5

1. echocardiography
2. electrocardiography
3. diagnostic pericardiocentesis
4. MS
5. antianginals
6. inotropics
7. cardiac enzyme studies
8. phlebography
9. beta blockers
10. stress/exercise testing
11. phonocardiography
12. MI

WORKSHEET 6

1. cardia
2. atria
3. aortae, aortas
4. hemangiomata
5. myocardia
6. atheromatous
7. arterial
8. aortic
9. venous
10. aneurysmal

CHAPTER 9
Hematic and Lymphatic Systems

WORKSHEET 1

A
1. eosinophil

2. basophil
3. neutrophil
4. hematophil, hemophil

B 1. erythrocytosis
2. leukocytosis
3. agranulocytosis
4. granulocytosis
5. thrombocytosis
6. lymphocytosis
7. reticulocytosis

C 1. erythrocytopenia
2. leukocytopenia
3. thrombocytopenia
4. granulocytopenia
5. lymphocytopenia

D 1. lymphadenitis
2. lymphadenopathy
3. lymphadenoma

E 1. hematopoiesis
2. erythropoiesis
3. leukopoiesis
4. myelopoiesis
5. lymphopoiesis

F 1. immunologist
2. immunology

G 1. splenocele
2. splenitis
3. splenic
splenetic
4. splenocolic

WORKSHEET 2

1. fibrin
2. fibrinogen
3. plasma
4. serum
5. antigens
6. T-cells
7. microcyte
8. poikilocyte
9. macrocyte
10. phagocyte

WORKSHEET 3

1. lymphadenectomy
2. lymphadenotomy
3. splenectomy

4. splenolysis
5. splenotomy
6. thymectomy
7. thymolysis

WORKSHEET 4

1. enlargement of the spleen and liver
2. pertaining to the spleen and kidney
3. downward displacement of the spleen
4. displacement of the spleen
5. inflamed spleen associated with jaundice
6. tumor of the spleen
7. splenic pain
8. development of bone marrow tissue
9. a bone marrow tumor
10. producing or originating in bone marrow
11. inflammation of the thymus
12. lack of blood cell development by bone marrow
13. anemia due to red cell destruction

WORKSHEET 5

1. hemostatic
2. hemoglobin
3. erythrocyte sedimentation rate
4. hematocrit
5. Ig
6. PMN, seg, poly
7. prothrombin time
8. Monospot
9. bleeding time
10. complete blood count
11. fibrinolytic
12. anticoagulant

WORKSHEET 6

1. thymic
2. splenic
3. anemic
4. hemophilic
5. lymphedematous
6. nuclear
7. hematologist
8. immunologist
9. serologist
10. pathologist

CHAPTER 10
Musculoskeletal System

WORKSHEET 1

A 1. cephalic
2. cephalopelvic
3. cephalitis, encephalitis
4. cephalopathy

B 1. craniomalacia
2. craniocele
3. cranioplasty
4. craniotomy

C 1. cervical
2. cervicobrachial
3. cervicofacial

D 1. myelorrhagia
2. myelosarcoma
3. myelomalacia
4. myeloblastoma

E 1. costochondral
2. costalgia
3. suprasternal
4. sternoid

F 1. chondroblast
2. chondrology
3. chondroangioma
4. chondrosarcoma
5. arthritis
6. arthrotome
7. arthropathy
8. costochondral

G 1. pelvimeter
2. lumbodynia or lumbago
3. lumbocostal

H 1. pubofemoral
2. condyloid
3. condylectomy

I 1. myoma
2. myosclerosis
3. myoplasty
4. myorrhexis
5. myosteoma

WORKSHEET 2

1. subluxation

2. rickets
3. wryneck
4. claudication
5. muscular dystrophy
6. talipes
7. sequestrum
8. myasthenia gravis

WORKSHEET 3

1. phalangectomy
2. thoracotomy
3. thoracentesis or thoracocentesis
4. vertebrectomy
5. arthrodesis
6. arthroclasia
7. osteoplasty
8. osteoclast
9. myoplasty
10. amputation

WORKSHEET 4

1. greenstick fracture—bone partially bent and partially broken, as when a green stick breaks
2. simple fracture—broken bone, no external wound; also known as closed fracture
3. compound fracture—broken bone with external wound to the site of fracture; also known as open fracture
4. softening of the bones in children due to lack of vitamin D
5. metabolic disease marked by acute arthritis and inflammation of joints, usually begins in the knee or foot
6. kyphosis—humpback, hunchback
7. scoliosis—lateral curvature of the spine; usually consists of two curves
8. lordosis—swayback; forward curvature of the spine
9. Paget's disease—skeletal disease of elderly with chronic inflammation of bones, resulting in thickening and softening of the bones
10. Ewing's sarcoma—endothelial myeloma forming a fusiform swelling on a long bone

WORKSHEET 9

1. myelography
2. rachicentesis
3. skin biopsy
4. myotasis
5. chrysotherapy
6. corticosteroids
7. antihyperuricemics
8. L_3
9. EMG
10. arthrography
11. prosthesis
12. arthrodesis
13. amputation
14. HNP
15. thermography

CHAPTER 11
Urogenital System

WORKSHEET 1

A
1. nephrotic, nephric, nephritic
2. nephritis
3. nephrocardiac, nephrocardial
4. nephroptosis
5. nephrogenic
6. nephrolith
7. nephroma
8. pyonephrosis
   nephropyosis
9. nephrosclerosis
10. hydronephrosis
    nephrophydrosis

B
1. pyelectasis
2. pyelitis
3. pyelocystitis
4. pyelopathy

C
1. ureterectasis
2. ureterolith
3. ureteromegaly
4. ureteropyosis
   pyoureter

D
1. cystitis
2. cystocele
3. cystoscope
4. cystic

E
1. vesicolith
2. vesicocele
3. vesicoprostatic

F
1. urethrostenosis
2. urethrotome
3. urethroprostatic

G
1. urogenital
   genitourinary
2. urograph
3. urolith
4. urologist
5. uropathy
6. urocystitis

H
1. polyuria
2. hematuria
3. pyuria
4. glucosuria
   glycosuria
5. oliguria
6. anuria
7. nocturia
   nycturia

I
1. orchitis
2. orchiopathy
3. orchialgia
   orchidalgia
   orchiodynia
4. orchidic
5. orchiepididymitis

J
1. epididymitis
2. epididymoorchitis

K
1. vesiculogram
2. vesiculopathy
3. vesiculitis

L
1. prostatodynia
   prostatalgia
2. prostatitis
3. prostatorrhea
4. prostatic
5. prostatometer
6. prostatocystalgia

M
1. balanic
2. balanorrhea

WORKSHEET 2

1. ureter
2. urethra
3. renal pelvis
4. Bowman's capsule
5. tubule
6. glomerulus
7. glans penis

8. prepuce
9. seminiferous tubule
10. bladder
11. prostate
12. vas deferens

WORKSHEET 3

1. vasoepididymostomy
2. vasectomy
3. urethrorrhaphy
4. ureteropyeloplasty
5. nephroureterectomy
6. cystolithectomy
7. cystoplasty
   vesicoplasty
8. cystorrhaphy
9. nephrocystanastomosis
10. prostatectomy
11. prostatolithotomy
12. balanoplasty

WORKSHEET 4

1. chemical, microscopic, and physical tests performed on urine
2. condition of excessive bacteria in the urine
3. examination of bladder with cystoscope
4. accumulation of serous fluid, especially in tunica vaginalis testis
5. lack of sperm production
6. semen discharge with urine
7. stenosis of the preputial orifice so that the foreskin cannot be pushed back over the glans penis
8. failure of testicles to descend into scrotum
9. a cystic tumor of the epididymis containing sperm
10. absence of one or both testes

WORKSHEET 5

1. intravenous pyelography
2. urinalysis
3. blood urea nitrogen
4. uricosuric agent
5. gonadotropin
6. pH
7. ATN
8. diuretic
9. spermicidal preparation

10. semen analysis
11. resectoscopy
12. nephrotomography
13. retrograde pyelography
14. urethroscopy
15. cystography
16. UTI

WORKSHEET 6

1. meatal
2. testicular
3. tubal, tubular
4. medullary
5. scrotal
6. calyces
7. papillae
8. medullae
9. pelves
10. scrota

CHAPTER 12
Female Reproductive System

WORKSHEET 1

A
1. gynecomastia
2. gynecology
3. gynecologist
4. gynecic

B
1. cervical
2. cervicocolpitis, cervicovaginitis
3. cervicitis
4. cervicovesical

C
1. colporrhaphy
2. colposcope
3. colposcopy

D
1. vaginitis
2. vaginal
3. vaginogenic
4. vaginocele
5. vaginography
6. vaginomycosis
7. vaginoperineal
8. vaginotome
9. vaginovesical or vesicovaginal
10. vaginolabial

E
1. hysteromyoma
2. hysteropathy

Answer Key

3. hysterospasm
4. hysterorrhexis
5. hysterosalpingography
6. hysterovaginal

F 1. metrorrhagia
2. parametritis
3. endometriosis

G 1. uterocele
2. uterocervical
3. uterorectal
4. uterovesical

H 1. oophoritis
2. oophoralgia, oophorodynia
3. oophorocarcinoma
4. oophorosalpingitis

I 1. salpingocele
2. salpingitis
3. salpingography
4. salpingo-oophoritis

J 1. pseudocyesis
2. dystocia
3. hemosalpinx
4. multigravida
5. menarche

WORKSHEET 2

1. pyosalpinx
2. primipara
3. gestation
4. LMP
5. hydrocephalus
6. corpus luteum
7. dystocia
8. atresia
9. Down's syndrome
10. pruritus vulvae

WORKSHEET 3

1. vaginectomy, colpectomy
2. oophoropexy
3. oophorrhaphy
4. colpoplasty, vaginoplasty
5. hystero-oophorectomy
6. colpoperineoplasty, vaginoperineoplasty
7. panhysterectomy
8. episiorrhaphy, perineorrhaphy
9. hysterosalpingo-oophorectomy
10. amniocentesis

WORKSHEET 4

1. a wartlike growth of skin
2. painful or difficult menstruation
3. fibrous tissue myoma
4. a highly contagious bacterial infection of the genitourinary system
5. herpes simplex of the genitals (any inflammatory skin disease caused by a herpesvirus and characterized by formation of small vesicles in clusters)
6. a small sac, embedded in the ovary, that encloses an ovum
7. pelvic inflammatory disease
8. inflammation of the peritoneum
9. infestation with a parasite of the genus *Trichomonas*
10. an infectious, chronic, venereal disease, characterized by lesions which may involve any organ or tissue

WORKSHEET 5

1. cervices
2. ova
3. uteri
4. spermatozoa
5. pelves
6. labia
7. gynecologist
8. vaginal
9. hydrocephalic
10. vulvar

WORKSHEET 7

1. Pap test
2. miscarriage
3. amniocentesis
4. cryosurgery
5. colpocleisis
6. D&C
7. panhysterectomy
8. tubal ligation
9. CPD
10. LMP
11. abortion
12. laparotomy
13. ultrasonography
14. chorionic villus biopsy
15. estrogens

CHAPTER 13
Endocrine System

WORKSHEET 1

A   1. adrenitis
      2. adrenogenital
      3. adrenalectomy
      4. adrenocortical

B   1. glycogenic
      2. hyperglycemia
      3. hypoglycemia
      4. glycogenesis

C   1. pancreatitis
      2. pancreatogenic, pancreatogenous, pancreatogenesis
      3. pancreatolysis
      4. pancreatopathy

D   1. thyroglossal
      2. thyroadenitis
      3. thyroidectomy
      4. thyrocele

WORKSHEET 2

1. vasopressin
2. myxedema
3. adenohypophysis
4. hirsutism
5. cretinism
6. insulin
7. Addison's disease
8. exophthalmic goiter
9. hyperparathyroidism
10. neurohypophysis

WORKSHEET 3

1. thyroidectomy
2. thyrochondrotomy
3. parathyroidectomy
4. pancreatoduodenectomy
5. adrenalectomy
6. bilateral adrenalectomy

WORKSHEET 4

1. a group of serious symptoms caused by overactivity of the cortices of the adrenal glands

2. the state of being a dwarf; underdevelopment of the body
3. an excessive amount of insulin in the blood
4. a condition due to deficiency in thyroid secretion, resulting in a lowered basal metabolism; a lesser degree of cretinism
5. an enlargement of the thyroid gland
6. excess of glucose in the blood
7. a metabolic disorder resulting from decreased activity of the posterior lobe of the pituitary gland
8. primary adrenal hypofunction
9. acidosis due to excess of ketone bodies
10. a disorder of carbohydrate metabolism characterized by hyperglycemia and glycosuria, resulting from inadequate production or utilization of insulin

WORKSHEET 5

1. gonads
2. ova
3. striae
4. atrophies
5. myxoadenomata
6. cretinism
7. dwarfism
8. hirsutism
9. giantism or gigantism
10. endocrinologist

WORKSHEET 7

1. FBS
2. RAIU
3. corticosteroids
4. vasopressin
5. thyroid echogram
6. T_4
7. XX
8. insulin
9. serum glucose test
10. antihyperlipidemics
11. RAI
12. HDL
13. T_3
14. XY
15. VLDL

412   CHAPTER 14
Nervous System

WORKSHEET 1

A   1. encephalopathy
       2. encephalitis

B   1. cerebellar
       2. cerebral
       3. cerebrospinal
       4. cranial

C   1. neurocyte
       2. neuroblast
       3. neuritis
       4. neuralgia, neurodynia
       5. neurotoxin

D   1. ventriculography
       2. ventriculometry
       3. ventriculoscopy

WORKSHEET 2

1. anesthesia
2. ataxia
3. asthenia
4. aphasia
5. hemiplegia
6. apoplexy
7. dysrhythmias
8. clonic spasm
9. bradykinesia
10. tremor

WORKSHEET 3

1. craniotomy
2. cerebrotomy
3. craniectomy
4. cranioplasty
5. gangliectomy
    ganglionectomy
6. neuroplasty
7. neurorrhaphy
    neurosuture
8. neurotomy
9. neurotripsy
10. thalamotomy

WORKSHEET 4

1. herniation of the brain
2. radiograph of the brain
3. brain abscess; pus in the brain
4. softening of the cerebrum
5. hardening of the cerebrum
6. softening of the skull
7. protrusion through the skull
8. paralysis of spinal origin
9. hemorrhage of the spinal cord
10. nerve pain
11. softening of the nerve tissue
12. involuntary movement associated with a reflexive movement
13. tumor of meninges
14. herniation of meninges

WORKSHEET 5

1. myelography
2. pneumoencephalography
3. antidepressants
4. lumbar puncture
5. psychotropic drugs
6. TIA
7. opiate
8. tranquilizer
9. echoencephalography
10. analgesics
11. anticonvulsant
12. computerized tomography

WORKSHEET 6

1. meningococci
2. crania
3. cerebella
4. nuclei
5. sensory
6. peripheral
7. nuclear
8. neuroglial
9. spinal

CHAPTER 15
Special Senses

WORKSHEET 1

A   1. ophthalmic

2. ophthalmitis
3. ophthalmoplegia
4. ophthalmoscope
5. ophthalmology

B 1. corectasia
       corectasis
   2. corectopia

C 1. pupilloscopy
   2. pupillary
   3. pupillometer

D 1. keratoscope
   2. keratometer
   3. keratotome
   4. keratitis

E 1. scleritis
   2. scleromalacia
   3. scleroiritis
   4. sclerokeratitis

F 1. retinal
   2. retinitis
   3. retinoscope
   4. retinochoroiditis

G 1. iridic
   2. iridoplegia
   3. iridocyclitis
   4. iridocele
   5. iridomalacia
   6. iridodynia
       iridalgia

H 1. cyclokeratitis
   2. cycloplegia
   3. cyclochoroiditis

I 1. blepharedema
   2. blepharalgia, blepharodynia
   3. blepharoplegia
   4. blepharoptosis
   5. blepharospasm

J 1. dacryocystalgia
   2. dacryocystoptosis
   3. dacryocystocele
   4. dacryocystitis

K 1. emmetropia
   2. amblyopia
   3. hyperopia
   4. chloropia
   5. nyctalopia

L 1. hemianopsia
   2. achromatopsia
   3. heteropsia

M 1. otodynia
       otalgia
   2. otoscope
   3. otorrhagia
   4. otopyorrhea
   5. otitis

N 1. audiogram
   2. audiometer
   3. audiology

O 1. myringomastoiditis
   2. myringitis
   3. myringotome
   4. myringomycosis

P 1. anacusis
       anacusia
   2. presbycusis, presbyacusia,
       presbyacousia

WORKSHEET 2

1. papilledema
2. ectropion
3. exotropia
4. aphakia
5. achromatopsia
6. ectopia lentis
7. cerumen
8. parotid
9. tinnitus
10. vertigo
11. anacusis

WORKSHEET 3

1. ophthalmotomy
2. ophthalmophlebotomy
3. iridotomy
    irotomy
    iritomy
4. cyclectomy
5. dacryocystorhinostomy
6. ototomy
7. otoplasty
8. myringoplasty
    tympanoplasty
9. myringotomy
    tympanotomy

10. stapedectomy
11. stapediotenotomy
12. mastoidocentesis
13. mastoidectomy
14. labyrinthotomy

WORKSHEET 4

1. white, opaque corneal opacity
2. pathological changes in the retina due to hypertension
3. farsightedness
4. abnormal intolerance to light
5. involuntary movement of the eyes
6. marked difference in the refractive power of the two eyes
7. examination of the eustachian tube
8. measurement of hearing
9. closure of the external auditory meatus
10. originating in the ear
11. measurement of the scope of the field of vision
12. secretion and discharge of tears

WORKSHEET 5

1. tonometry
2. cycloplegic agents
3. audiometry
4. miotics/cholinergics
5. ophthalmodynamometry
6. gonioscopy
7. beta-adrenergic blocking agents
8. mydriatics
9. OD
10. AD
11. OS
12. AS
13. OU
14. otoscopy
15. retinoscopy

WORKSHEET 6

1. tympanic
2. meatal
3. antral
4. auricular
5. auditory
6. pinnae
7. antra

CHAPTER 16
Oncology

WORKSHEET 1

A 1. oncogenesis
   2. oncologist
   3. oncotic
   4. oncosis
   5. oncolysis

B 1. carcinectomy
   2. carcinogen
   3. carcinoid
   4. carcinolysis
   5. carcinophobia
   6. carcinosarcoma

C 1. adipoma, lipoma, steatoma
   2. fibrocytoma
   3. leiomyoma
   4. meningioma
   5. neuroma
   6. lymphangioma
   7. adenoma

D 1. chondrosarcoma
   2. osteosarcoma
   3. hemangiosarcoma
   4. lymphangiosarcoma
   5. leiomyosarcoma
   6. rhabdomyosarcoma

WORKSHEET 2

1. proliferation
2. staging
3. sarcoma
4. carcinoma
5. neoplasm
6. grading
7. lymphomas
8. metastasis

WORKSHEET 3

1. a protuberance from a mucous membrane which is generally attached to a thin stalk
2. a neoplasm that is cancerous as opposed to benign
3. growing rapidly
4. resembling a fibroma

5. reproducing rapidly and repeatedly as by cell division
6. movement of malignant cells from one area of the body to another
7. malignancy of hematopoietic tissue
8. malignant tumor of epithelial origin (black tumor)

WORKSHEET 4

1. myxomata
2. carcinomata
3. sarcomata
4. carcinogenic
5. carcinolytic
6. carcinomatous
7. carcinophobic
8. fibromatous
9. lymphomatous
10. melanomatous
11. sarcomatous

Abbreviation	Meaning
AB	abortion
ABC	aspiration biopsy cytology
ABG	arterial blood gasses
A.C., a.c.	acromioclavicular (joint)
	before meals
AC	air conduction
Acc	accommodation
ACG	angiocardiography
ACS	American Cancer Society
ACTH	adrenocorticotropic hormone
AD	right ear (auris dextra)
ad lib.	as desired
adeno-CA	adenocarcinoma
ADH	antidiuretic hormone
AE	above the elbow
AFB	acid-fast bacillus
AFP	alpha-fetoprotein
A/G	albumin/globulin ratio
AGN	acute glomerulonephritis
AHF	antihemophilic factor VIII
AHG	antihemophilic globulin factor VIII
AK	above the knee
ALL	acute lymphocytic leukemia
AMA	American Medical Association
AMI	acute myocardial infarction
ANS	autonomic nervous system
AP	anterior-posterior; anteroposterior
AP view	anteroposterior view (radiology)
ARDS	adult respiratory distress syndrome
AS	aortic stenosis
	left ear (auris sinistra)
ASD	atrial septal defect
ASHD	arteriosclerotic heart disease
Astigm	astigmatism
ATN	acute tubular necrosis
AV	atrioventricular
BA	barium enema
BaE	barium enema
baso	basophil
BBB	bundle-branch block
BE	below the elbow
B.I.D., b.i.d.	twice a day

Common Medical Abbreviations

Abbreviation	Meaning
BIN, bin	twice a night
BK	below the knee
BM	bowel movement
BMR	basal metabolic rate
BNO	bladder neck obstruction
BP	blood pressure
BPH	benign prostatic hyperplasia
	benign prostatic hypertrophy
BUN	blood urea nitrogen
bx	biopsy
C.	Celsius, centigrade
$\bar{c}$	with
C-1	first cervical vertebra
C-2	second cervical vertebra
C-3	third cervical vertebra
CA, Ca	cancer
CAD	coronary artery disease
CAT Scan	computerized axial tomography
CBC	complete blood count
CC	cardiac catheterization
	chief complaint
cc.	cubic centimeter
CCU	coronary care unit
CDC	Centers for Disease Control
CDH	congenital dislocation of the hip
CEA	carcinoembryonic antigen
CHF	congestive heart failure
CLL	chronic lymphocytic leukemia
cm.	centimeter
CNS	central nervous system
CO_2	carbon dioxide
COLD	chronic obstructive lung disease
contra	against
COPD	chronic obstructive pulmonary disease
CP	cerebral palsy
CPD	cephalopelvic disproportion
CPR	cardiopulmonary resuscitation
CS, C-section	cesarean section
CSF	cerebrospinal fluid
CT scan	computerized tomography scan
CV	cardiovascular

418

Abbreviation	Meaning
CVA	cerebrovascular accident
CVD	cardiovascular disease
CWP	childbirth without pain
CXR	chest x-ray; chest radiograph
cysto	cystoscopic examination
D	diopter (lens strength)
d	day (24 hours)
db	decibel
/d	per day
D&C	dilation and curettage
DDS	Doctor of Dental Surgery
D&E	dilation and evacuation
DES	diethylstilbestrol
Derm.	dermatology
DI	diabetes insipidus
	diagnostic imaging
diff	(white cell) differential
DM	diabetes mellitus
DNA	deoxyribonucleic acid
DO	Doctor of Osteopathy
DOB	date of birth
DPT	diphtheria-pertussis-tetanus
DUB	dysfunctional uterine bleeding
DVT	deep vein thrombosis
Dx	diagnosis
EBV	Epstein-Barr virus
ECG, EKG	electrocardiogram
ECF	extracellular fluid
EDC	estimated or expected date of confinement
EEG	electroencephalogram
EENT	eye, ear, nose, and throat
Em	emmetropia
EMG	electromyogram
ENT	ear, nose, and throat
EOM	extraocular movement
eosin	eosinophil
ESR	erythrocyte sedimentation rate
EST	electric shock therapy
ET	esotropia
et	and
F.	Fahrenheit
FACP	Fellow of the American College of Physicians
FACS	Fellow of the American College of Surgeons
FBS	fasting blood sugar
FDA	Food and Drug Administration
FEF	forced expiratory flow
FEKG	fetal electrocardiogram
FEV	forced expiratory volume
FHR	fetal heart rate
FHT	fetal heart tone

Abbreviation	Meaning
FS	frozen section
FSH	follicle-stimulating hormone
FTI	free thyroxine index
FTND	full-term normal delivery
FUO	fever of undetermined origin
FVC	forced vital capacity
Fx	fracture
GB	gallbladder
GC	gonorrhea
GH	growth hormone
GI	gastrointestinal
Gm., gm.	gram
gr.	grain
GTT	glucose tolerance test
Gtt., gtt.	drops
GU	genitourinary
Gyn	gynecology
H	hypodermic
h	hour
HCG	human chorionic gonadotropin
HCl	hydrochloric acid
HCT, Hct	hematocrit
HD	hip disarticulation
	Hodgkin's disease
HDL	high-density lipoprotein
Hg	mercury
HGB, hgb, Hb	hemoglobin
HHS	Department of Health and Human Services (replaced HEW)
HNP	herniated nucleus pulposus (herniated disk)
HP	hemipelvectomy
h.s.	at bedtime
HSG	hysterosalpingography
ht, hct	hematocrit
hypo	hypodermically
ICF	intracellular fluid
ICU	intensive care unit
I&D	incision and drainage
ID	intradermal
Ig	immunoglobulin
IH	infectious hepatitis
IM	intramuscular
IOP	intraocular pressure
IPPB	intermittent positive-pressure breathing
I.Q.	intelligence quotient
IS	intercostal space
IU	international unit
IUD	intrauterine device
I.V.	intravenously
IVC	intravenous cholangiography
IVP	intravenous pyelogram

420	Abbreviation	Meaning
	KD	knee disarticulation
	kg.	kilogram
	KUB	kidney, ureter, bladder
	l	liter
	L-1	first lumbar vertebra
	L-2	second lumbar vertebra
	L-3	third lumbar vertebra
	L&A	light and accommodation
	LAT, lat.	lateral
	lb.	pound
	LDL	low-density lipoprotein
	LE	left eye
	LH	luteinizing hormone
	LLQ	left lower quadrant
	LMP	last menstrual period
	LP	lumbar puncture
	LPN	Licensed Practical Nurse
	LRQ	lower right quadrant
	LUQ	left upper quadrant
	lymphs	lymphocytes
	M	meter
	m	minim
	mcg.	microgram
	MCH	mean corpuscular hemoglobin
	MCHC	mean corpuscular hemoglobin concentration
	MCV	mean corpuscular volume
	M.D.	Doctor of Medicine
	mets	metastases
	MH	marital history
	MI	myocardial infarction
	mix. astig.	mixed astigmatism
	ml.	milliliter
	mm.	millimeter
	mono	monocyte
	MS	mitral stenosis
		multiple sclerosis
		musculoskeletal
	MSH	melanocyte-stimulating hormone
	MVP	mitral valve prolapse
	myop.	myopia
	NB	newborn
	NPH	neutral protamine Hagedorn (insulin)
	NPO	nothing by mouth
	NSAID	nonsteroidal anti-inflammatory drug
	O_2	oxygen
	OA	osteoarthritis
	OB	obstetrics
	OC	oral contraceptive
	OD	right eye (oculus dexter)

Abbreviation	Meaning
od	once a day
OHS	open heart surgery
OR	operating room
Ortho, ORTH	orthopedics; orthopaedics
OS	left eye (oculus sinister)
os	mouth
Oto.	otology
OU	both eyes (oculi unitas)
	each eye (oculus uterque)
OV	both eyes
oz.	ounce
P	pulse
PA	posteroanterior
PA view	posteroanterior view (radiology)
P.A.	pernicious anemia
Pap	Papanicolaou
paren.	parenterally
PAT	paroxysmal atrial tachycardia
Path	pathology
PBI	protein-bound iodine
P.C., p.c.	after meals
PCV	packed cell volume (hematocrit)
PD	postprandial (after meals)
P.E.	physical examination
per	through or by
PGH	pituitary growth hormone
pH	hydrogen ion concentration
PID	pelvic inflammatory disease
PKU	phenylketonuria
PMN	polymorphonuclear neutrophil
PMP	previous menstrual period
PND	paroxysmal nocturnal dyspnea
PNS	peripheral nervous system
P.O.	orally
poly	polymorphonuclear neutrophil
PP	postprandial
p.r.n.	as required
PT	prothrombin time
P.T.	Physical Therapy
PTH	parathyroid hormone
PVC	premature ventricular contraction
q	every
q.d.	every day
q.h.	every hour
q. 2h.	every two hours
Q.I.D., q.i.d.	four times a day
qm	every morning
qn	every night
qns	quantity not sufficient

422	Abbreviation	Meaning
	R.	respiration
	RA	rheumatoid arthritis
	rad; rem	radiation absorbed dose; roentgen-equivalent-man
	RAI	radioactive iodine
	RATx	radiation therapy
	RBC	red blood cell; red blood count
	RBE	relative biological effects
	RD	respiratory disease
	RE	right eye
	REM	rapid eye movement
	Rh.	blood factor
	RLQ	right lower quadrant
	R.N.	Registered Nurse
	RNA	ribonucleic acid
	ROM	range of motion
	RP	retrograde pyelogram
	RU	routine urinalysis
	RUQ	right upper quadrant
	Rx	prescription
	$\bar{s}$	without
	S-A	sinoatrial (node)
	SD	shoulder disarticulation
	seg	polymorphonuclear neutrophil
	SH	serum hepatitis
	SLE	systemic lupus erythematosus
	SOB	short(ness) of breath
	sos	if necessary
	sp. gr.	specific gravity
	SR	sedimentation rate
	ss.	half
	ST	esotropia
	st	stage (i.e., staging of a disease)
	staph	staphylococcus
	Stat.	immediately
	STD	skin test dose
	strep	streptococcus
	subcu., SC	subcutaneous
	T	temperature
	T-1	first thoracic vertebra
	T-2	second thoracic vertebra
	T-3	third thoracic vertebra
	T_3	triiodothyronine
	T_4	thyroxine
	T&A	tonsillectomy and adenoidectomy
	TB	tuberculosis
	TDT	tone decay test
	THA	total hip arthroplasty
	THR	total hip replacement
	TIA	transient ischemic attack
	T.I.D., t.i.d.	three times a day

Abbreviation	Meaning	**423**
TKA	total knee arthroplasty	
TKR	total knee replacement	
TNM	(primary) tumor, (regional lymph) nodes, (remote) metastasis	
top.	topically	
TPN	total parenteral nutrition	
TPR	temperature, pulse, and respiration	
TPUR	transperineal urethral resection	
tr., tinct.	tincture	
TSH	thyroid-stimulating hormone	
TTH	thyrotrophic hormone	
TUR, TURP	transurethral resection (for prostatectomy)	
Tx	tumor cannot be assessed	
U.	units	
UA	urinalysis	
UC	uterine contractions	
UGI	upper gastrointestinal	
UHF	ultrahigh frequency	
ULQ	upper left quadrant	
ung.	ointment	
URI	upper respiratory infection	
URQ	upper right quadrant	
USP	United States Pharmacopeia	
UTI	urinary tract infection	
UV	ultraviolet	
VA	visual acuity	
VC	vital capacity	
VD	venereal disease	
VF	visual field	
VHD	ventricular heart disease	
VLDL	very-low-density lipoprotein	
VSD	ventricular septal defect	
WBC	white blood cell; white blood count	
Wt.	weight	
w/v	weight by volume	
x	multiplied by	
XP	xeroderma pigmentosa	
XT	exotropia	
XX	female sex chromosomes	
XY	male sex chromosomes	

APPENDIX C

Index of Genetic Disorders

MEDICAL WORD ELEMENT/ENGLISH TERM

Medical Word Element	Pronunciation	Meaning	Page Numbers
a-	ăh	without, not, lack of	39
ab-	ăb	from, away from	40
-ac	ăk	pertaining to	28
acr/o-	ăk-rō	extremity	305
ad-	ăd	to, toward, near	40
acromi/o	ā-krō-mē-ō	acromion, projection of scapula	214
aden/o	ăd-ē-nō	gland	68, 183
adenoid/o	ăd-ē-noid-ō	adenoid	125
adip/o	ăd-ĭ-pō	fat	68
adren/o	ăd-rē-nō	adrenal glands	306
adrenal/o	ă-drĕn-ăl-ō	adrenal glands	306
agranul/o	ā-grăn-ū-lō	without granules	183
-al	ăl	pertaining to	28
albumin/o	ăl-bū-mĭn-ō	white protein, albumin	37, 246
-algesia	ăl-gē-sē-ah	pain	333
-algia	ăl-jē-ah	pain	14
alveol/o	ăl-vē-ŏl-ō	alveolus (pl. alveoli)	125
ambi-	ăm-bĭ	both, both sides	36
ambly/o	ăm-blē-ō	dull, dim	356
amphi-	ăm-fĭ	on both sides	36
an-	ăn	without, not, lack of	39
an/o	ā-nō	anus, opening of the rectum	97
andr/o	ăn-drō	male	245, 306
angi/o	ăn-jē-ō	vessel	152
ankyl/o	ăng-kĭ-lō	stiff joint, fusion or growing together of parts	214
ante-	ăn-tē	before, in front of	36
anter/o	ăn-tĕr-ō	before, in front of, anterior	36, 55
anthrac/o	ăn-thrah-kō	coal	126
anti-	ăn-tĭ	against	41
aort/o	ā-ŏr-tō	aorta	152
aque/o	ā-kwē-ŏ	water	356
ar-	ăr	without, not, lack of	39
-ar	ĕr	pertaining to	28

Index of Medical Word Elements

Medical Word Element	Pronunciation	Meaning	Page Numbers
-arche	ăr-kē	beginning	274
arteriol/o	ăr-tĕr-ĭ-ŏl-ō	little artery, arteriole	152
arthr/o	ăr-thrō	joint	212
-ary	ĕr-ē	pertaining to	28
-asthenia	ăs-thē-nē-ăh	without strength	334
atel/o	ăt-ē-lō	incomplete, imperfect	126
ather/o	ăth-ĕr-ō	fatty deposit, fatty degeneration	152
atri/o	ā-trē-ō	atrium	152
audi/o	aw-dē-ō	hearing	357
bacteri/o	băk-tē-rē-ō	bacteria	246
balan/o	bah-lăn-ō	glans penis	245
bas/o	bā-sō	basic or alkaline	183
bi-	bī	two	38
bil/i	bĭl-ē	biliary system	97
-blast	blăst	germ cell, embryonic, primitive	185, 216
blast/o	blăs-tō	embryonic, primitive, germ cell	183, 385
blephar/o	blĕf-ah-rō	eyelid	356
brachi/o	brăk-ē-ō	arm	213
brady-	brăd-ē	slow	41
bronch/o	brŏng-kō	bronchus (pl. bronchi)	125
bronchi/o	brŏng-kē-ō	bronchus (pl. bronchi)	125
bucc/o	bŭk-ō	cheek	95
calc/o	kăl-kō	calcium	306
calcane/o	kal-kā-nē-ō	calcaneum, heel bone	214
-capnia	kăp-nē-ah	carbon dioxide, CO_2	126
carcin/o	kăr-sĭn-ō	cancer	385
cardi/o	kăr-dē-ō	heart	2, 152
carp/o	kăr-pō	wrist, carpus	213
-cele	sĕl	hernia, swelling	14
celi/o	sē-lē-ō	belly, abdomen	96
-centesis	sĕn-tē-sĭs	surgical puncture	13
cephal/o	sĕf-ăl-ō	head	211
cerebell/o	sĕr-ē-bĕl-lō	cerebellum	332
cerebr/o	sĕr-ē-brō	cerebrum	332
cervic/o	sĕr-vĭ-kō	neck, cervix	212, 272
cheil/o	kī-lō	lip	95

Medical Word Element	Pronunciation	Meaning	Page Numbers
chem/o	kē-mō	chemical, drug	385
chlor/o	klŏr-ō	green	38
-chlorhydria	klŏr-hǐ-drē-ah	hydrochloric acid	98
chol/e	kō-lē	bile, gall	97
cholangi/o	kō-lăn-jē-ō	bile vessel	97
cholecyst/o	kō-lē-sǐs-tō	gallbladder	97
choledoch/o	kō-lē-dō-kō	bile duct	97
chondr/o	kŏn-drō	cartilage	214
choroid/o	kō-roid-ō	choroid	356
-chrome	krōm	color	247
chrom/o	krōm-ō	color	183
circum-	sĕr-kŭm	around	40
cirrh/o	sǐr-rō	yellow, tawny	38, 97
-clasis	klăh-sǐs	a breaking (of), refracture	14
-clast	klăst	to break	216
col/o	kō-lō	colon	96
colp/o	kŏl-pō	vagina	272
condyl/o	kŏn-dǐ-lō	condyle	215
coni/o	kō-nē-ō	dust	126
contra-	kŏn-trah	against	41
cor/e	kō-rē	pupil	357
core/o	kō-rē-ō	pupil	357
corne/o	kŏr-nē-ō	cornea	356
coron/o	kŏr-ō-nō	heart	152
cost/o	kŏs-tō	ribs	212
crani/o	krā-nē-ō	skull bones, cranium, skull	212, 332
-crine	krǐn or krīn	to secrete	98, 307
cry/o	krī-o	cold	385
crypt/o	krǐp-tō	hidden	68, 246
-cusis	kū-sǐs	hearing	358
cutane/o	kū-tā-nē-ō	skin	68
cyan/o	sī-ăn-ō	blue	38
cycl/o	sī-klō	ciliary body	356
-cyesis	sī-ē-sǐs	pregnancy	274
cyst/o	sǐs-tō	bladder, sac of fluid	245, 385
cyt/o	sī-tō	cell	2, 55
dacry/o	dăk-rē-ō	tear	356
dacryoaden/o	dăk-rē-ō-ăd-ĕn-ō	tear gland	356
dactyl/o	dăk-tǐ-lō	digit (finger or toe)	213
dent/o	dĕnt-ō	tooth	95
derm/o	dĕr-mō	skin	69
dermat/o	dĕr-mah-tō	skin	69
-desis	dē-sǐs	binding, stabilization, fusion	13, 216
dextr/o	dĕks-trō	to the right of	37
di-	dī	two	38
dia-	dē-ah	through, across	40
diplo-	dǐp-lō	double	39
-dipsia	dǐp-sē-ăh	thirst	307

Medical Word Element	Pronunciation	Meaning	Page Numbers
dist/o	dĭs-tō	distant	55
dors/o	dŏr-sō	back	37, 55
duoden/o	dū-ŏd-ē-nō	duodenum	96
-dynia	dĭn-ē-ăh	pain	14
dys-	dĭs	bad, painful, difficult	41
ec-	ĕk	out, out from	40
-ectasis	ĕk-tăh-sĭs	dilation, expansion	14
ecto-	ĕk-tō	outside	40
-ectomy	ĕk-tŏ-mē	excision, removal	13
embol/o	ĕm-bōl-ō	embolus, plug	152
-emesis	ē-mĕ-sĭs	vomit	98
-emia	ē-mē-ăh	blood condition (of)	14
emmetr/o	ĕm-ē-trō	correct measure	356
encephal/o	ĕn-sĕf-ah-lō	brain	332
endo-	ĕn-dō	in, within	40
enter/o	ĕn-tĕr-ō	intestines	96
eosin/o	ē-ō-sĭn-ō	red, rosy, dawn-colored	183
epi-	ĕp-ĭ	upon, over, in addition to	37, 55
epididym/o	ĕp-ĭ-dĭd-ĭ-mō	epididymis	245
epiglott/o	ĕp-ĭ-glŏt-ō	epiglottis	125
episi/o	ē-pĭz-ē-ō	vulva	273
-er	ĕr	one who	28
erythem/o	ĕr-ĭ-thē-mō	red	69
erythr/o	ē-rĭth-rō	red	2, 38, 69
erythrocyt/o	ē-rĭth-rō-sī-tō	red cell	183
esophag/o	ē-zŏf-ah-gō	esophagus	95
-esthesia	ĕs-thē-zē-ah	feeling, sensation	333
eu-	ū	good, easy	41
ex-	ĕks	out, out from	40
exo-	ĕks-ō	outside	40
extern/o	ĕks-tĕrn-ō	outside	56
extra-	ĕks-trah	outside	40
femor/o	fĕm-ō-rō	femur, thigh bone	213
fibul/o	fĭb-ū-lō	fibula	214
galact/o	gă-lăk-tō	milk	273
gangli/o	găng-glē-ō	ganglion (knot)	333
ganglion/o	găng-glē-ŏn-ō	ganglion (knot)	333
gastr/o	găs-trō	stomach	2, 96
-gen	jĕn	to produce	14
-genesis	jĕn-ē-sĭs	origin, beginning process	247
gingiv/o	jĭn-jĭ-vō	gum	95
glauc/o	glaw-kō	gray	38
gli/o	glī-ō	glue	333
-globin	glō-bĭn	protein	185
glomerul/o	glō-mĕr-ū-lō	glomerulus	245
gloss/o	glŏs-ō	tongue	95

Medical Word Element	Pronunciation	Meaning	Page Numbers
gluc/o	gloo-kō	sugar, sweetness	246, 306
glucos/o	gloo-kō-sō	sugar	246
glyc/o	glī-kō	sugar, sweetness	246, 306
gonad/o	gō-năd-ō	sex glands	306
-gram	grăm	a writing, record	14, 70, 153
granul/o	grăn-ū-lō	granule	183
-graph	grăf	instrument used for recording	14, 70, 153
-graphy	gră-fē	process of recording	14, 70
-gravida	grăv-ĭ-dah	pregnancy	274
gynec/o	jĭn-ē-kō-gĭ-nē-kō	woman, female	273
hem/o	hēm-o	blood	183
hemangi/o	hē-măn-jē-ō	blood vessel	152
hemat/o	hĕm-ah-tō	blood	183
hemi-	hĕm-ē	half, partial	39
hepat/o	hĕp-ah-tō	liver	97
heter/o	hĕt-ĕr-ō	different	41, 183
hidr/o	hĭ-drō	sweat	41, 69
hist/o	hĭs-tō	tissue	56, 69
home/o	hō-mē-ō	likeness, resemblance	306
homo-	hō-mō	same	41, 183
humer/o	hū-mĕr-ō	humerus	212
hydr/o	hĭ-drō	water	41
hyper-	hĭ-pĕr	over, above, excessive, beyond	39, 56
hypo-	hĭ-pō	under, below, beneath, less	37, 39, 56
hyster/o	hĭs-tĕr-ō	uterus, womb	273
-ia	ē-ah	condition (of), process	28
-iasis	ī-ā-sĭs	abnormal condition, formation of, presence of	98
-ic	ĭk	pertaining to	28
-ical	ĭk-ăl	pertaining to	28
ichthy/o	ĭk-thē-ō	dry, scaly	69
-icle	ĭk-ăl	small, little, minute	29
ile/o	ĭl-ē-ō	ileum	96
ili/o	ĭl-ē-ō	ilium	213
im-	ĭm	not	39
immun/o	ĭm-ū-nō	safe, protected	183
in-	ĭn	not	39
infra-	ĭn-frah	under, below, beneath, after	37, 56
inter-	ĭn-tĕr	between	37
intra-	ĭn-trah	in, within	40
ir/o	ĭr-ō	iris	356
irid/o	ĭr-ĭ-dō	iris	356
-is	ĭs	forms noun from root	28
is/o	ī-sō	equal	183

Medical Word Element	Pronunciation	Meaning	Page Numbers
ischi/o	ĭs-kē-ō	ischium	213
-ism	ĭzm	condition, state of being	28
-ist	ĭst	one who specializes	29
-itis	ī-tĭs	inflammation	15
jejun/o	jĕ-joo-nō	jejunum	96
kary/o	kăr-ē-ō	nucleus	183
kerat/o	kĕr-ăh-tō	cornea; hornlike; hard; horny substance	69, 356, 385
kinesi/o	kĭ-nē-sē-ō	movement	333
-kinesia	kĭ-nē-zē-ăh	movement	333
labi/o	lā-bē-ō	lip	95, 273
labyrinth/o	lăb-ĭ-rĭn-thō	labyrinth, inner ear, maze	357
lacrim/o	lăk-rĭ-mō	tear	356
lact/o	lăk-tō	milk	69, 273
lamin/o	lăm-ĭ-nō	lamina	212, 215
lapar/o	lăp-ăr-ō	abdominal wall, abdomen	96
laryng/o	lah-rĭng-ō	larynx	125
later/o	lăt-ĕr-ō	side	37, 56
leiomy/o	lī-ō-mī-ō	smooth (visceral) muscle	215, 385
-lepsy	lĕp-sē	seizure	334
leuc/o-	loo-kō	white	38
leuk/o	loo-kō	white	38
leukocyt/o	loo-kō-sī-tō	white cell	184
lingu/o	lĭng-gwō	tongue	95
lip/o	lĭ-pō	fat	68
-lith	lĭth	stone, calculus	16, 98, 247
-lithiasis	lĭth-ī-ah-sĭs	presence, condition, or formation of calculi	247
lob/o	lō-bō	lobe	125
-logy	lō-jē	study of	15
lumb/o	lŭm-bō	loins	213
lymph/o	lĭm-fō	lymph, lymph tissue	184
-lysis	lĭ-sĭs	separate, destroy, break down	14
macro-	măk-rō	large	39
mal-	măl	ill, bad, poor	41
-malacia	măh-lā-shē-ăh	softening	15, 216
mamm/o	mă-mō	breast	69, 273
-manometer	măn-ŏm-ĕt-ĕr	instrument to measure pressure	153
mast/o	măs-tō	breast	69, 273
mastoid/o	măs-toi-dō	mastoid process	357
medi-	mē-dē	middle	37, 56

Medical Word Element	Pronunciation	Meaning	Page Numbers
medull/o	mĕd-ū-lō	medulla	333
-megaly	meg-ăh-lē	enlargement	15
melan/o	mĕl-ah-nō	black	38, 69
mening/o	mĕ-nĭng-gō	meninges, brain covering	333
meningi/o	mĕ-nĭn-jē-ō	meninges, brain covering	333
men/o	mĕn-ō	menses, menstruation	273
mes/o	mĕs-ō	middle	37
meta	mĕt-ah	after, beyond, over, change	41
metacarp/o	mĕt-ah-kăr-pō	metacarpus, bones of the hand	213
-meter	mē-tĕr	measure, instrument for measuring	15
metr/o	mĕ-trō	uterus, womb	273
-metry	mĕt-rē	act of measuring, to measure	15
micro-	mī-krō	small	39
mid-	mĭd	middle	37
mono-	mŏn-ō	one	38, 184
morph/o	mŏr-fō	shape	184
multi-	mŭl-tē	many, much	39
my/o	mī-ō	muscle	215
myc/o	mī-kō	fungus	69
-mycosis	mī-kō-sĭs	fungal infection	358
myel/o	mī-ē-lō	bone marrow, spinal cord	184, 215, 333
myring/o	mĕ-rĭng-gō	tympanic membrane, eardrum	357
narc/o	năr-kō	sleep	333
nas/o	nā-zō	nose	124
nat/a	nā-tă	birth	273
ne/o	nē-ō	new	385
nephr/o	nĕf-rō	kidney	2, 245
neur/o	nū-rō	nerve, neuron	333
neutr/o	nū-trō	neutral dye	184
noct/o	nŏk-tō	night	246
nucle/o	nū-klē-ō	nucleus	56
ocul/o	ŏk-ū-lō	eye	356
odont/o	ō-dŏn-tō	tooth	95
-oid	oid	resemble	15
-ole	ŏl	small, little, minute	29
olig/o	ō-lĭ-gō	scanty	246
-oma	ō-măh	tumor	15
onc/o	ŏng-kō	tumor, mass	385
onych/o	ŏn-ĭ-kō	nail	69
oo/o	ō-ō	egg, ovum	273
oophor/o	ō-ŏf-ō-rō	ovary	273
ophthalm/o	ŏf-thăl-mō	eye	356
-opia	ō-pē-ah	vision	358

Medical Word Element	Pronunciation	Meaning	Page Numbers
-opsia	ŏp-sē-ah	vision	358
opt/o	ŏp-tō	eye	356
orch/o	ŏr-kō	testes	245
orchi/o	ŏr-kē-ō	testes	245
orchid/o	ŏr-kǐ-dō	testes	245
or/o	ŏr-ō	mouth	95
orth/o	ŏr-thō	straight	126, 215
-ory	ŏr-ē	pertaining to	28
-osis	ō-sǐs	abnormal condition, increase	15, 185
-osmia	ŏz-mē-ah	smell	126
oste/o	ŏs-tē-ō	bone	2, 215
ot/o	ō-tō	ear	357
-ous	ŭs	pertaining to	28
ovari/o	ō-vǎr-ē-ō	ovary	273
ox/o	ŏks-ō	oxygen, O_2	126
oxy/o	ŏk-sǐ-ō	oxygen, O_2	152
pachy/o	pǎk-ē-ō	thick, heavy	69
pan-	pǎn	all	41
pancreat/o	pǎn-krē-ǎ-tō	pancreas	97, 306
papill/o	pǎp-ǐ-lō	nipple-like protuberance or elevation	385
para-	pǎr-ah	near, beside, beyond, abnormal	40
-para	pǎr-ah	to bear	274
parathyroid/o	pǎr-ah-thī-roi-dō	parathyroid glands	306
-paresis	pah-rē-sǐs	partial or incomplete paralysis	15, 334
patell/o	pah-tĕl-ō	patella, kneecap	214
-pathy	pǎh-thē	disease	15
pector/o	pĕk-tō-rō	chest	126
ped/i	pĕd-ē	foot	214
pelv/i	pĕl-vē	pelvis	213
-penia	pē-nē-ǎh	decrease, deficiency, lack of	15, 185
peri-	pĕr-ǐ	around	40, 56
perine/o	pĕr-ǐ-nē-ō	perineum	273
peritone/o	pĕr-ǐ-tō-nē-ō	peritoneum	98
-pexy	pĕk-sē	fixation, suspension	13
phag/o	fǎg-ō	swallow, eat	184
-phagia	fā-jē-ah	eating, ingesting, swallowing	15, 98, 307
phak/o	fā-kō	lens	357
phalang/o	fǎl-ǎn-jō	phalanges, bones of fingers and toes	213
pharyng/o	fah-rǐng-gō	pharynx, throat	95, 125
-phasia	fā-zē-ah	speech	15, 334
-phil	fǐl	to love, attraction for	185
-philia	fǐl-ē-ǎh	attraction for, to love	16
phleb/o	flĕb-ō	vein	153

Medical Word Element	Pronunciation	Meaning	Page Numbers
-phobia	fō-bē-ăh	fear	15
-phonia	fō-nē-ah	voice	127
-phoresis	fō-rē-sĭs	borne, carried	185
phren/o	frĕn-ō	diaphragm, mind	126
-phylaxis	fĭ-lăk-sĭs	protection	307
-physis	fĭ-sĭs	growth, to grow	216, 307
pil/o	pĭ-lō	hair	69
-plakia	plăk-ē-ăh	plate	386
-plasia	plā-zē-ăh	formation, development, growth	16, 386
-plasm	plāzm	formation, growth, development	386
-plasty	plăs-tē	formation, plastic repair, surgical repair	13, 216
-plegia	plē-jē-ăh	paralysis, stroke	15, 334
pleur/o	ploo-rō	pleura	126
-pnea	nē-ah	breathing	127
pneum/o	nū-mō	lung, air	125
pneumat/o	nū-mah-tō	air, breath	125
pneumon/o	nū-mŏn-ō	lung, air	125
pod/o	pō-dō	foot	214
-poiesis	poi-ē-sĭs	formation, production	16, 185
poikil/o	poi-kĭ-lō	varied, irregular	184
polio-	pō-lē-ō	gray	38
poly-	pŏl-ē	many, much	39
-porosis	pō-rō-sĭs	pores or cavities	216
post-	pōst	after, backward, behind	37
poster/o-	pōs-tĕr-ō	after, backward, back, behind, posterior	37, 56
-prandial	prăn-dē-ăl	pertaining to a meal	98
pre-	prē	before, in front of	36
presby/o	prĕs-bē-ō	old age, elderly	357
primi-	prĭ-mĭ	first	38
pro-	prō	before, in front of	36
proct/o	prŏk-tō	anus, rectum	96
prostat/o	prŏs-tah-tō	prostate	246
proxim/o	prŏk-sĭm-ō	near	56
pseudo-	soo-dō	false	41
-ptosis	tō-sĭs	prolapse, falling, dropping	16
-ptysis	tĭ-sĭs	spitting	127
pub/o	pū-bō	pubis anterior	213
pulmon/o	pŭl-mŏn-ō	lung	125
pupill/o	pū-pĭ-lō	pupil	357
purpur/o	pŭr-pū-rō	purple	38
py/o	pī-ō	pus	246
pyel/o	pī-ē-lŏ	renal pelvis	245
pylor/o	pī-lō-rō	pylorus	96
-pyorrhea	pī-ō-rē-ah	discharge of pus, purulent discharge	358

Medical Word Element	Pronunciation	Meaning	Page Numbers
quad-	kwŏd	four	39
quadri-	kwŏd-rĭ	four	39
rach/o	rāk-ō	vertebrae, spinal column	212
rachi/o	răk-ē-ō	vertebrae, spinal column	212
rect/o	rĕk-tō	rectum	97
ren/o	rē-nō	kidney	245
reticul/o	rē-tĭk-ū-lō	net, mesh (immature RBC)	184
retin/o	rĕt-ĭ-nō	retina	357
retro-	rĕt-rō	after, backward, behind	37
rhabd/o	răb-dō	rod	215
rhabdomy/o	răb-dō-mĭ-ō	striated (skeletal) muscle	215, 385
rhin/o	rī-nō	nose	125
-rrhage	rĭj	burst forth (of)	16
-rrhagia	rā-jē-ăh	burst forth (of)	16
-rrhaphy	ră-fē	suture	13
-rrhea	rē-ăh	discharge, flow	16, 98
-rrhexis	rek-sĭs	rupture	16
rube/o	roo-bē-ō	red	38
salping/o	săl-pĭn-gō/ săl-pĭn-jō	fallopian tubes, oviducts, uterine tubes, eustachian tube	273, 357
-salpinx	săl-pĭnks	fallopian tubes, oviducts, uterine tubes	273
sarc/o	săr-kō	flesh	385
scirrh/o	skĭr-rō	hard	385
scler/o	sklē-rō	sclera, hard	41, 70, 357
-sclerosis	sklĕ-rō-sĭs	abnormal condition (of) hardening	16
-scope	skōp	instrument to view or examine	16
-scopy	skō-pē	visual examination	16, 216
seb/o	sĕb-ō	sebum	70
semi-	sĕm-ē	half, partial	39
sial/o	sī-ăh-lō	saliva, salivary gland	95
sider/o	sĭd-ĕr-ō	iron	184
sigmoid/o	sĭg-moi-dō	sigmoid colon	97
sinistr/o	sĭn-ĭs-trō	left	37
sinus/o	sī-nŭs-ō	sinus, cavity	125
somat/o	sō-măt-ō	body	306
-spasm	spăzm	involuntary contraction, twitching	16
spermat/o	spĕr-mah-tō	sperm	246

Medical Word Element	Pronunciation	Meaning	Page Numbers
spher/o	sfē-rō	globe, round	184
sphincter/o	sfĭngk-tĕr-ō	sphincter	96
sphygm/o	sfĭg-mō	pulse	153
spir/o	spī-rō	breathe	126
splen/o	splē-nō	spleen	98, 184
spondyl/o	spŏn-dĭ-lō	vertebrae, backbone	212
squam/o	skwā-mō	scale	70
staped/o	stā-pē-dō	stapes	357
-stasis	stā-sĭs	standing still, control, stop	16, 185, 386
steat/o	stē-ă-tō	fat, fatty	70
-stenosis	stĕ-nō-sĭs	constriction, narrowing	16, 153
stern/o	stĕr-nō	sternum, breastbone	212
steth/o	stĕth-ō	chest	126
stomat/o	stō-mah-tō	mouth	95
-stomy	stō-mē	mouth, forming a new opening	13
sub-	sŭb	under, beneath, below	37
super-	soo-pĕr	above	40
supra-	soo-prah	above	40, 56
sym-	sĭm	union, together	41
syn-	sĭn	union, together	41
tachy-	tăk-ē	rapid	41
-taxia	tăk-sē-ah	muscular coordination	334
ten/o	tĕn-ō	tendon	215
tend/o	tĕnd-ō	tendon	215
tendin/o	tĕn-dĭn-ō	tendon	215
-tension	tĕn-shŭn	pressure	153
test/o	tĕs-tō	testes	245
thalam/o	thăl-ăh-mō	thalamus, chamber	333
thel/o	thē-lō	nipple	70
-therapy	thĕr-ăh-pē	treatment	70, 386
therm/o	thĕr-mō	heat	385
thorac/o	thō-rah-kō	chest	126, 212
-thorax	thō-răks	chest	127
thromb/o	thrŏm-bō	clot	153, 184
thrombocyt/o	thrŏm-bō-sĭ-tō	platelet, thrombocyte	184
thym/o	thī-mō	thymus	184, 306
thyr/o	thī-rō	thyroid	306
thyroid/o	thī-roi-dō	thyroid	306
tibi/o	tĭb-ē-ō	tibia	214
-tic	tĭk	pertaining to	28
-tocia	tō-sē-ah	childbirth, labor	274
-tome	tōm	instrument to cut	13
-tomy	tō-mē	incision, cut into	13
ton/o	tŏn-ō	tone	333
tonsill/o	tŏn-sĭ-lō	tonsil	95, 125
-toxic	tŏks-ĭk	poison	16, 307

Medical Word Element	Pronunciation	Meaning	Page Numbers
tox/o	tŏks-ō	poison	385
trache/o	trā-kē-ō	trachea	125
trans-	trănz	through, across	40, 56
trich/o	trĭk-ō	hair	70
tri-	trī	three	39
-tripsy	trĭp-sē	crush	14
-trophy	trō-fē	nourishment, development	307, 334
-tropia	trō-pē-ah	turning	358
-tropin	trō-pĭn	stimulate	307
tympan/o	tĭm-pah-nō	tympanic membrane, eardrum	357
-ula	ūlā	small, little, minute	29
-ule	yool	small, little, minute	29
ultra-	ul-trah	beyond, excess	40
ungu/o	ŭng-gwō	nail	70
uni-	yoo-nē	one	38
ur/o	ū-rō	urine	245
ureter/o	ū-rē-tĕr-ō	ureter	245
urethr/o	ū-rē-thrō	urethra	245
-uria	ū-rē-ah	urine	247, 307
uter/o	ū-tĕr-ō	uterus, womb	273
vagin/o	vă-jĭn-ō	vagina	272
vas/o	vah-sō	vas deferens, vessel	152, 246
ven/o	vē-nō	vein	153
ventricul/o	vĕn-trĭk-ū-lō	ventricles, little belly	333
ventr/o	vĕn-trō	belly, belly-side	56
venul/o	vĕn-ū-lō	venule	153
vertebr/o	vĕr-tē-brō	vertebrae, backbone	212
vesic/o	vĕs-ĭ-kō	bladder	245
vesicul/o	vĕ-sĭk-ū-lō	seminal vesicle	246
viscer/o	vĭs-ĕr-ō	organ	56
vulv/o	vŭl-vō	vulva	273
xanth/o	zăn-thō	yellow	38, 70
xer/o	zē-rō	dry	70
-y	ē	condition, process	28

English Term	Medical Word Element	Pronunciation	Page Numbers
abdomen	celi/o	sē-lē-ō	96
	lapar/o	lăp-ăr-ō	96
abdominal wall	lapar/o	lăp-ăr-ō	96
abnormal	para-	păr-ăh	40
abnormal condition	-iasis	ī-ā-sĭs	98
(of)	-osis	ō-sĭs	15, 185
	-sclerosis	sklĕ-rō-sĭs	16
above	hyper-	hĭ-per	39, 56
	super-	soo-per	40
	supra-	soo-prah	40, 56
acromion	acromi/o	ā-krō-mē-ō	214
across	-dia	dē-ăh	40
	trans-	trănz	40, 56
adenoid	adenoid/o	ăd-ē-noid-ō	125
adrenal glands	adren/o	ăd-rē-nō	306
	adrenal/o	ă-drĕn-ăl-ō	306
after	infra-	ĭn-frăh	56
	meta-	mĕt-ăh	41
	post-	pōst	37
	postero-	pōs-ter-ō	37
	retro-	rĕt-rō	37
against	anti-	ăn-tĭ	41
	contra-	kŏn-trăh	41
air	pneum/o	nū-mō	125
	pneumat/o	nū-măh-tō	125
	pneumon/o	nū-mŏn-ō	125
albumin	albumin/o	ăl-bū-mĭn-ō	246
alkaline	bas/o	bā-sō	183
all	pan-	păn	41
alveolus (pl. alveoli)	alveol/o	ăl-vē-ōl-ō	125
anterior	anter/o	ăn-ter-ō	55
anus	an/o	ā-nō	97
	proct/o	prŏk-tō	96
aorta	aort/o	ā-or-tō	152
arm	brachi/o	brăk-ē-ō	213
around	circum-	sĕr-kŭm	40
	peri-	pĕr-ĭ	40, 56
arteriole	arteriol/o	ar-tēr-ĭ-ōl-ō	152
artery (little)	arteriol/o	ar-tēr-ĭ-ōl-ō	152
atrium	atri/o	ā-trē-ō	152
attraction for	-phil	fĭl	185
	-philia	fĭl-ē-ăh	16
away from	ab-	ăb	40
back	dors/o	dor-sō	37, 55
	poster/o	pŏs-tēr-ō	56
backbone	spondyl/o	spŏn-dĭl-ō	212
	vertebr/o	vĕr-tĕ-brō	212
backward	post-	pōst	37
	postero-	pōs-tĕr-ō	37

English Term	Medical Word Element	Pronunciation	Page Numbers
backward	retro-	rĕt-rō	37
bacteria	bacteri/o	băk-tē-rē-ō	246
bad	dys-	dĭs	41
	mal-	măl	41
basic	bas/o	bā-sō	183
before	ante-	ăn-tē	36
	anter/o	ăn-tĕr-ō	36, 55
	pre-	prē	36
	pro-	prō	36
beginning	-arche	ăr-kē	274
beginning process	-genesis	jĕn-ē-sĭs	247
behind	post-	pōst	37
	postero-	pōs-tĕr-ō	37, 56
	retro-	rĕt-rō	37
belly	celi/o	sē-lē-ō	96
	ventr/o	vĕn-trō	56
belly-side	ventr/o	vĕn-trō	56
below	hypo-	hĭ-pō	37, 39, 56
	infra-	ĭn-frăh	37, 56
	sub-	sŭb	37
beneath	hypo-	hĭ-pō	37
	infra-	ĭn-frah	37, 56
	sub-	sŭb	37
beside	para-	păr-ăh	40
between	inter-	ĭn-tĕr	37
beyond	hyper-	hĭ-pĕr	56
	meta-	mĕt-ah	41
	para-	păr-ăh	40
	ultra-	ŭl-trah	40
bile	chol/e	kō-lē	97
bile duct	choledoch/o	kō-lē-dō-kō	97
bile vessel	cholangi/o	kō-lăn-jē-ō	97
biliary system	bil/i	bĭl-ē	97
binding	-desis	dē-sĭs	13, 216
birth	nat/a	nā-tă	273
black	melan/o	mĕl-ah-nō	38, 69
bladder	cyst/o	sĭs-tō	245, 385
	vesic/o	vĕs-ĭ-kō	245
blood	hem/o	hēm-ō	183
	hemat/o	hĕm-ăh-tō	183
blood condition (of)	-emia	ē-mē-ăh	14
blood vessel	hemangi/o	hē-măn-jē-ō	152
blue	cyan/o	sī-ăn-ō	38
body	somat/o	sō-măt-ō	306
bone	oste/o	ŏs-tē-ō	2, 215
bone marrow	myel/o	mī-ē-lō	184, 215, 333
borne	-phoresis	fō-rē-sĭs	185
both	ambi-	ăm-bĭ	36
both sides	ambi-	ăm-bĭ	36
brain	encephal/o	ĕn-sĕf-ah-lō	332
brain covering	mening/o	mĕ-nĭng-gō	333
	meningi/o	mĕ-nĭn-jē-ō	333

English Term	Medical Word Element	Pronunciation	Page Numbers
contraction, involuntary	-spasm	spăzm	16
control	-stasis	stā-sĭs	386
cornea	corne/o	kŏr-nē-nō	356
	kerat/o	kĕr-ah-tō	356
correct measure	emmetr/o	ĕm-ē-trō	356
cranium	crani/o	krā-nē-ō	212
crush	-tripsy	trĭp-sē	14
cut into	-tomy	tō-mē	13
dawn-colored	eosin/o	ē-ō-sĭn-ō	183
decrease	-penia	pē-nē-ăh	15, 185
deficiency	-penia	pē-nē-ăh	15
destroy	-lysis	lĭ-sĭs	14
development	-plasia	plā-zē-ăh	16, 386
	-plasm	plăzm	386
	-trophy	trō-fē	307, 334
diaphragm	phren/o	frĕn-ō	126
different	heter/o	hĕt-ĕr-ō	41, 183
difficult	dys-	dĭs	41
digit (finger or toe)	dactyl/o	dăk-tĭ-lō	213
dilation	-ectasis	ĕk-tăh-sĭs	14
dim	ambly/o	ăm-blē-ō	356
discharge	-rrhea	rē-ăh	16, 98
discharge of pus	-pyorrhea	pī-ō-rē-ah	358
disease	-pathy	păh-thē	15
distant	dist/o	dĭs-tō	55
double	diplo-	dĭp-lō	39
dropping	-ptosis	tō-sĭs	16
drug	chem/o	kē-mō	385
dry	ichthy/o	ĭk-thē-ō	69
	xer/o	zē-rō	70
dull	ambly/o	ăm-blē-ō	356
duodenum	duoden/o	dū-ŏd-ē-nō	96
dust	coni/o	kō-nē-ō	126
ear	ot/o	ō-tō	357
eardrum	myring/o	mē-rĭng-gō	357
	tympan/o	tĭm-pah-nō	357
easy	eu-	ū	41
eat	phag/o	făg-ō	184
eating	-phagia	fā-jē-ăh	15, 98, 307
egg	oo/o	ō-ō	273
elderly	presby/o	prĕz-bē-ō	357
embolus	embol/o	ĕm-bōl-ō	152
embryonic	-blast	blăst	185, 216
	blast/o	blăs-tō	183, 385
enlargement	-megaly	meg-ăh-lē	15
epididymis	epididym/o	ĕp-ĭ-dĭd-ĭ-mō	245
epiglottis	epiglott/o	ĕp-ĭ-glŏt-ō	125
equal	is/o	ī-sō	183
esophagus	esophag/o	ē-zŏf-ah-gō	95

English Term	Medical Word Element	Pronunciation	Page Numbers
eustachian tube	salping/o	săl-pĭn-gō/ săl-pĭn-jō	357
examination, visual	-scopy	skō-pē	16
excess	ultra-	ŭl-trah	40
excessive	hyper-	hī-per	39, 56
excision	-ectomy	ĕk-tō-mē	13
expansion	-ectasis	ĕk-tăh-sĭs	14
extremity	acr/o	ăk-rō	305
eye	ocul/o	ŏk-ū-lō	356
	ophthalm/o	ŏf-thăl-mō	356
	opt/o	ŏp-tō	356
eyelid	blephar/o	blĕf-ah-rō	356
falling	-ptosis	tō-sĭs	16
fallopian tubes	salping/o	săl-pĭng-gō	273
	-salpinx	săl-pĭnks	274
false	pseudo-	soo-dō	41
fat	adip/o	ăd-ĭ-pō	68
	lip/o	lĭ-pō	68
	steat/o	stē-ăh-tō	70
fatty	steat/o	stē-ăh-tō	70
fatty degeneration	ather/o	ăth-ĕr-ō	152
fatty deposit	ather/o	ăth-ĕr-ō	152
fear (of)	-phobia	fō-bē-ăh	15
feeling	-esthesia	ĕs-thē-zē-ah	333
female	gynec/o	gĭ-nĕ-kō	273
femur	femor/o	fĕm-ō-rō	213
fibula	fibul/o	fĭb-ū-lō	214
finger	dactyl/o	dăk-tĭ-lō	213
first	primi-	prĭ-mĭ	38
fixation	-pexy	pĕk-sē	13
flesh	sarc/o	săr-kō	385
flow	-rrhea	rē-ăh	16, 98
foot	ped/i	pĕd-ē	214
	pod/o	pō-dō	214
formation	-iasis	ī-ā-sĭs	14, 98
	-plasia	plā-zē-ăh	16, 386
	-plasm	plăzm	386
	-plasty	plăs-tē	13, 216
	-poiesis	poi-ē-sĭs	16, 185
formation of calculi	-lithiasis	lĭth-ĭ-ă-sĭs	247
forming a new opening	-stomy	stō-mē	13
four	quad-	kwŏd	39
	quadri-	kwŏd-rĭ	39
from	ab-	ăb	40
front	anter/o	ăn-tĕr-ō	55
fungus	myc/o	mĭ-kō	69
fungal infection	-mycosis	mĭ-kō-sĭs	358
fusion	-desis	dē-sĭs	13, 216

English Term	Medical Word Element	Pronunciation	Page Numbers
gall	chol/e	kō-lē	97
gallbladder	cholecyst/o	kō-lē-sĭs-tō	97
ganglion (knot)	gangli/o	găng-glē-ō	333
	ganglion/o	găng-glē-ōn-ō	333
germ cell	-blast	blăst	185, 216
	blast/o	blăs-tō	183
gland	aden/o	ăd-ēn-ō	68, 183
glans penis	balan/o	bah-lăn-ō	245
globe	spher/o	sfē-rō	184
glomerulus	glomerul/o	glō-mĕr-ū-lō	245
glue	gli/o	glē-ō	333
good	eu-	ū-	41
granule	granul/o	grăn-ū-lō	183
gray	glauc/o	glaw-kō	38
	polio-	pō-lē-ō	38
green	chlor/o	klŏr-ō	38
growth	-physis	fĭ-sĭs	307
	-plasia	plā-zē-ăh	16, 386
	-plasm	plăzm	386
gum	gingiv/o	jĭn-jĭ-vō	95
hair	pil/o	pī-lō	69
	trich/o	trĭk-ō	70
half	hemi-	hĕm-ē	39
	semi-	sĕm-ē	39
hard	kerat/o	kĕr-ăh-tō	356
	scirrh/o	skĭr-rō	385
	scler/o	sklē-rō	41, 70, 357
hardening	-sclerosis	sklĕ-rō-sĭs	16
head	cephal/o	sĕf-ăl-ō	211
hearing	audi/o	aw-dē-ō	357
	-cusis	kū-sĭs	358
heart	cardi/o	kăr-dē-ō	2, 152
	coron/o	kŏr-ō-nō	152
heat	therm/o	thĕr-mō	385
heavy	pachy/o	păk-ē-ō	69
heel bone	calcane/o	kăl-kā-nē-ō	214
hernia	-cele	sĕl	14
hidden	crypt/o	krĭp-tō	68, 246
horny, hornlike, horny substance	kerat/o	kĕr-ăh-tō	69, 356, 385
humerus	humer/o	hū-mĕr-ō	212
hydrochloric acid	-chlorhydria	klŏr-hĭ-drē-ah	98
ileum	ile/o	ĭl-ē-ō	96
ilium	ili/o	ĭl-ē-ō	213
ill	mal-	măl	41
imperfect	atel/o	ăt-ē-lō	126
in	endo-	ĕn-dō	40
	intra-	ĭn-trah	40
in addition to	epi-	ĕp-ĭ	55

English Term	Medical Word Element	Pronunciation	Page Numbers
in front of	ante-	ăn-tē	36
	anter/o	ăn-tĕr-ō	36
	pre-	prē	36
	pro-	prō	36
incision	-tomy	tō-mē	13
incomplete	atel/o	ăt-ē-lō	126
increase	-osis	ō-sĭs	15, 185
inflammation	-itis	ī-tĭs	15
ingesting	-phagia	fā-jē-ăh	15, 98
inner ear	labyrinth/o	lăb-ĭ-rĭn-thō	357
instrument to cut	-tome	tōm	13
instrument for measuring	-meter	mē-tĕr	15
instrument to measure pressure	-manometer	măn-ŏm-ĕt-ĕr	153
instrument to view or examine	-scope	skōp	16
instrument used for recording	-graph	grăf	14, 70, 153
intestines	enter/o	ĕn-tĕr-ō	96
involuntary contraction	-spasm	spăzm	16
iris	ir/o	ĭr-ō	356
	irid/o	ĭr-ĭ-dō	356
iron	sider/o	sĭd-ĕr-ō	184
irregular	poikil/o	poi-kĭ-lō	184
ischium	ischi/o	ĭs-kē-ō	213
jejunum	jejun/o	jē-joo-nō	96
joint	arthr/o	ăr-thrō	212
kidney	nephr/o	nĕf-rō	2, 245
	ren/o	rē-nō	245
kneecap	patell/o	pah-tĕl-ō	214
labor	-tocia	tō-sē-ah	274
labyrinth	labyrinth/o	lăb-ĭ-rĭn-thō	357
lack of	a-	ah	39
	an-	ăn	39
	ar-	ăr	39
	-penia	pē-nē-ăh	15
lamina	lamin/o	lăm-ĭ-nō	212, 215
large	macro-	măk-rō	39
larynx	laryng/o	lah-rĭng-ō	125
left	sinistr/o	sĭn-ĭs-trō	37
lens	phak/o	fā-kō	357
less	hypo-	hī-pō	56
likeness	home/o	hō-mē-ō	306
lip	cheil/o	kī-lō	95
	labi/o	lā-bē-ō	95, 273
little	-icle	ĭk-ăl	29
	-ole	ŏl	29
	-ula	ūlā	29

English Term	Medical Word Element	Pronunciation	Page Numbers
little	-ule	yool	29
little belly	ventricul/o	vĕn-trĭk-ū-lō	333
liver	hepat/o	hĕp-ăh-tō	97
lobe	lob/o	lō-bō	125
loins	lumb/o	lŭm-bō	213
lung	pneum/o	nū-mō	125
	pneumon/o	nū-mŏn-ō	125
	pulmon/o	pŭl-mŏn-ō	125
lymph	lymph/o	lĭm-fō	184
lymph tissue	lymph/o	lĭm-fō	184
male	andr/o	ăn-drō	245, 306
many	multi-	mŭl-tē	39
	poly-	pŏl-ē	39
mass	onc/o	ŏng-kō	385
mastoid process	mastoid/o	măs-toi-dō	357
maze	labyrinth/o	lăb-ĭ-rĭn-thō	357
measure	-meter	mē-tĕr	15
measuring (act of)	-metry	mĕt-rē	15
medulla	medull/o	mĕd-ū-lō	333
meninges	mening/o	mĕ-nĭng-gō	333
	meningi/o	mĕ-nĭn-jē-ō	333
menses	men/o	mĕn-ō	273
menstruation	men/o	mĕn-ō	273
mesh (immature RBC)	reticul/o	rē-tĭk-ū-lō	184
metacarpus (bones of the hand)	metacarp/o	mĕt-ah-kăr-pō	213
middle	medi-	mē-dē	37, 56
	mes/o-	mĕs-ō	37
	mid-	mĭd	37
milk	galact/o	gă-lăk-tō	273
	lact/o	lăk-tō	69
mind	phren/o	frĕn-ō	126
minute	-icle	ĭk-ăl	29
	-ole	ŏl	29
	-ula	ūlā	29
	-ule	yool	29
mouth	or/o	ŏr-ō	95
	stomat/o	stō-mah-tō	95
	-stomy	stō-mē	13
movement	kinesi/o	kĭ-nē-sē-ō	333
	-kinesia	kĭ-nē-zē-ăh	333
much	multi-	mŭl-tē	39
	poly-	pŏl-ē	39
muscle	my/o	mī-ō	215
muscular coordination	-taxia	tăk-sē-ah	334
nail	onych/o	ŏn-ĭ-kō	69
	ungu/o	ŭng-gwō	70
narrowing	-stenosis	stĕ-nō-sĭs	16, 153

English Term	Medical Word Element	Pronunciation	Page Numbers
near	ad-	ăd	40
	proxim/o	prŏk-sĭm-ō	56
neck	cervic/o	sĕr-vĭ-kō	212, 272
nerve	neur/o	nū-rō	333
net (immature RBC)	reticul/o	rē-tĭk-ū-lō	184
neuron	neur/o	nū-rō	333
neutral dye	neutr/o	nū-trō	184
new	ne/o	nē-ō	385
night	noct/o	nŏk-tō	246
nipple-like protuberance or elevation	papill/o	păp-ĭ-lō	385
nipple	thel/o	thē-lō	70
nose	nas/o	nā-zō	124
	rhin/o	rī-nō	125
not	a-	ah	39
	an-	ăn	39
	ar-	ăr	39
	im-	ĭm	39
	in-	ĭn	39
nourishment	-trophy	trō-fē	307, 334
nucleus	kary/o	kăr-ē-ō	183
	nucle/o	nū-klē-ō	56
old age	presby/o	prĕs-bē-ō	357
on both sides	amphi-	ăm-fĭ	36
one	mono-	mŏn-ō	38, 184
	uni-	yoo-nē	38
one who	-er	ĕr	28
one who specializes	-ist	ĭst	29
organ	viscer/o	vĭs-ĕr-ō	56
origin	-genesis	gĕn-ĕ-sĭs	247
out	ec-	ĕk	40
	ex-	ĕks	40
out from	ec-	ĕk	40
	ex-	ĕks	40
outside	ecto-	ĕk-tō	40
	exo-	ĕks-ō	40
	extern/o	ĕks-tĕr-nō	56
	extra-	ĕks-trah	40
ovary	oophor/o	ō-ŏf-ō-rō	273
	ovari/o	ō-văr-ē-ō	273
over	epi-	ĕp-ĭ	55
	hyper-	hī-pĕr	39
	meta-	mĕt-ah	41
oviduct(s)	salping/o	săl-pĭng-gō	273, 357
	-salpinx	săl-pĭnks	274
ovum	oo/o	ō-ō	273
oxygen, O_2	ox/o	ŏks-ō	126
	oxy/o	ŏks-ĭ-ō	152
pain	-algesia	ăl-gē-sē-ah	333
	-algia	ăl-jē-ah	14

English Term	Medical Word Element	Pronunciation	Page Numbers
pain	-dynia	dĭn-ē-ăh	14
painful	dys-	dĭs	41
pancreas	pancreat/o	păn-krē-ăt-ō	97, 306
paralysis	-plegia	plē-jē-ăh	15, 334
paralysis, partial or incomplete	-paresis	pah-rē-sĭs	15, 334
parathyroid glands	parathyroid/o	păr-ah-thī-roi-dō	306
partial	hemi-	hĕm-ē	39
	semi-	sĕm-ē	39
patella	patell/o	pah-tĕl-ō	214
pelvis	pelv/i	pĕl-vē	213
perineum	perine/o	pĕr-ĭ-nē-ō	273
peritoneum	peritone/o	pĕr-ĭ-tō-nē-ō	98
pertaining to	-ac	ăk	28
	-al	ăl	28
	-ar	ĕr	28
	-ary	ĕr-ē	28
	-ic	ĭk	28
	-ical	ĭk-ăl	28
	-ory	ŏr-ē	28
	-ous	ŭs	28
	-tic	tĭk	28
pertaining to a meal	-prandial	prăn-dē-ăl	98
phalanges (bones of fingers and toes)	phalang/o	făl-ăn-jō	213
pharynx	pharyng/o	fah-rĭng-gō	95, 125
plastic repair	-plasty	plăs-tē	13, 216
plate	-plakia	plăk-ē-ah	386
platelet	thrombocyt/o	thrŏm-bō-sī-tō	184
pleura	pleur/o	ploo-rō	126
plug	embol/o	ĕm-bŏl-o	152
poison	-toxic	tŏks-ĭk	16, 307
	tox/o	tŏks-ō	385
poor	mal-	măl	41
pores	-porosis	pō-rō-sĭs	216
posterior	poster/o	pŏs-tĕr-ō	56
pregnancy	-cyesis	sī-ē-sĭs	274
	-gravida	grăv-ĭ-dah	274
presence of	-iasis	ī-ā-sĭs	14, 98
presence of calculi	-lithiasis	lĭth-ī-ă-sĭs	247
pressure	-tension	tĕn-shŭn	153
primitive	-blast	blăst	185, 216
	blast/o	blăs-tō	183
process	-ia	ē-ăh	28
	-y	ē	29
production	-poiesis	poi-ē-sĭs	16, 185
prolapse	-ptosis	tō-sĭs	16
prostate	prostat/o	prŏs-tăh-tō	246
protected	immun/o	ĭm-ū-nō	183
protection	-phylaxis	fĭ-lăk-sĭs	307
protein	-globin	glō-bĭn	185

English Term	Medical Word Element	Pronunciation	Page Numbers
sugar	glyc/o	glĭ-kō	246, 306
surgical puncture	-centesis	sĕn-tē-sĭs	13
surgical repair	-plasty	plăs-tē	13, 216
suspension	-pexy	pĕk-sē	13
suture	-rrhaphy	răf-ē	13
swallow	phag/o	făg-ō	184
swallowing	-phagia	fā-jē-ăh	15, 98
sweat	hidr/o	hĭ-drō	41, 69
sweetness	gluc/o	gloo-kō	306
	glyc/o	glĭ-kō	306
swelling	-cele	sĕl	14
tawny	cirrh/o	sĭr-rō	97
tear	dacry/o	dăk-rē-ō	356
	lacrim/o	lăk-rĭ-mō	356
tear gland	dacryoaden/o	dăk-rē-ō-ăd-ĕn-ō	356
tendon	ten/o	tĕn-ō	215
	tend/o	tĕnd-ō	215
	tendin/o	tĕn-dĭn-ō	215
testes	orch/o	ŏr-kō	245
	orchi/o	ŏr-kē-ō	245
	orchid/o	ŏr-kĭ-dō	245
	test/o	tĕs-tō	245
thalamus	thalam/o	thăl-ah-mō	333
thick	pachy/o	păk-ē-ō	69
thigh bone	femor/o	fĕm-ō-rō	213
thirst	-dipsia	dĭp-sē-ăh	307
three	tri-	trĭ	39
throat	pharyng/o	făr-ĭng-ō	125
thrombocyte	thrombocyt/o	thŏm-bō-sĭ-tō	184
through	-dia	dē-ah	40
	trans-	trănz	40
thymus	thym/o	thĭ-mō	184, 306
thyroid	thyr/o	thĭ-rō	306
	thyroid/o	thĭ-roi-dō	306
tibia	tibi/o	tĭb-ē-ō	214
tissue	hist/o	hĭs-tō	56, 69
to	ad-	ăd	40
to bear	-para	păr-ah	274
to break	-clast	klăst	216
to grow	-physis	fĭ-sĭs	216
to love	-phil	fĭl	185
	-philia	fĭl-ē-ăh	16
to measure	-metry	-mĕt-rē	15
to produce	-gen	jĕn	14
to secrete	-crine	krĭn or krĭn	98, 307
to the left of	sinistr/o	sĭn-ĭs-trō	37
to the right of	dextr/o	dĕks-trō	37
	syn-	sin	41
toe	dactyl/o	dăk - tĭ - lō	41
together	sym-	sĭm	41
tone	ton/o	tŏn-ō	333

Index

An "F" following a page number indicates a figure. A "T" following a page number indicates a table.